Health Informatics

This series is directed to healthcare professionals leading the transformation of healthcare by using information and knowledge. For over 20 years, Health Informatics has offered a broad range of titles: some address specific professions such as nursing, medicine, and health administration; others cover special areas of practice such as trauma and radiology; still other books in the series focus on interdisciplinary issues, such as the computer based patient record, electronic health records, and networked healthcare systems. Editors and authors, eminent experts in their fields, offer their accounts of innovations in health informatics. Increasingly, these accounts go beyond hardware and software to address the role of information in influencing the transformation of healthcare delivery systems around the world. The series also increasingly focuses on the users of the information and systems: the organizational, behavioral, and societal changes that accompany the diffusion of information technology in health services environments.

Developments in healthcare delivery are constant; in recent years, bioinformatics has emerged as a new field in health informatics to support emerging and ongoing developments in molecular biology. At the same time, further evolution of the field of health informatics is reflected in the introduction of concepts at the macro or health systems delivery level with major national initiatives related to electronic health records (EHR), data standards, and public health informatics.

These changes will continue to shape health services in the twenty-first century. By making full and creative use of the technology to tame data and to transform information, Health Informatics will foster the development and use of new knowledge in healthcare.

More information about this series at https://link.springer.com/bookseries/1114

Mussaad Al-Razouki • Sophie Smith
Editors

Hybrid Healthcare

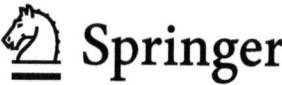 Springer

Editors
Mussaad Al-Razouki
Business Development
Kuwait Life Sciences Company
Kuwait City, Kuwait

Sophie Smith
Executive
Nabta Health
Dubai, United Arab Emirates

ISSN 1431-1917   ISSN 2197-3741   (electronic)
Health Informatics
ISBN 978-3-031-04835-7   ISBN 978-3-031-04836-4   (eBook)
https://doi.org/10.1007/978-3-031-04836-4

This Springer imprint is published by the registered company Springer Nature Switzerland AG
The registered company address is: Gewerbestrasse 11, 6330 Cham, Switzerland

Contents

About the Editors

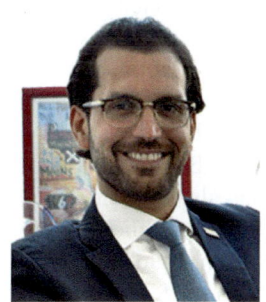

Mussaad Al-Razouki has over 17 years of experience in venture capital and private equity investment with a focus on healthcare and technology, shifting from an excellence in clinical practice and research to the management and financing of healthcare and education systems. A graduate of Columbia Business School, Dr. Razouki is the first-ever Arab national to receive an MBA with a focus on Healthcare Management and Finance. Dr. Razouki is a member of the Hermes Honors Society of Columbia Business School, an honor bestowed on the top 1000 global alumni of the university. An Oral and Maxillofacial surgeon by training, Dr. Razouki has completed clinical rotations at New York Presbyterian Hospital of Columbia University Medical Center, Harlem Hospital, Cleveland University Hospital of Case Western Reserve University, and Mass General Hospital of Harvard University. Dr. Razouki graduated with Cum Laude Honors from Creighton University with a Bachelors in Biology (Ethology) and TPP (Theology, Philosophy, and Political Science).In 2007, Dr. Razouki joined the world's largest and oldest strategic consulting firm, Booz Allen Hamilton, which at the time was operating in over 100 countries across six continents with four billion dollars in revenue. Dr Razouki had the honor of working with all six GCC Ministers of Health and completed health and public sector projects across the GCC, Lebanon, and Egypt.In 2009, Dr. Razouki was selected to join the Office of Tony Blair to lead the development of the Kuwait 2030 Vision for Health, Education, and Entrepreneurship together with the Council of Ministers of Kuwait. Dr. Razouki was also selected to head the Prime Minister's Early Warning System Committee on Health and played an integral part in the establishment of the Kuwait Talent Bank, which would go on to form the backbone of the Kuwait Youth Parliament and the future Ministry of State for Youth Affairs.In 2011, Dr. Razouki and his partners completed the purchase of a Kuwait based healthcare development company, which was rebranded as Kleos Healthcare. Today, Kleos is widely recognized as a regional thought leader on Middle East healthcare, with a variety of projects in its pipeline ranging from developing a Medical Takaful Insurance Company to working on a 750 mn USD government PPP.In 2012, Dr. Razouki co-founded Dubai based Glambox.me, one of the region's leading e-commerce platforms that later on completed a ~1.4 mn USD Series A funding round (which at the time was the largest Series A round in the history of Middle East entrepreneurship) with notable MENA VC firms including STC Ventures, MBC Ventures, and R&R ventures, as well as a subsequent 3.5 USD Series B round and a successful exit in 2017.Dr. Razouki has also invested in multiple digital platforms in New York and Silicon Valley, including most notably, Instavest.com, a global leader in personalized FinTech valued at 12 mn USD which manages over $250 mn worth of assets, and ShiftSmart, a leading San Francisco startup focusing on improving employee development and retention for the growing Sharing Economy valued at 5 mn USD.In 2015, Dr. Razouki was the first-ever Kuwaiti doctor to complete the "Reforming of Public Systems: Health, Higher Education and Finance" Executive Education course at the prestigious Grande École, Paris Institute of Political Studies ("Sciences Po").Dr. Razouki believes that the future of healthcare is approaching the singularity of coalescing the physical world with the digital. As a result, Dr. Razouki has incubated, funded, and developed multiple local, regional, and international digital health platforms including the 2014 LTE MENA winner for best mobile application—AbiDoc—the region's first online appointment booking platform and call center and Kuwait's largest network of private hospitals, clinics, and doctors, MEDtrip—the world's top medical tourism platform with offices in Denver, Colorado and Cebu, Philippines, Sihatech—Saudi Arabia's largest digital health application company, Nabta Health, the MENA region's first women's health application, and Cera Care, a London based digital health company focused on excellence in elder care across Europe, which was awarded the Healthcare Startup of the Year 2016 at the Healthcare Startup Awards, from over 1000 entries and is currently valued at 200 mn GBP (a 6667% ROI).In 2015, Dr. Razouki was presented with the Kuwait e-Award for best eHealth application by His Highness Sheikh Sabah Al-Ahmed Al-Jaber Al-Sabah, the Emir of Kuwait. Dr. Razouki was also selected by Stanford Medicine as part of a group of 20 global authors to write a chapter on digital health investing in the Springer published book: Digital Health: Scaling Healthcare to the World. He is the only author from the Arab World.During 2015, Dr. Razouki was also an Industry Expert Board Member at Al Ayadi Al Baytha Health Company, a 50 mn USD fully owned company of Al Khabeer Capital, which is one of Saudi Arabia's largest and most active private equity investors with over three billion dollars of assets under management. Dr. Razouki worked together with the turnaround team at Al Khabeer and the asset's management to unlock unrealized value in one of Saudi Arabia's fastest growing medical services companies.In 2016, Dr. Razouki was selected by the Abdul Rahman Al Sumait Award Executive Committee to represent the science community in Kuwait and present at the first-ever meeting of the committee. The Committee is co-chaired by His Excellency Sheikh Sabah Khalid Al Hamad Al Sabah, Kuwait's Minister of Foreign Affairs and Mr. Bill Gates. At one million USD, it is the largest science prize awarded for scientific achievement in Africa. Dr. Razouki was also nominated as one of the top five venture capital investors in the Middle East and North Africa by Arabian Business. Dr. Razouki also won two awards at the seventh annual Middle East Healthcare Leadership Awards for both Middle East Public-Private Partnership of the Year for the Jaber Hospital PPP Sustainable Hospital Project and Healthcare Entrepreneur of the Year. Dr. Razouki also won the prestigious Best Startup Award at the 2016 ArabNet Riyadh StartUp Battle Field competition as well as the winner of the 2017 Startup Championship MENA, for Sihatech. Dr. Razouki was also selected to participate in the prestigious World Economic Forum Global Health and Healthcare Community Meeting in 2016 as part of the Future Trends

in Health Task Force which was Chaired by Dr. Melanie
Walker, Advisor to the President of the World Bank, Dr.
Jim Young Kim. Dr. Razouki was the only participant
from Kuwait and had the honor of having seven out of
the 10 final key technological trends and themes accepted
in the final outcome report of the forum. Dr. Razouki was
also selected by the World Economic Forum and the
International Finance Corporation (IFC) as one of the
100 top entrepreneurs shaping the 4th Industrial
Revolution in the MENA region.In 2017, Dr. Razouki
was appointed to the Advisory Board of Popular Science
Magazine. An outlet for eminent scientists such as
Charles Darwin and Thomas Edison's writings and ideas
in the nineteenth century, Popular Science is the most
prestigious science magazine in the world and was first
launched in 1872.Dr. Razouki was also appointed by the
Kuwait Foundation for the Advancement of Sciences to
the Board of Trustees of the Jaber Al Ahmed Center for
Molecular Imaging and Nuclear Medicine (JAC), the
MENA region's first center of excellence and Type II
facility dedicated to the production of common radio-
pharmaceuticals for applications in positron emission
tomography. Dr. Razouki is also a Chairman of the
Executive Committee.Dr. Razouki is also the Principal
Author of the annual Middle East Science Report, first
presented at the World Bank Meeting on Youth and
Technology in Algiers (Video Start Time 1:08), the
region's premiere publication on the state of science in
the MENA region capturing the progress of scientific
thought and research across 50 of the region's top universities and research institutions as well as interviewing
over 100 of the region's top scientific minds. Dr. Razouki
has also been invited to lecture at top universities and
events including Cambridge University, Columbia
University, Harvard University, and the Cleveland Clinic.
Dr. Razouki has also spoken at the World Economic
Forum on the Middle East (Dead Sea, 2017) and the
World Bank: Youth, Technology and Finance Conference
in Algiers during 2018.In 2017, Dr. Razouki and his partners also closed the largest successful Series A in the history of technology entrepreneurship in the Kingdom of
Saudi Arabia by securing 5 million Saudi Riyals to sup-
port the growth of the Saudi Internet Health Application
Technology Company (www.Sihatech.com) from Waed
Aramco Entrepreneurship and existing strategic investor

Waseel ASP. As a co-founder of Nabta Health, Dr. Razouki is the proud winner of the People's Choice Award at ArabNet (Kuwait, 2017) as well as the winner of StartUp Championship at the STEP Conference (Dubai 2018) where Nabta was chosen by a panel of judges from over 200 ventures across the MENA region. Nabta Health was also awarded the best Scientific Paper at the Innovation Arabia Forum (Dubai, 2018).In 2018, Dr. Razouki was also recognized as one of the top 100 Leaders who Inspire in an inaugural book on Kuwait developed in coordination with the United National Development Program (UNDP). Dr. Razouki also contributed a chapter on Growth Hacking Healthcare, as part of the Springer published book: Digital Health Entrepreneurship.In 2019, Dr. Razouki established BaitCare as Kuwait's Leading Home Care Company focused on Physiotherapy, Post Stroke Rehabilitation, Post Surgery Rehabilitation, Nursing, and Sports Therapy. That same year, Dr. Razouki was honored by CNBC by the inclusion of both Sihatech and Nabta Health as the only two companies from the MENA region to be part of the 100 Most Promising Technology Ventures in the world. Dr. Razouki was elected as the Treasurer of the inaugural Kuwaiti Society of Science, Technology and Innovation, the country's most prestigious social gathering of STEM professionals. Dr. Razouki was also nominated for a third time by Arabian Business as Investor of the Year and Mentor of the Year at the 2019 Arabian Business Awards in Dubai. Dr. Razouki was also included in the HIMSS Future50 International List aimed at identifying and bringing together the top 50 Healthcare IT leaders in Europe, Middle East, Africa, and Asia Pacific. Dr. Razouki was also selected to be part of the first-ever Kuwait Knowledge Index, a joint initiative between the World Bank and the General Secretariat of the Supreme Council for Planning of Kuwait.In 2020, Dr. Razouki was selected to represent the State of Kuwait on the Board of Directors of the Arab Company for Drug Industries and Medical Appliances (ACDIMA), a Pan-Arab Public-Private Partnership established by Arab Economic Unity Council on March 6th, 1976 with a paid-up capital of 60 million KD (roughly one billion dollars in 2020). ACDIMA maintains strategic ownership in fifteen large-cap Middle East and North Africa pharmaceutical manufacturers including the Saudi Pharmaceutical Industries & Medical Appliances Corporation (SPIMACO), a Saudi Joint Stock company with a fully paid-up capital of 1.2 billion Saudi Riyals, and the Gulf Pharmaceutical Industries Manufacturers (Julphar) of the UAE, an ADX listed company with a market cap of around one billion AED. ACDIMA shareholders include the MENA regions top sovereign wealth funds including the Kuwait Investment Authority, the Public Investment Authority of Saudi Arabia, the Qatar Investment Authority, the Libyan Foreign Investment Company, the Jordan Investment Corporation, as well as direct governmental ownership by the Arab Republic of Egypt, the Republic of Algeria, the Republic of Tunisia, the Kingdom of Bahrain, the State of Palestine, the Syrian Arab Republic, the Republic of Yemen, the Republic of Sudan, the Sultanate of Oman, and the United Arab Emirates. Also in late 2020, Dr. Razouki was appointed to the Founding Committee of the Kuwait Innovation Center (KIC), an initiative of the Kuwait Foundation for the Advancement of Sciences (KFAS) established after the announcement of His Highness the Emir of Kuwait, the late Sheikh Sabah Al-Ahmed Al-Jaber Al-Sabah: "To create an ideal environment for innovation and attracting Kuwaiti intellectuals, inventors, and innovators and entrepreneurs whose ideas contribute to supporting the Kuwaiti economy, and through which provide many more job opportunities." The mission of KIC is to further foster the socio-economic development of Kuwait by promoting and advancing entrepreneurship and scalable startups that are able to further enhance the national innovation ecosystem. Thus, the main role of the center is to support entrepreneurs, with an emphasis on the youth, and companies to guide them through the various phases of the innovation lifecycle. The committee will also oversee the establishment of a $200 million Arab Technology Innovation Fund, which will be the third-largest venture capital fund focused on the Middle East and North Africa region. In 2021, Dr. Razouki was selected by His Excellency, Mr. Abdul Aziz Dakheel Al Dakheel the Head of His Highness the Prime Minister's Diwan to lead a committee on setting a new strategy for the Prime Minister's Office of Kuwait as well as develop a new permanent technical and advisory unit to spearhead the implementation of the 2021–2024 strategy. Dr. Razouki is the current

Chief Investment and Business Development Officer of Kuwait Life Sciences Company (KLSC) where he is part of a team that manages over 150 million dollars in assets under management including local, regional, and international investments on behalf of the Kuwait Investment Authority (KIA), the sovereign wealth fund of the State of Kuwait. Dr. Razouki is the youngest ever chief executive at a KIA owned company, the National Technology Enterprises Company. National Technology Enterprises Company (NTEC) was incorporated in November of 2002, by the Kuwait Council of Ministers as a fully owned company by the Kuwait Investment Authority (KIA), the sovereign wealth fund of the State of Kuwait. Capitalized at 100 million Kuwait Dinars (KD) which is equivalent to approximately $350 million US Dollars, NTEC aims to play a vital role in servicing major stakeholders in Kuwait and the Middle East region with their technology requirements and currently manages over one billion dollars in assets.Dr. Razouki is considered a thought leader within the life sciences industry and has championed the building of strong pillars of the local life sciences ecosystem including the region's premier pharmaceutical licensing and distribution platform; NewBridge—a 100 mn USD revenue company operating across all 22 MENA countries including Iraq, Iran, and Turkey as well as South Africa, Clinart—the region's top Clinical Research Organization (CRO) and host of the first-ever Phase II Clinical Trial in the history of Kuwait at the Dasman Diabetes Institute which achieved a successful exit to CTI in Q3 2020, eCore—the region's top active pharmaceutical ingredients licensor and distributor, the Life Sciences Academy—the region's first-ever training and development company focused on the healthcare and life sciences industry as well as Innomedics—one of Kuwait's top medical device distribution companies that pioneered the distribution of personalized digital health products in the region.Dr. Razouki has a number of inventions and patents registered with the Sabah Al Ahmed Center for the Gifted and Creative including Alberti—a Physical Therapy and MSK Robot with Artificial Intelligence, Equifoam—a Reactive Protective Equestrian Technology, Spider Duster—an Automated Building Window Washing Robot, iToilet—an IoT connected bathroom based laboratory, and Cyniq—a Solar Powered, WiFi, and WiTricity enabled beach umbrella.Dr. Razouki is also a former advisor to the central Kuwaiti government where he worked with senior government leaders during the administration of HE the Prime Minister, Sheikh Naser Al Mohammad Al Sabah and Deputy Prime Minister for Economic Affairs, Sheikh Ahmed Al Fahad Al Sabah on Healthcare, Education, and Entrepreneurial reforms as part of Kuwait's 100-billion-dollar Development Plan. Dr. Razouki continues to work closely with the Council of Ministers of Kuwait and is currently advising the government on the development of the Sabah Al Ahmad National Genome Center together with the Kuwait Foundation for the Advancement of Sciences, a National Pharmaceutical Quality Control Laboratory, and the 1 bn USD Jaber Hospital project, a 1168 facility which will be the largest single healthcare structure in the Middle East.

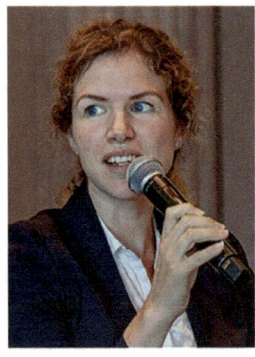

Sophie Smith is the Founder and CEO of Nabta Health (2017–present), a hybrid healthcare platform for women, empowering women in emerging markets to detect, diagnose, and treat non-communicable diseases. Smith is credited with coining the term "hybrid healthcare" and conceptualizing the hybrid healthcare model, which builds on principles of integrated care through the application of three core concepts: patient centricity, augmented intelligence, and decentralization.Smith has 11 years of industry experience as a technologist and serial impact entrepreneur. Prior to founding Nabta, Smith worked for Accenture as a technology consultant for 4 years and then founded several impact startups over 3 years including myZindagi (a doctor-finding platform based in Pakistan) and Le Plastics (a plastic recycling company based in Sierra Leone). Smith's lifetime ambition is to make healthcare affordable and accessible for all women.Smith read History at the University of Cambridge (2007–2010) and completed an MBA with the Quantic School of Business and Technology (2018).

Chapter 1
Introduction: What Is Hybrid Healthcare?

Mussaad Al-Razouki and Sophie Smith

Abstract Hybrid Healthcare is a term coined by Dr. Mussaad Al-Razouki and Sophie Smith to signify the transition of the traditional healthcare system into a digitally enabled system that still maintains a much needed humanistic presence in the physical space. Healthcare is an industry that cannot and should not be fully digitized. Digital technology must be embraced as part of a hybrid approach that puts the emphasis on the patient and the prevention of disease.

Keywords Hybrid healthcare · Digital health · Evidence based medicine
COVID-19 · Code of Hammurabi · Employer based healthcare

Silver Linings

In today's modern medical marketplace, healthcare businesses are usually divided into 'traditional' and 'digital' varieties. Traditional modalities of care are considered technical, rigid in nature, and are unerringly evidence-based. They involve quantitative methodologies along with established medical toolkits such as diagnostics (radiological and in the lab), population health and best practice guidelines (e.g. the National Institute for Healthcare and Excellence in the United Kingdom also known as NICE), and clinically validated data inputs. Digital modalities of care are still considered by many in the traditional medical establishment to be snake oil—flexible in nature, dismissive of best practice, and usually focused on intangibles such as access, patient experience, and patient engagement.

M. Al-Razouki (✉)
Business Development, Kuwait Life Sciences Company, Kuwait City, Kuwait
e-mail: mussaad@klsc.com.kw

S. Smith
Executive, Nabta Health, Dubai, United Arab Emirates
e-mail: sophie@nabtahealth.com

This book is about showing that the future of healthcare is a hybrid of the traditional and the digital; of in-person, provider-led healthcare systems, and virtual, patient-led, technology-enabled systems in which individuals are ultimately the architects of their own care. The next 15 chapters and 253 pages have been compiled over 18 months by 19 different authors from 13 different countries including China, India, Germany, Kuwait, Switzerland, the United Arab Emirates, United States, and the United Kingdom.

In our post COVID-19 era, we find that the word hybrid has entered the global zeitgeist, especially when it comes to the return to work and the discussion of hybrid workplaces or hybrid movie releases in theatres and in homes. Even though we started work on this book back in 2019, we are pleased to see the acceleration in the use of the word hybrid in healthcare.

Today, healthcare must be delivered by both traditional *and* digital means. The future of quality healthcare is firmly set in the coalescence of the digital world with not just the physical world, but the biological one as well (what is known as "the singularity"). The healthcare industry and all its stakeholders must be open to embracing a hybrid approach if they are to truly scale their businesses and drive positive changes in global population health.

Since antiquity, healthcare has been firmly rooted in the physical world. Doctors in Ancient Athens or biblical Babylon would visit with patients the same way they do today, the only difference would be that history's healers were usually motivated to keep their patients, their community, healthy, as opposed to the current fee for service model of 'sickcare.'

As of this date of publication, the scourge of COVID-19 has infected over 500 million people worldwide resulting in close to 6.3 million deaths, with ~86 million infections and 1 million deaths in the United States alone (with ~400,000 of those deaths occurring despite the availability of a COVID-19 vaccine since June 2021). What began in earnest as a seasonal pandemic quickly morphed into a once-in-a-century pandemic that changed the way we work, play and live, perhaps forever. The pandemic catapulted many industries—airlines, cinemas, cruise ships, hotels, live events, and more—onto the razor's edge of disruption. To cope with new, contact-based challenges, companies set up hybrid workplaces (for example; allowing employees to work from home or at the office) and began utilizing hybrid technological infrastructure (for example; storing company data on local and remote cloud-based servers).

This rapid evolution of behaviors was also seen, to an extent, in the healthcare industry. Pharmaceutical companies around the world collaborated to produce life-saving vaccines in a record 12 months. A plethora of digital health platforms focused on wellness and mental health were spawned. Prior to the pandemic, healthcare was one of the slowest industries to adopt the technologies of the twenty-first century. Even now, in a post-pandemic world of data rich social media profiles, the elusive electronic medical record escapes us. While consumers can easily transact everything from a home sharing vacation to buying an actual home online, most hospitals are still struggling with optimizing OR scheduling software or adopting computer order physician entry (CPOE) systems.

During the COVID-19 pandemic, the consumer's home became the epicenter of corporate focus, welcoming home cinema experiences, food delivery, and even IoT-enabled fitness solutions. While the home continues to be neglected from a healthcare perspective, the pandemic has ensured that the industry is ripe for a transition to hybrid healthcare. The intersection of the traditional healthcare system with new digital technologies will enable the rise of a robust hybrid healthcare ecosystem; one that encourages accountability, efficiency and cost-effectiveness through its three pillars of patient centricity, augmented intelligence, and decentralization.

The COVID-19 pandemic might have been a step backwards for humanity but its silver lining is that it has secured a great leap forward in the form of hybrid healthcare.

From Tablet to Tablet

Today, some 4000 years after Hammurabi's famous coded tablet, digital health entrepreneurs must consider hybrid models both of healthcare finance and healthcare delivery. Coding the digital realm and placing a touch screen tablet in a clinician or patient's hands is not enough. The haptic halo of human touch must remain omnipresent, despite the decentralized delivery mechanisms. To embrace the future head on, healthcare executives, clinicians, academics and entrepreneurs must dare to cross the digital divide and also plunge headfirst into the archaic world of traditional healthcare delivery.

Indeed, in a hybrid healthcare world, there will no longer need to be a four-tiered caste system of primary, secondary, tertiary and quaternary care. All patients will be of primary importance, while second to none technology is utilized to provide a holistic three dimensional experience.

This book will introduce various new-age modalities of healthcare including electronic medical records, online health marketplaces, digital diagnostics and therapeutics, as well recent developments in genetic therapy, robotic surgery, machine learning and artificial intelligence, cloud biology, the blockchain, and population health (including big data and personalized/precision medicine). The final chapters of the book will cover contemporary examples of hybrid healthcare such as retail medicine as well as other futuristic hybrid healthcare models focused on care delivery and clinical research. Finally, the book will also consider the topic of privacy in a semi-automated hybrid healthcare world and what consequences this may have for both health system regulators and clinical providers.

Hybrid for Humanity

There are over seven billion people that share our planet. It takes roughly seven trillion dollars per year to keep our global population (relatively) healthy, with over 50% of that spend occurring in the United States. As the world population skyrockets past the 10 and 15-billion-person mark in the next few decades, healthcare expenditure will not be able to keep up. Healthcare systems around the world, already struggling to cope with the growing prevalence of non-communicable diseases, will collapse.

Hybrid healthcare has the ability to take on the challenges of a rapidly growing, increasingly unhealthy global population by exponentially increasing its base and pace of delivery using the power of digital technologies, data collection, and analytics. Traditionally, the art and science of medicine (and some would say even the very nature of life itself), has relied on the constant yin and yang of 'trial and error'. Allowing for rapid experimentation, the likes of which we saw during the pandemic for the first time since World War II - across marketing funnel(s), product development, sales segments, and other areas of healthcare - will help the most diligent digital health entrepreneurs find the most efficient way(s) to scale their businesses.

And healthcare has always been about scale. Our burgeoning population means digital healthcare entrepreneurs will need to employ a hybrid healthcare approach to address the pain points of future generations. The belated promise of prevention in healthcare, a pyrrhic battle until the recent widespread use of smartphones, will also only be realized by digital means. The Holy Grail of Healthcare, that is precision or personalized medicine, will be seized by technological innovations that are designed to plug into a hybrid healthcare ecosystem.

Hybrid healthcare companies must focus on low-cost alternatives to traditional marketing if they are to realize efficiencies sufficient to serve the needs of our growing population. For example, they should look to use social media, viral marketing, psychographics, and targeted advertising, instead of wasting valuable runway dollars on offline advertising. Ironically, a viral digital health venture may be the best cure. Magical spagyric self-care apps and philosopher stone platforms will not simply or spontaneously self-generate ex-nihilo. We must work together, digital and traditional, if we are to survive.

In the dog-eat-dog world of entrepreneurship, there is no such thing as luck. The digital enablers that fuel hybrid healthcare; these miraculous tools of medicine, are the result of thousands of man-hours of analog and artificial intelligence. To paraphrase Thomas Jefferson, the harder you work, the luckier you get. This is hybrid healthcare.

Part I
Technologies Enabling Hybrid Healthcare

Chapter 2
Towards Artificial and Human Intelligence in Hybrid Healthcare

Anthony Chang, Tatiana Moreno, William Feaster, and Louis Ehwerhemuepha

Abstract Artificial Intelligence (AI) in hybrid healthcare has a wide application that begins with the application of machine learning (ML) algorithms and incorporates different cognitive technologies in either a research or clinical medical settings. The ultimate goal of AI is allowing patient portals, electronic health records, and even diagnostic and therapeutic equipment to not only mimic human cognition, but eventually one day surpass all of humanity's cognitive abilities combined. Indeed, the most elementary use case of AI in healthcare is the use of ML and other cognitive disciplines for diagnosing diseases and then mapping those diagnostic outcomes with a contemporary (or perhaps even a novel or tailored) treatment plan. Deep learning (also known as deep structured learning or hierarchical learning) is part of a broader family of machine learning methods based on learning data representations, as opposed to task-specific algorithms. In the hybrid healthcare context, this means gathering all the data (ever) recorded in patient Electronic Health Records (EHRs) and forming a digital knowledge base that includes various patient demographic, personal and clinical data, as well as all the past diagnoses, clinical decisions and treatment outcomes. The dream potential is that such AI systems will one day unlock a new era of personalized medicine that would go beyond the capability of an entire task force of specialists. As patient data skyrockets into the superfluous stratosphere of deep data lakes, AI will be as essential a tool to a doctor as the stethoscope once was.

A. Chang (✉) · T. Moreno · W. Feaster
The Sharon Disney Lund Medical Intelligence and Innovation Institute (MI3) at CHOC
Children's, Orange, CA, USA

L. Ehwerhemuepha
The Sharon Disney Lund Medical Intelligence and Innovation Institute (MI3) at CHOC
Children's, Orange, CA, USA

School of Computational and Data Science, Chapman University, Orange, CA, USA

© The Author(s), under exclusive license to Springer Nature
Switzerland AG 2022
M. Al-Razouki, S. Smith (eds.), *Hybrid Healthcare*, Health Informatics,
https://doi.org/10.1007/978-3-031-04836-4_2

Keywords Artificial Intelligence (AI) · Machine Learning (ML) · Deep Learning Algorithms · Virtual Healthcare · Convolution Neural Networks (CNNs) · Swarm Intelligence · Natural Language Processing (NLP) · Digital Medicine and Wearable Technology

Introduction to Artificial Intelligence

Artificial Intelligence Defined

Human intelligence is the ability to apply complex cognitive processes to acquire knowledge and to accomplish set objectives [1]. One of the most recent theories about human intelligence was developed by Howard Gardner in 1983 where he proposed the theory of multiple intelligences [2]. He identified eight different kinds of human intelligence deferring from the approach of Charles Spearman on "General Intelligence" [2, 3]. Artificial intelligence (AI) is the science of creating intelligent machines and computer programs to comprehend human intelligence with minimal to no human intervention [4]. The term was first used by John McCarthy in 1956 and Alan Turing, several years later, wrote the seminal paper on machines simulating human behavior and performing tasks that require intelligence [5, 6].

Why Artificial Intelligence Now?

Recent advances in artificial intelligence (AI) has fueled a technological revolution and unlocked a new wave of opportunity and innovation in digital medicine [4, 7]. Indeed, AI forms an important cornerstone of the future of hybrid healthcare. The emergence of AI in healthcare has been a result of the large volume of Big Data, the rise of sophisticated algorithms specifically in machine and deep learning, and the increase in storage capacity and computational power with cloud computing (more on this in Chap. 4) and graphic processing units (GPUs) [8]. The availability of vast amounts of data in healthcare has made AI in this context more relevant. While the great volume of data has allowed for the construction of intricate machine and deep learning models, the future of AI and its success will rest on the quality and integrity of biomedical data.

Current State of AI: Limitations of Humans and AI

The introduction of artificial intelligence into the medical field has prompted a lack of physician confidence and comfortability with AI due to a deficiency of knowledge in this area. While there is a "black box" mentality among many clinicians in regards to AI, it is integral to not only educate clinicians on the fundamentals of machine learning and AI, but also reinforce the predominant goal of attaining both human cognition and artificial intelligence in synergy within the medical field.

Advances in the use of deep learning algorithms such as convolutional neural networks and variational autoencoders for analyses of radiological images [9, 10] has led to a common misconception on how artificial intelligence might one day replace human intervention (in this case, the radiologist) in a clinical setting. While AI may outperform humans in areas of image interpretation and data analytics, it does not presently have the capacity of surpassing humans in areas of cognition and operation. Complex decision making and operational procedures in a clinical setting are best managed by healthcare providers and can be improved by augmenting both human and artificial intelligences. Clinicians' experience is unlikely to be replaced by artificial intelligence in the near future but instead their consolidation will drive a flourishing healthcare system. This is why we advocate a hybrid approach to incorporating healthcare into the decision making/diagnostic tree of a clinical organization. Together, human IQ and machine AI are much more powerful than when operating in silos.

Of course, there are various limitations in both human cognition and artificial intelligence; thus the coalescence between human and machine can mitigate the impact of these constraints and optimize both resources. Human bias coupled with machine impartiality and human contextual familiarity coupled with machine velocity will drive the future of medicine. Figure 2.1 delineates the advantages and weaknesses of human and machine on a singular level. It is noteworthy to mention the disadvantages of human and machine are balanced by the assets of one another. For example, a machine's lack of cognition is counterbalanced by human cognition, and humans' brute time consumption is met with machine velocity. The imperfections of both man and machine are clearly neutralized by the presence of both. Humans working with machines are better than either working in isolation. The difference between human and machine is simply but directly declared by Dr. Stuart G. Walesh as he states "The computer is incredibly fast, accurate and stupid. Man is unbelievably slow, inaccurate and brilliant. The marriage of the two is a challenge and opportunity beyond imagination." [11]

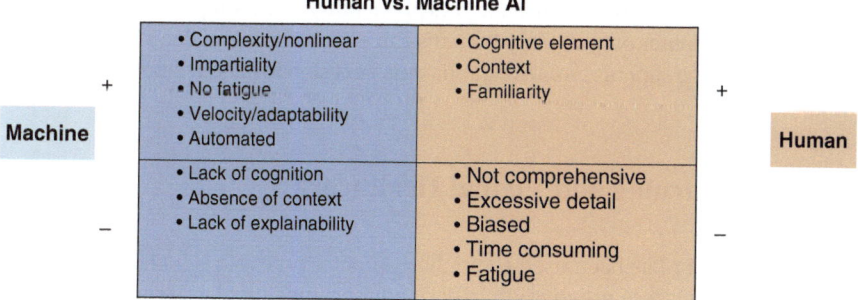

Fig. 2.1 Demonstration of the positive and negative aspects of human cognition and artificial intelligence

Health Care Data

Electronic Health Records (EHR) and Clinical Decision Support

The emergence and utilization of EHR systems in healthcare facilities has resulted in the proliferation of large amounts of electronic medical data. We also have a new tsunami of data fast approaching the healthcare system thanks to all the connected devices, both personal wearables (or even sensors that may one day be injected into our bodies) and large scale medical devices. The management of this medical data has been plagued with issues of which accessibility for advanced analytics is most pronounced. However, the digitalization of medical records or the electronic medical records (EMR), is what catalyzed the synchronization of advanced analytics and artificial intelligence with traditional health care [12]. The widespread use of electronic health record data coupled with advanced analytics software has revolutionized the visualization and interpretation of this substantial data. Analytics platforms including Qlik and Tableau have set the foundation for the exploration and visual analysis of large quantities of patient record data and detected relevance in vast amounts of this unstructured data [13]. The strides made in healthcare data visualization propelled the rapid growth of artificial intelligence research in medicine. The emergence and utilization of EMR systems in healthcare facilities has also advanced the progression of AI in medicine including various platforms hosting multi-site electronic health records data to facilitate data analysis [14]. This large volume of electronically captured data has enabled the application of various branches of artificial intelligence in medicine.

Although the EHR has catalyzed the emergence of AI and machine learning algorithms for clinical support, this system is introducing vast amounts of data to be interpreted and time consuming data entry which is a clerical burden for physicians [15]. To combat clinical fatigue, artificial intelligence has played a key role in abating physician burnout and working as a clinical support tool to provide higher value of care to patients [15]. Ultimately, AI has the capability of automating routine functions including updating patient records or billing through robotic process automation (RPA) [15]. Through the use of RPA, physicians will have more time to spend with patients face-to-face, and it is key to note RPA and AI cannot replace clinicians due to machine's lack of cognition and explainability to develop a plan of action in response to computer output. Only humans can use machine and deep learning algorithms as decision support tools to establish the next step in patient care management.

Machine Learning and Virtual Healthcare

Machine learning has been used to predict patients' probable ICU length of stays, chronic kidney disease progression, risk of adult asthma, to classify high-risk pediatric severe sepsis cases, and countless others [16–19]. Machine learning is an application of artificial intelligence which has been prevalent in the medical field allowing for the pursuance of diverse research projects. Research using de-identified EHR data from the University of California San Francisco Medical Center from 2011–2016 has been done to develop a machine learning algorithm to detect severe sepsis in pediatric patients up to 4 h before onset [19]. Early detection of severe sepsis in pediatric patients is vital for an effective treatment plan. The use of boosted ensembles of decision trees for predicting severe sepsis has outperformed existing pediatric organ dysfunction and inflammatory response scoring systems [19]. This machine learning algorithm is another vital opportunity for clinical decision support and not only aims to flag all high-risk patients but also limit the number of falsely reported cases of pediatric severe sepsis to control alert fatigue. It is in the best interest of hospitals to utilize and implement these indispensable tools for better allocation of resources, to improve patient care, and to circumvent adverse clinical outcomes.

Not only has artificial intelligence and machine learning been applied to predictive modeling but also has contributed to virtual healthcare. The development of virtual assistants have emerged in medicine to help resolve the issue of insufficient clinical workforce to handle patients with chronic symptoms [20]. While it is imperative to recognize virtual health assistants are not meant to replace in person visits with health care providers, virtual interaction with medical assistants can use patient data to individualize support for these patients in real-time [20]. Diabetes rates are globally increasing, and the assistance of a virtual medical assistant can aid patients that are struggling with diabetes management [20]. Utilizing virtual educational and medical visits does not replace but augments patients' access to more support systems and improve upon patient's psychosocial well-being and metabolic control [20].

Image Classification Through Convolution Neural Networks (CNNs) and Swarm Intelligence

With the digitalization of medical records over the past 50 years there has been a prevalent issue regarding the sheer size of this data and how to extrapolate relevant information. The large volume of medical data has given rise to new machine and deep learning algorithms with the capability of analyzing and providing relevant classification and predictive elements. There have been recent strides in deep learning and artificial intelligence in image recognition. Convolution Neural Networks (CNNs) have been useful for image recognition where different features from an image are extracted by applying various filters over the image.

Specific case studies have explored the accuracy of deep learning convolution neural networks (CNN) in detecting the presence of thoracic diseases such as lung cancer and tuberculosis in patients [21]. The detection of these possible thoracic diseases is made possible through the use of a CNN developed to detect 14 diverse pathologies some including pulmonary masses, pneumonia, and nodules in frontal-view chest radiographs [21].

Using the ChestX-ray [8] largest open source dataset consisting of over 100,000 anonymized chest X-ray images provided by the NIH Clinical Center [22], researchers were able to develop an algorithm named CheXNeXt to not only detect 14 clinically relevant pathologies but also highlight the specific areas of the X-ray image where each pathology was determined to reside [21]. The algorithm's predictive performance was compared to nine practicing cardiothoracic specialty radiologists, and CheXNeXt achieved statistically comparable performance to these practicing radiologists in determining ten pathologies, and achieved statistically significantly higher performance in detecting atelectasis. However, the radiologists achieved a statistically significantly higher performance detecting cardiomegaly, emphysema, and hiatal hernias than the algorithm [21]. While CheXNeXt did perform worse on three pathologies in comparison to the practicing radiologists, it is noteworthy to mention the algorithm labeled 420 chest X-ray images in 1 min and 30 s whereas radiologists were able to accomplish this task in 240 min on average [21].

The findings from this study illuminate the relevance of the necessary desegregation of human and machine in medicine. There are always areas in which human intelligence outperforms artificial intelligence and vice versa; therefore, it is crucial to remove this divide to exponentially progress in all aspects of healthcare. While great strides have been made in machine vision using convolution neural networks, computers still lack context and the ability to provide a spectrum of possibilities relating to diagnosis classification. For example, a machine is able to provide binary classification of the presence or absence of a specific disease or diagnosis but lacks human cognition and explainability to provide a large spectrum of output delineating a more sophisticated diagnosis and plan of action. Thus, the rapidity of machines to process information coalesced with the experience of humans is the recipe guiding the future evolution of medicine.

Swarm Intelligence

As usual, we look to biological systems when developing a new paradigm or an advancement in computing—in this case, swarm intelligence. Swarm intelligence is the approach to complex problem solving by sharing information within members of a large group or community [23–25]. We may be able to achieve a hybrid human-machine swarm intelligence if such group/community is made of both humans and machine sharing information under an appropriate framework.

Research at Stanford University School of Medicine in Artificial Swarm Intelligence (ASI) has been done to address a key question of whether a small group of radiologists working together in real-time could outperform machine learning systems that can currently surpass individual physician performance [26]. A software platform called swarm.ai was developed and allowed groups of humans to form closed-loop swarms where they have the capability of thinking together in real time as a unified system [26]. The swarm.ai platform user interface allows users to manipulate a "graphical puck" driving it to select an answer by positioning their "graphical magnet" with respect to the puck.

The swarm.ai platform was used in a study conducted by eight radiologists connected by AI swarming algorithms to diagnose a set of fifty chest X-rays. Ultimately, when comparing the CheXNeXt machine learning algorithm with individual radiologist performance and ASI performance, the ASI significantly outperformed both in terms of binary classification, mean absolute error and area under the ROC curve. This example of ASI delineates the stark outperformance of the union of human and machine in comparison to both working in seclusion, and reaffirms the necessity of human cognition.

Exploring Natural Language Processing (NLP)

Over 80% of healthcare data is unstructured ranging from medical video data from medical imaging devices to clinical notes. Many healthcare systems do not have the capacity to handle, manage, and process this information [27]. Natural Language Processing (NLP) has bridged the gap between human language and computer to process and understand unstructured data (Fig. 2.2).

A case study using NLP automated a clinical extraction system used to obtain detailed epilepsy information from unstructured clinical notes and to derive epilepsy surgery candidacy scores which were validated using expert manual chart

Fig. 2.2 Natural language process schematic diagram

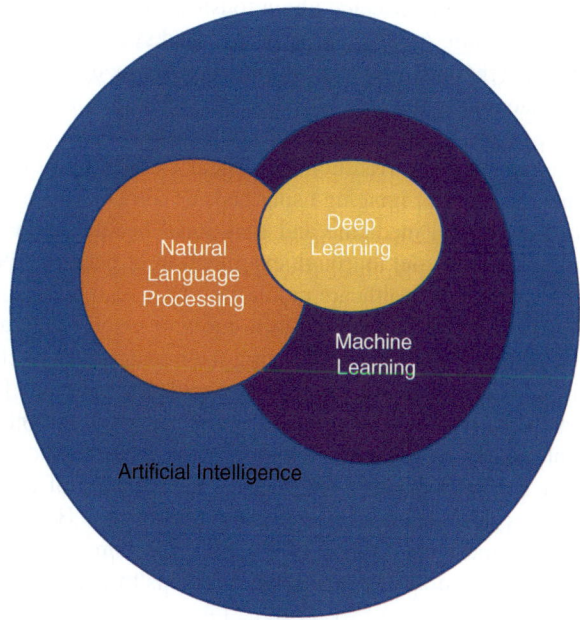

review [28]. This EHR-integrated NLP application was developed to flag patients most in need of surgery using retrospective neurologic data from the Cincinnati Children's Hospital Medical Center (CCHMC) [28]. This application was able to detect eligible patients for surgical consultation up to 2 years prior to their actual referral [28]. These dynamic epilepsy surgery candidacy scores would aid clinicians in deciphering which patients are optimal candidates for surgery at an earlier period. Natural Language Processing is another key instance of the consolidation of artificial and human intelligence to organize vast amounts of data with the purpose of propelling rapid diagnoses and decreasing unfavorable patient outcomes.

This case study elucidates the union of man and machine through an application predicting a patients' candidacy for epileptic surgery. The application then flags these patients thus providing the clinician with an extra layer of vital information in determining the most suitable next step in a patient's treatment plan. For NLP to be effective the synergy of human cognition with machine intelligence is vital. While machine intelligence can provide classifications and diagnosis predictions through clinical notes, physician action is what drives patient treatment and care. Humans and the AI machine are the backbone of the capability and efficacy of NLP.

Future of AI in Medicine

Digital Medicine and Wearable Technology

Traditional healthcare has been transformed through innovations in digital medicine. The prevalence and ubiquitousness of technology have led to a progression in digital health. An abundance of digitized systems including sensors detecting heart rate and rhythm, smartwatches measuring blood pressure, glucose tracking systems, and measuring oxygen saturation through use of an oximeter to observe sleep apnea have incorporated AI systems to provide health information in the hands of the average person [29]. Traditional physical examination of patients combined with the incorporation of imaging using bedside ultrasound imaging is yet another example of how digital medicine and traditional healthcare may syndicate to provide the most accurate and thorough examination of patients [29]. Wearable biosensors for the purpose of healthcare monitoring have also come to fruition since the influx of smartphones, and this real-time monitoring has the capability of providing vital information on health, improving the management of chronic illness and notifying health care professionals of any health irregularities [30]. Not only does digital medicine refer to the pervasiveness of medical content in the hands of all patients but also is prevalent on a larger scale in a healthcare environment. A Stanford research team looking to improve the accuracy of the surgical removal of breast tumors developed a system using Microsoft's HoloLens headsets to replicate a three-dimensional image of the patient's tumor onto the surgical site [31]. This three-dimensional image allows surgeons to use the reflections of the hologram to remove all of the tumor while leaving intact as much health tissue as possible [31]. Digitized applications to improve medical capabilities and content, commerce and instant connectivity is the fundamental goal and future of AI in digital medicine.

Ultimately, the future of our hybrid healthcare system is dependent on the unification of human and artificial intelligence. While there have been abundant strides in the technological automation of various healthcare practices, it is of paramount importance to understand the two leading contributors in the progress of the efficiency and efficacy of patient care are both human and machine. This was clearly shown in a study using deep learning-assisted diagnosis of cerebral aneurysms where the augmentation of both human/physician intelligence and that of artificial intelligence exceeded the use of either alone [32]. The growth in digital medicine and rise in wearable and implantable technology benefits from embedded AI to organize, store, and analyze the large volumes of data generated. Generative artificial intelligence algorithms like Generative Adversarial Networks will circumvent the issue of small sample sizes data in cases where only a small amount of data is available or when dealing with human labeled data specifically in small patient populations or rare disease. While many view AI as dehumanizing medicine it is vital to recognize AI's role in relieving clinicians' burden with big data and allowing clinicians' more time for patient interaction. The ability of machines to process vast amounts of data in minutes linked with years of physician experience is what will drive revolutionary advancements in medicine. The combination of AI and traditional medicine will be a norm rather than an exception and the best healthcare systems will have effectively integrated technology in medicine; thus, the unification of digital medicine, AI, and EMR data will be the hallmark of a thriving hybrid healthcare system.

References

1. Hunt E. Human intelligence. Cambridge University Press; 2010.
2. Gardner H. Frames of mind: the theory of multiple intelligences. Paris: Hachette UK; 2011.
3. Spearman C. "General intelligence". Objectively Determined and Measured. In: Jenkins JJ, Paterson DG, editors, Studies in individual differences: The search for intelligence. Appleton-Century-Crofts. 1961:59–73.
4. Hamet P, Tremblay J. Artificial intelligence in medicine. Metabolism. 2017;69:S36–40.
5. Bush V, et al. As we may think. Atl Mon. 1945;176(1):101–8.
6. Turing A. Computing machinery and intelligence. Mind. 1950;59(236):433.
7. Komorowski M, Celi LA, Badawi O, Gordon AC, Faisal AA. The artificial intelligence clinician learns optimal treatment strategies for sepsis in intensive care. Nat Med. 2018;24(11):1716.
8. Dilsizian SE, Siegel EL. Artificial intelligence in medicine and cardiac imaging: harnessing big data and advanced computing to provide personalized medical diagnosis and treatment. Curr Cardiol Rep. 2014;16(1):441.
9. Thrall JH, Li X, Li Q, et al. Artificial intelligence and machine learning in radiology: opportunities, challenges, pitfalls, and criteria for success. J Am Coll Radiol. 2018;15(3):504–8.
10. Hosny A, Parmar C, Quackenbush J, Schwartz LH, Aerts HJWL. Artificial intelligence in radiology. Nat Rev Cancer. 2018;18(8):500–10.
11. Fripp J, Fripp M, Fripp D. Speaking of science. Newnes; 2000.

12. AOCNP DCC. The evolution of the electronic health record. Clin J Oncol Nurs. 2015;19(2):153.
13. Siddiqui T, Alkadri M, Khan NA. Review of programming languages and tools for big data analytics. Int J Adv Res Comput Sci. 2017;8(5):1112–8.
14. Evans RS. Electronic health records: then, now, and in the future. Yearb Med Inform. 2016;25(S01):S48–61.
15. Martin A. Using AI and NLP to alleviate Physician Burnout. 2019.
16. Rojas JC, Carey KA, Edelson DP, Venable LR, Howell MD, Churpek MM. Predicting intensive care unit readmission with machine learning using electronic health record data. Ann Am Thorac Soc. 2018;15(7):846–53.
17. Kumar M. Prediction of chronic kidney disease using random forest machine learning algorithm. Int J Comput Sci Mob Comput. 2016;5(2):24–33.
18. Nir-Paz R, Almogy G, Keren A, et al. 2223. Real-time prediction of respiratory pathogen infection based on machine learning decision support tool. In: Open forum infectious diseases, vol. 6; 2019. p. S758–9.
19. Le S, Hoffman J, Barton C, et al. Pediatric severe sepsis prediction using machine learning. Front Pediatr. 2019;7:413.
20. Ramchandani N. Virtual coaching to enhance diabetes care. Diabetes Technol Ther. 2019;21(S2):S2–48.
21. Rajpurkar P, Irvin J, Ball RL, et al. Deep learning for chest radiograph diagnosis: A retrospective comparison of the CheXNeXt algorithm to practicing radiologists. PLoS Med. 2018;15(11):e1002686.
22. Wang X, Peng Y, Lu L, Lu Z, Bagheri M, Summers RM. Chestx-ray8: hospital-scale chest X-ray database and benchmarks on weakly-supervised classification and localization of common thorax diseases. In: Proceedings of the IEEE conference on computer vision and pattern recognition; 2017. p. 2097–106.
23. Blum C, Merkle D. Swarm intelligence in optimization. In: Blum C, Merkle D, editors. Swarm Intell; 2008. p. 43–85.
24. Bonabeau E, Dorigo M, de RDF MD, Theraulaz G, Théraulaz G, et al. Swarm intelligence: from natural to artificial systems. Oxford University Press; 1999.
25. Krause J, Ruxton GD, Krause S. Swarm intelligence in animals and humans. Trends Ecol Evol. 2010;25(1):28–34.
26. Rosenberg L, Lungren M, Halabi S, Willcox G, Baltaxe D, Lyons M. Artificial swarm intelligence employed to amplify diagnostic accuracy in radiology. In: 2018 IEEE ninth annual information technology, electronics and mobile communication conference (IEMCON); 2018. p. 1186–91.
27. Kong H-J. Managing unstructured big data in healthcare system. Healthc Inform Res. 2019;25(1):1.
28. Wissel BD, Greiner HM, Glauser TA, et al. Prospective validation of a machine learning model that uses provider notes to identify candidates for resective epilepsy surgery. Epilepsia. 2019 61 39–48.
29. Topol EJ. A decade of digital medicine innovation. Sci Transl Med. 2019;11(498):eaaw7610.
30. Kim J, Campbell AS, de Ávila BE-F, Wang J. Wearable biosensors for healthcare monitoring. Nat Biotechnol. 2019;37(4):389–406.
31. White T. High-tech health: how digital medicine is improving patient care. Stanford Med. 2018. Stanford Med. http://stanmed.stanford.edu/2018fall/digital-medicine-improve-patient-care.html
32. Park A, Chute C, Rajpurkar P, et al. Deep learning—assisted diagnosis of cerebral aneurysms using the HeadXNet model. JAMA Netw Open. 2019;2(6):e195600.

Chapter 3
Hybrid Healthcare Enhanced by Blockchain

Wendy Charles

Abstract As hybrid healthcare organizations strive to combine traditional in-person treatment models with digital health technologies, there is a need to manage data and technologies more effectively and efficiently. Blockchain technology is increasingly implemented in healthcare and may enhance functions to allow healthcare providers more capabilities and flexibility as they desire to utilize more features of digital health. At its most basic, blockchain is a time-stamped sequential list of data linked together using cryptography and managed by a distributed cluster of computers: a "distributed ledger technology." This chapter introduces blockchain concepts as they are applied to healthcare and the hybridization of digital health in interpersonal healthcare delivery. There is a detailed focus on blockchain features that can assist organizations in meeting the Final Rule of the 21st Century Cures Act for patient-centered access and value-based care information. This chapter also offers basic guidelines as to when a blockchain might best meet an organization's needs, as well as step-by-step decisions organizations should consider when implementing blockchain. Healthcare leaders and providers are provided with a nuanced understanding of blockchain's current potential and how this technology may assist with hybrid healthcare.

Keywords Blockchain · Digital health · Digital front door · Hybrid health · Smart contracts

Blockchain is an innovative method of managing data by combining several traditional methods of record keeping and automation. Blockchain concepts were first described in a 2008 white paper attributed to the pseudonym "Satoshi Nakamoto," [1] a person or group that has not been definitively identified to this day. The first notions of blockchain examined a peer-to-peer electronic financial environment that

W. Charles (✉)
BurstIQ, Englewood, CO, USA

University of Colorado Denver, CO, USA
e-mail: wendy.charles@cuanschutz.edu

© The Author(s), under exclusive license to Springer Nature
Switzerland AG 2022
M. Al-Razouki, S. Smith (eds.), *Hybrid Healthcare*, Health Informatics,
https://doi.org/10.1007/978-3-031-04836-4_3

does not require a central intermediary, such as a bank, for registering financial transactions. As a result of this interest, a cryptocurrency, bitcoin, was developed and communicated over a blockchain-based network [2]. At the time of this writing in 2020, the use of blockchain-based networks are now used in widespread applications across most large industries, including electronic technologies used for healthcare [3, 4]. This chapter introduces blockchain concepts and describes emerging applications in the hybridization of interpersonal care interactions and digital health.

Introduction to Blockchain

While the term blockchain is gaining popularity, many of the core features and terms may seem novel to a healthcare audience. This section introduces several fundamental concepts as applied to healthcare technologies.

Core Features

Ledgers

Comparable to an old-fashioned accounting log book, blockchain technology stores information on a single ever-growing ledger [5] instead of using a database that stores in prescribed fields or columns and rows. The ledger does not allow previous entries to be changed or deleted, but new entries are added to the ledger each time information is created, retrieved, or appended [6]. This allows for a clear audit trail and removes common data disputes when data are missing or erroneous.

When entries are created, they are verified as correct, placed order, and held in a queue [7]. Each type of blockchain platform uses performance optimization techniques for how many entries can be created and held in the queue before they are bundled together as a "block" [7]. When bundled together in a block, there is much more security to preserve the integrity of individual entries.

Security

The next core feature of blockchain is cryptography—a method of protecting information by ensuring that each transaction is digitally signed [8]. Cryptography using public and private key pairs ensures privacy when shared because stakeholders can only access information for which they have the correct keys. Each new entry is also summarized as a "one-way cryptographic hash." A hash is defined by the U.S. National Institute of Standards and Technology [9] as a unique and unpredictable output of the same size/length to any type of input (e.g., a word, string of text, file, or even block). The calculations are extremely sophisticated so that the hash output could not be reverse-engineered to determine the input. There is also a single hash that represents a cryptographic signature of all contents of the block, including information about when the block was created as well as additional information about the blockchain validation structure [9]. This block "summary" hash also helps to verify that blocks shared in a network are undamaged and unaltered [9]. Changing the content within a block would also change its block signature hash.

Block signature hashes comprise the technology for how blocks are linked together to form a "chain." The block signature hash is saved in the header of the next block created. If modifying the content of a block, this would then require all subsequent blocks to change their signature hashes because they contain the signature hashes of the previous blocks [8]. Therefore, changing any information within a block could create an easily-detected break in the chain and would lead to rejection of altered blocks [9]. While this design feature allows blockchains to be very secure, there are circumstances where contents of a block could be retroactively modified. Such retroactive tampering requires tremendous computing power or a collaboration within the platform governance structure. Therefore, blockchains are theoretically (or technically) not "immutable" and NIST instead describes blockchain technology as "tamper resistant" and "tamper evident" [9].

Shared Distribution

To protect information stored on a blockchain, ledgers are distributed across many computers or servers referred to as "nodes" [9]. There can be a few as three nodes or thousands of nodes. In general, the distribution of blockchains across nodes provides protection against modification or loss. If the ledger in each node remains identical to the ledgers in other participating nodes, the blockchain is believed to maintain integrity [8]. This feature is particularly pertinent to the protection of health information with consideration that health information stored on a central server is prone to accidental modification / deletion or server downtimes. Further, health servers are vulnerable to cyber-attacks, malware, or even ransom [6, 10].

Consensus

Because nodes communicate with each other instead of passing information through a central authority, it is important to ensure that the nodes agree about the authenticity and validity of new blocks. Therefore, blockchain platforms rely on different decision-making tools to reach "consensus" [11]. Once consensus has been reached, the block is transmitted to all the nodes to update their ledgers to maintain consistency. There are many consensus models—each with their own positive and negative attributes—depending on the particular uses and needs of the platform [9].

Permissioning

The concept of blockchain "permissioning" determines whether any person can join a blockchain or whether participation is restricted to known and invited users. While there are a number of variations, there are two high-level categorizations of blockchains: "permissioned" and "permissionless."

Permissionless blockchains allow anyone to join and perform actions for the network without advanced permission, such as Bitcoin and Ethereum platforms, and are popular for transacting cryptocurrency [12]. Network participants are pseudonymous in that they are only identified by a public key (similar to a public user ID). Also, transactions on permissionless networks are transparent and visible to all participants on the network and all stakeholders have equal access to audit transactions [8]. Scalability of ledger size and privacy are concerns for permissionless chains and thus are not used for health information [13].

Permissioned blockchain networks restrict involvement to specific people or organizations [9] to protect the privacy of information and identity of participants. These platforms have also been designed to manage data volume, speed, and scalability needed for health-related applications [14–16]. These private networks, such as Hyperledger suite of products [17], are typically maintained by consortia or individual organizations, and are designed to feature granular or fine-grained permissions [18]. Information within blocks can be encrypted so that only the owners of the cryptographic keys can access information within an area [8]. Therefore, the governance structure ensures oversight not just of the authenticity of blocks but also provides systematic checks and privacy validations of the entire network [9].

There is also an option that is essentially a hybrid of permissionless and permissioned networks. Data is stored in a private location but the public chain provides additional data integrity and protection. In fact, some health-oriented blockchains have chosen to pursue this option because they are concerned that a permissioned blockchain would be too centralized and less trustworthy. As an example of health companies that have a private area on the Ethereum platform, Dentacoin is a blockchain company designed to improve affordability in the dental industry [8] and ConsenSys Health offers an enterprise-level blockchain for multiple healthcare solutions [14].

Smart Contracts

Code can be added to blockchain ledgers to automate and regulate how data are used. These pieces of code are called "smart contracts" and execute automatically when specified conditions are met [19]. While not particularly "smart" or technically a "contract," smart contracts can implement terms, obligations, payments, and even financial penalties as specified in a traditional contract [19] operating the same way, indefinitely [8]. Smart contracts are not necessarily included in every block-chain, but have many valuable uses in healthcare [8].

For example, smart contracts can automate access controls involving protected health information for transparent regulatory and audit purposes [19, 20]. The auto-mation afforded by smart contracts is a critical principle for healthcare efficiency that will be described later regarding how blockchain can enhance capabilities for hybrid health.

Healthcare Enhanced by Blockchain

Hybrid healthcare enlists the multi-faceted efforts healthcare organizations are put-ting forward to include digital health technologies and traditional in-person treat-ment models to put patients at the center of healthcare delivery [21]. Ideally, blockchain need not replace existing technology but should be added to enhance the capabilities of the existing digital health technologies [10]. There are a wide range of blockchain-based hybrid health configurations being developed and this section explains how blockchain can be a valuable component of hybrid healthcare.

Aggregation of Patient Information

Blockchain networks have remarkable and unique capabilities to integrate disparate and complicated data sources [10]. As examples for hybrid health, blockchain is very useful when there is need to bring together multiple sources of medical infor-mation, treatment, and other factors that can influence medical decisions [22]. When integrating information, organizations can choose to store data on the blockchain ("on-chain") or "off-chain" where the blockchain points to central servers or data repositories called "data lakes" [23]. When data are stored off-chain, the blockchain is not used for storage but only to verify data integrity [13]. While most healthcare data are currently stored off-chain, healthcare organizations are increasingly experi-menting with storing data on-chain to ensure more protection against data tamper-ing and to allow more functionality without having to reformat or recode raw data.

As an example of an organization processing health information on-chain, Intermountain Healthcare, a non-profit 22-hospital, 180-clinic healthcare system used the BurstIQ blockchain to integrate surgical information from electronic health records (nature of surgery, surgeons, time to close, adverse events), billing informa-tion, scheduling, surgical supply usage, and inventory [24]. By mapping these data sources and querying the ledger, administrator could identify and visualize outliers on multiple combinations of parameters to standardize surgical costs and care. As a result of this unique functionality, the hospital system saved $90 million dollars over four years and used blockchain-based dashboards to educate surgeons about practices used by their peers [24].

Patient Control and Engagement with Health Information

In conventional healthcare delivery, health information is often maintained by a single healthcare organization or system without full patient access to incentivize continued care through that system [8]. Unfortunately, this tendency has prevented patients from being able to identify and correct errors in their health information and to actively engage with their providers [8]. In an effort to improve digital medical record access, the Final Rule of the 21st Century Cures Act implemented in 2020, the Office of the National Coordinator's (ONC) Health Information Technology promotes innovation in healthcare delivery systems. This Rule requires ready access to digital medical records using modern computers and smart phone based software apps to gain considerably more healthcare information [25]. A goal is to prevent waste from duplicating testing when other medical providers are not aware of previous testing and diagnostics.

While no specific technology solutions are required, organizations are looking to blockchain technologies to make healthcare information more accessible [26]. First, blockchain is being used as one of the technologies to improve interoperability to connect medical stakeholders without requiring complex and expensive layers of data mediators. Blockchain has already been used to create Health Insurance Portability and Accountability Act (HIPAA)-compliant cost-effective health information exchanges. For instance, in 2018, the State of Colorado integrated the three largest health information exchanges by adding quality records to a blockchain [15]. This level of access to digital health records allows for complete and cost-effective exchanges [8].

An additional key consideration of health information access involves ensuring patient authorization of how their health information will be used or disclosed [10]. Patients increasingly want to provide and rescind access to their health information and under their own terms [8]. Therefore, to authorize health information more readily with other physicians and care providers [26], blockchain offers unique capabilities for managing authorization at a granular or fine-grained level [14, 27]. As a real-world example, the country of Estonia implemented a layer of blockchain underneath their electronic health record system [28, 29]. With a user-friendly interface, patients login to see how their health information is accessed and can easily add or remove permissions using blockchain-based controls. This type of granular consent also manages patients' consent for research, advanced directives, and other healthcare decisions [30]. Medical providers and researchers can review patients' decisions stored in this digital trusted environment and act on them accordingly, confident that they are adhering to patient wishes [10].

Digital Front Doors

The 21st Century Cures Act is also driving toward a value-driven digital health system. The ONC specified that patients must be granted access to considerably more care health ecosystem information to acquire information about care quality and costs [25, 26]. Similar to consumers' experiences with online travel and shopping, the goal is to promote transparency of services and quality to enable patients to have more perceived patient and payer choice [25]. This shift will provide patient with patients with the transparency to make more informed decisions as healthcare consumers [26].

This regulation is compelling hybrid healthcare to be much more than an "office visit." A new concept—a "digital front door"—exceeds capabilities of a patient portal and instead serves as a comprehensive strategy for engaging patients and providers at multiple points of their healthcare journey [31]. Digital front doors may not necessarily introduce new technologies but can leverage blockchain to enhance communication and engagement. As a prominent example of a digital front door, the National Health Services in the United Kingdom is building a digital front door with the ultimate goal of connecting more clinical practices [32]. This technology will provide patients with a wide range of digital options: to book appointments, pre-registration, order prescriptions, track symptoms, perform virtual visits, and specify organ donation preferences [32, 33]. While different types of technologies can be used, blockchain is being explored as one of the underlying technologies that can integrate all of these sources of information allowing a digital front door to connect far more options in a single user interface. A digital front door also offers efficiencies resulting from automating tasks that had customarily been human-based manual tasks [31]. Specifically, using blockchain-based smart contracts, there is automation of time-intensive processes, such as making referrals to specialists, or providing answers to routine questions. Digital front doors have been shown to reduce no-shows, increase efficiency with billing/payment plans, productivity and, hence, revenue [31].

Integration of Internet of Things

Internet-based digital tools allow for a transition from capturing snapshots of disease in a doctor's office to real-time continuous monitoring [34]. When biosensors are designed with characteristics more easily adapted to the human body, such as watches, belts, bendable strips, or glasses, there is greatly increased compliance [35] These advances in medical Internet of Things (IoT) devices, have led to portable, off-the-shelf electrocardiograms, electroencephalograms, and kinematic motion sensors to track patients' health remotely [36]. These devices are also currently being deployed for remote depression and anxiety management and diabetes management [36].

Blockchain has a unique capability of bringing together raw disparate sources of these medical IoT devices with the treatment network [10] so that physicians have more capability of monitoring patients remotely [36]. Because blockchain-based integration of IoT devices has been shown to be cost-effective, this technology is increasingly implemented in wider monitoring applications [10].

Automation of Alerts and Diagnoses

When using medical IoT sensors for monitoring, the vast amounts of accumulated data present an ongoing challenge—there is too much data for a medical provider to review and manage [37]. Therefore, blockchain-based smart contracts are also automated to create physician alerts as a patient's health is worsening [36]. As an example of a sensor integrated with electronic health records using blockchain, a diabetic patient can connect a glucose monitor that can alert the physician when the results are too high [37]. Smart contracts can also generate texts to patients and providers [37].

A blockchain-based data collection strategy can store information from multiple disparate sources and create larger data sets for training artificial intelligence algorithms. This strategy is being applied to create new neural networks and other artificial intelligence strategies for diagnosis [22] or reading radiology images [37]. This technology is also anticipated to provide benefit for cancer patients to plan personalized care and determine individual treatment plans based on different disease trajectories [36].

Implementation Considerations

Needs and Values

Before planning to launch a blockchain solution, it is necessary to understand the needs and values of your organization.

When a Blockchain Is Helpful

Blockchain offers many features that improve data aggregation and integrity, but should only be considered when the problem cannot be achieved by readily available technologies. Stated another way, health professionals should ask "how can blockchain benefit us?" instead of asking "how can we use blockchain?" [9].

To help organizations assess the business value of adding blockchain, the World Economic Forum [38] offers useful grids and guidelines in "Blockchain Beyond the Hype: A Practical Framework for Business Leaders." This report asks organizations to consider a number of business questions and work through a flowchart of needs, such as needs for intermediaries or levels of access. Another report published by the World Economic Forum [39] provides a list of blockchain dimensions, capabilities and value drivers to consider. For example, if a business identifies the need to improve profitability and quality, the blockchain value drivers are automation, traceability, speed/efficiency, control, security, and evidence of tampering [39].(page 8).

These grids are very helpful for identifying blockchain capabilities that correspond to their values.

The National Institute of Standards and Technology [9] offers a flowchart to assist organizations determine when blockchain may be helpful for a collaborative effort. A blockchain may be useful when:

- Multiple organizations or individuals need a shared, consistent data source.
- There is uncertain trust among all parties.
- More than one organization or individual needs to contribute or review data.
- There is an audit log of all activities accessible to all parties.
- There is a need for shared leadership where there is not a single central authority [9] (page 42).

Implementation

After making a decision to move forward with blockchain in hybrid healthcare, the implementation is context- and case-specific [21]. The following are recommended steps:

1. *Provide education.* Blockchain technology is subject to varying degrees of misunderstandings and hype [10]. Therefore, discussions about blockchain may require considerable stakeholder and organization education, as some individuals may not understand the inherent differences of blockchain from cryptocurrency [38, 40, 41].
2. *Stay open-minded about platforms.* After stakeholders have granted permission to gather information about blockchain solutions, start with a platform-agnostic approach.

   Blockchain technologies such as Hyperledger Fabric, Ethereum, Quorum, Corda, etc. all have strengths and weaknesses [42]. Some are better suited to meet a specific need than others and it is difficult to design programming to make up for inherent weaknesses. The specific blockchain platform and programming capabilities should be selected only after considering all of the organization's needs.
3. *Fit within existing ecosystem.* Determine how blockchain will be integrated into an organization's existing healthcare ecosystem. My employer, for example, performs the following sub-steps with organizations to identify organizations' needs:

   a. Create user profiles about what the individual user roles will perform [43].
   b. Identify which regulatory requirements may apply to the nature of data and intended use of the blockchain. This is an area where many technology companies have not had much training or experience, yet healthcare organizations must ensure that the final product will meet the requirements for compliance. We advocate "compliance by design" thinking [44] to build compliance into the initial documentation and design.

    c. Map the flow of information between stakeholders and determine which steps can be automated by smart contracts and at which time or event triggers.

    d. Create comprehensive journey mapping of each step of the user experience and data flow so that the electronic systems, user steps, and data rules are clearly documented and understood.

    e. Design a system architecture map that shows the relationships between the layers of applications, interfaces, smart contracts, data storage, and blockchains.

4. *Make collaborative decisions early.* If implementing a blockchain across organizations, there is a need to make technical and operational decisions early. Blockchain consortia should determine how to share responsibilities for liability, maintenance, and decision-making [41]. There should also be careful planning about how to manage users, data and risks [9].

5. *Participate actively in the review and testing.* There is an iterative process with building and testing to ensure that features meet the organization's needs. It is much easier to modify an undesirable outcome early in the programming stages.

6. *Update business documentation.* As part of implementation and training, business processes should be evaluated and updated, as necessary, to describe training, risk assessments, and maintenance.

Challenges

As with the development and implementation of any technology used to enhance hybrid health, blockchain involves some challenges that should be taken into considerations when considering blockchain technologies.

Immature Technologies

Because blockchain is a newer technology and there are few large scale implementations published, healthcare organizations may be risk averse and may decline to be early adopters [45]. While evidence about blockchain uses in healthcare is continuing to accrue, there isn't enough evidence available yet to predict many outcomes or best practices [46]. In fact, Lazar et al. [47] noted there is minimal evidence yet to project clear strategic visions about blockchain's future uses in healthcare. Specifically, it is currently unknown as to whether there will be synergistic benefits or risks, unexpected values or costs, or escalating acceptance or tensions [48]. In general, more evidence should be collected and published before blockchain can be implemented with confidence.

Interoperability

While blockchain has potential to integrate sources of health information from electronic health records, there are currently obstacles for interoperability with health record systems. While these challenges may be mitigated by the requirements of the Twenty-first Century Cures Act [49], there is not currently a standard for designing blockchain-based application programming interfaces [50]. In addition, while blockchain can easily connect data from remote patient monitoring systems, there is uncertainty about how to manage or integrate data. While a dashboard or other user-interface could be created to visualize all information collected on a blockchain platform, there is not currently a way to include the quantity or quality of information into an existing electronic health record display [51]. Working groups within the International Organization of Standardization [52] and the Institute of Electrical and Electronics Engineers [53] have been working towards common standards for both blockchain and electronic health record systems.

Security and Privacy Regulations

Because blockchain offers enhancements for managing healthcare information, few regulatory mechanisms are in place to offer clear direction for healthcare compliance. In fact, a survey of governments indicted that regulatory constraints were the largest obstacle for blockchain adoption [54]. In the absence of clear direction, blockchain uses for health information are following HIPAA for electronic data exchanges and for safeguards of protected health information [10, 15, 55]. For data generated about European Union citizens, there is need for electronic systems to adhere to the General Data Protection Regulation [56], which has a provision for the right to be forgotten. There are mechanisms by which a blockchain can adhere to these regulations in a compliant manner [57], but it is important for organizations to develop training, policies and risk mitigation strategies as well as ongoing evaluations [48]. Likewise, regulators need to acquire appropriate skill sets and training in blockchain to understand how a blockchain can operate in a healthcare environment [10].

Future Research

More research on blockchain is necessary to understand the effectiveness for use as a hybrid health solution for care delivery. Blockchain developers and healthcare organizations should jointly create more evidence-based practices about implementations and uses. Extensive research is currently being conducted about privacy-preserving frameworks [58], security parameters [59], implementation strategies [12], adding medical IoT devices to electronic medical records [60], governance strategies [41], and dozens of other applications [3, 54, 61, 62]. Kazgan [45] notes, though, that data validation studies of clinical outcomes are particularly valuable. When involving patients in an interventional study, patients' feedback about usability and feature desirability should be collected, when possible [63].

Conclusions

Blockchain technology is still in an early stage of development for healthcare, but was designed from well-established cryptographic principles [9]. While only a few uses of blockchain were offered in this chapter to describe the hybrid of interpersonal healthcare delivery and technology applications, the number of blockchain-based opportunities is increasingly rapidly. As more evidence is collected to demonstrate effectiveness, efficiency, and satisfaction of using blockchain in hybrid healthcare, health organizations. Health professionals interested in advancing hybrid health solutions are encouraged to learn about blockchain and understand its strengths and limitations.

References

1. Nakamoto S. Bitcoin: a peer-to-peer electronic cash system. 2008. https://bitcoin.org/bitcoin.pdf. Accessed 18 May 2018.
2. Vaughn BE. Enterprise, history, and change. In: Metcalf D, Bass J, Hooper M, Cahana A, Dhillon V, editors. Blockchain in healthcare: innovations that empower patients, connect professionals and improve care. Orlando: Merging Traffic; 2019. p. 151–66.
3. Ornes S. Core concept: blockchain offers applications well beyond Bitcoin but faces its own limitations. Proc Natl Acad Sci U S A. 2019;116:20800–3. https://doi.org/10.1073/pnas.1914849116.
4. Crosby M, Nachiappan N, Pattanayak P, Verma S, Kalyanaraman V. Blockchain technology: beyond Bitcoin. Appl Innov Rev. 2016;2:6–10.
5. Bennett K, Decker C. Certified blockchain business foundations: official exam study guide: Blockchain Training Alliance, Inc. 2019. https://blockchaintrainingalliance.com/collections/blockchain-exam-prep-guides/products/cbbf-official-exam-study-guide. Accessed 22 Jan 2019.
6. Li H, Zhu L, Shen M, Gao F, Tao X, Liu S. Blockchain-based data preservation system for medical data. J Med Syst. 2018;42:141. https://doi.org/10.1007/s10916-018-0997-3.
7. Ribitzky R, St Clair J, Houlding DI, CT MF, Ahier B, Gould M, et al. Blockchain Healthc Today. 2018;1 https://doi.org/10.30953/bhty.v1.24.
8. Engelhardt MA. Hitching healthcare to the chain: an introduction to blockchain technology in the healthcare sector. Technol Innov Manag Rev. 2017;7:22–34. https://doi.org/10.22215/timreview/1111.
9. Yaga D, Mell P, Roby N, Scarfone K. Blockchain technology overview. Gaithersburg (MD): National Institute of Standards and Technology. 3 Oct 2018. Report No.: NISTIR 8202.
10. Brodersen C, Kalis B, Leong C, Mitchell E, Pupo E, Truscott A. Blockchain: securing a new health interoperability experience. In: Accenture Consulting L, editor. August ed. Dublin; 2016.

11. Tosh DK, Shetty S, Liang X, Kamhoua C, Njilla L. Consensus protocols for blockchain-based data provenance: challenges and opportunities. In: Chakrabarti S, editor. 2017 IEEE 8th Annual Ubiquitous Computing, Electronics and Mobile Communication Conference (UEMCON); 2017 Oct 19–21; New York, NY. Piscataway (NJ): IEEE; 2017. p. 469–74.
12. Labazova O, editor. Towards a framework for evaluation of blockchain implementations. Fortieth International Conference on Information Systems; 15–18 Dec 2019, Munich, Germany. New York (NY): Bepress/Elsevier, Inc; 2019.
13. Carter G, White D, Nalla A, Shahriar H, Sneha S. Toward application of blockchain for improved health records management and patient care. Blockchain Healthc Today. 2019. 2. https://doi.org/10.30953/bhty.v2.37.
14. Passerat-Palmbach J, Farnan T, Miller R, Gross MS, Flannery HL, Gleim B. A blockchain-orchestrated federated learning architecture for healthcare consortia. 2019. https://arxiv.org/abs/1910.12603. Accessed 1 Nov 2019.
15. Vendituoli M. Colorado health data organizations partner with startup to pilot blockchain-based platform. 2018. https://www.bizjournals.com/denver/news/2018/08/15/colorado-health-data-organizations-partner-with.html. Accessed 8 Oct 2019.
16. Tith D, Lee J-S, Suzuki H, Wijesundara WMAB, Taira N, Obi T, et al. Application of blockchain to maintaining patient records in electronic health record for enhanced privacy, scalability, and availability. Healthc Inform Res. 2020;26:3–12. https://doi.org/10.4258/hir.2020.26.1.3.
17. Campbell RE. Transitioning to a Hyperledger Fabric quantum-resistant classical hybrid public key infrastructure. J Br Blockchain Assoc. 2019;2:4. https://doi.org/10.31585/jbba-2-2-(4)2019.
18. Shahaab A, Lidgey B, Hewage C, Khan I. Applicability and appropriateness of distributed ledgers consensus protocols in public and private sectors: a systematic review. IEEE Access. 2019;7:43622–36. https://doi.org/10.1109/ACCESS.2019.2904181.
19. Bell L, Buchanan WJ, Cameron J, Lo O. Applications of blockchain within healthcare. Blockchain Healthc Today. 2018. 1. https://doi.org/10.30953/bhty.v1.8.
20. Chamber of Digital Commerce. "Smart contracts" legal primer. Washington; 2018, Feb 22.
21. Ewert B. Focusing on quality care rather than 'checking boxes': How to exit the labyrinth of multiple accountabilities in hybrid healthcare arrangements. Public Admin. 2018; https://doi.org/10.1111/padm.12556.
22. Wang WM, Cheung CF, Lee WB, Kwok SK. Knowledge-based treatment planning for adolescent early intervention of mental healthcare: a hybrid case-based reasoning approach. Expert Syst. 2007;24:232–51. https://doi.org/10.1111/j.1468-0394.2007.00431.x.
23. Vazirani AA, O'Donoghue O, Brindley D, Meinert E. Implementing blockchains for efficient health care: systematic review. J Med Internet Res. 2019;21:e12439. https://doi.org/10.2196/12439.
24. Tinianow A. Blockchain technology is already improving lives at 22 hospitals. 2019. https://www.forbes.com/sites/andreatinianow/2019/09/23/blockchain-technology-is-already-improving-lives-at-22-hospitals/#3e1eabc06c7d. Accessed 25 Sep 2019.
25. Department of Health and Human Services. 21st Century Cures Act: Interoperability, information blocking, and the ONC Health IT Certification Program. Fed Regist. 2020;85 FR 25642,25642-61. https://www.govinfo.gov/content/pkg/FR-2020-05-01/pdf/2020-07419.pdf.
26. ONC's cures act final rule. 2020. https://www.healthit.gov/curesrule/overview/about-oncs-cures-act-final-rule. Accessed 20 Mar 2020.
27. Zhang X, Poslad S, editors. Blockchain support for flexible queries with granular access control to electronic medical records (EMR). IEEE International Conference on Communications (ICC); 20–24 May 2018; Kansas City, MO. Piscataway (NJ): IEEE; 2018. p. 2018.
28. Aaviksoo A. Building blockchain powered trusted digital health services. Estonia. In: Cenaj T, editor. Converge2Xcelerate 2019. Boston, MA: Stamford (CT): Partners in Digital Health; 2020.
29. Heston TF. A case study in blockchain healthcare innovation. Int J Curr Res. 2017;9:60587–8.

30. Benchoufi M, Porcher R, Ravaud P. Blockchain protocols in clinical trials: transparency and traceability of consent. F1000Res. 2018;6:–66. https://doi.org/10.12688/f1000research.10531.5.
31. A digital front door strategy: what it is, isn't, and why you need one. 2019. https://www2.relatient.net/a-digital-front-door-strategy-what-it-is-isnt-and-why-you-need-one/. Accessed 14 Mar 2020.
32. Best J. The NHS app: opening the NHS's new digital "front door" to the private sector. BMJ. 2019;367:l6210. https://doi.org/10.1136/bmj.l6210.
33. Martich GD, Bertram R, Schueller S. Getting beyond the hype with apps and making it a reality. 2019. https://www.chartis.com/forum/wp-content/uploads/2019/07/WP_Appsolute-Necessity.pdf. Accessed 14 Mar 2020.
34. Fagherazzi G, Ravaud P. Digital diabetes: perspectives for diabetes prevention, management and research. Diabetes Metab. 2018;45:322–9. https://doi.org/10.1016/j.diabet.2018.08.012.
35. Lim H-R, Kim HS, Qazi R, Kwon Y-T, Jeong J-W, Yeo W-H. Advanced soft materials, sensor integrations, and applications of wearable flexible hybrid electronics in healthcare, energy, and environment. Adv Mater. 2019;1901924 https://doi.org/10.1002/adma.201901924.
36. Rahman A, Rashid M, Le Kernec J, Philippe B, Barnes SJ, Fioranelli F, et al. A secure occupational therapy framework for monitoring cancer patients' quality of life. Sensors (Basel). 2019;19:–5258. https://doi.org/10.3390/s19235258
37. Spencer P. The digital front door: why total cost of care risk is not inevitable. Healthc Financ Manage. 2018;72. https://www.hfma.org/topics/hfm/2018/january/57410.html
38. Mulligan C, Zhu Scott J, Warren S, Rangaswami JP. Blockchain beyond the hype: a practical framework for business leaders. Geneva (Switzerland): World Economic Forum; 23 Apr 2018.
39. Warren S, Deshmukh S, Whitehouse S, Treat D, Worley A, Herzig J, et al. Building value with blockchain technology: how to evaluate blockchain's benefits. Geneva (Switzerland): World Economic Forum; 16 Jul 2019.
40. Morkunas VJ, Paschen J, Boon E. How blockchain technologies impact your business model. Bus Horiz. 2019;62:295–306. https://doi.org/10.1016/j.bushor.2019.01.009.
41. Sulkowski AJ. Blockchain, business supply chains, sustainability, and law: the future of governance, legal frameworks, and lawyers? Del J Corp L. 2018;43 https://doi.org/10.2139/ssrn.3262291.
42. Bass J. The truth about blockchain and its application to health care. Healthc Financ Manage. 2019. https://www.hfma.org/Content.aspx?id=63125
43. McLellan S, Muddimer A, Peres SC. The effect of experience on System Usability Scale ratings. J Usability Stud. 2012;7:56–67.
44. Charles W, Marler N, Long L, Manion S. Blockchain compliance by design: regulatory considerations for blockchain in clinical research. Front Blockchain. 2019;2 https://doi.org/10.3389/fbloc.2019.00018.
45. Kazgan M. Real challenge in digital health entrepreneurship: changing human behavior. In: Wulfovich S, Meyers A, editors. Digital health entrepreneurship. Cham: Springer; 2019. p. 7–16.
46. Schmid A, Cacace M, Götze R, Rothgang H. Explaining health care system change: problem pressure and the emergence of "hybrid" health care systems. J Health Polit Policy Law. 2010;35:455–86. https://doi.org/10.1215/03616878-2010-013.
47. Lazar MA, Pan Z, Ragguett R-M, Lee Y, Subramaniapillai M, Mansur RB, et al. Digital revolution in depression: a technologies update for clinicians. Pers Med Psychiatry. 2017;4–6:1–6. https://doi.org/10.1016/j.pmip.2017.09.001.
48. McDermott AM, Hamel LM, Steel D, Flood PC, Mkee L. Hybrid healthcare governance for improvement? Combining top-down and bottom-up approaches to public sector regulation. Public Admin. 2015;93:324–44. https://doi.org/10.1111/padm.12118.
49. 21st Century Cures Act. Pub L.114–225, 130 Stat. 1033 (December 13, 2016).
50. Agbo CC, Mahmoud QH, Eklund JM. Blockchain technology in healthcare: a systematic review. Healthcare. 2019;7:56. https://doi.org/10.3390/healthcare7020056.

51. Bellini V, Petroni A, Palumbo G, Bignami E. Data quality and blockchain technology. Anaesth Crit Care Pain Med. 2019;38:521–2. https://doi.org/10.1016/j.accpm.2018.12.015.
52. International Organization for Standardization. ISO/TC 307: blockchain and distributed ledger technologies. Standards catalogue. 2019. https://www.iso.org/committee/6266604/x/catalogue/p/0/u/1/w/0/d/0. Accessed 29 June 2019.
53. IEEE Standards Association. P2418.6 - Standard for blockchain for healthcare and life sciences. 2019. https://standards.ieee.org/project/2418_6.html. Accessed 29 June 2019.
54. Justinia T. Blockchain technologies: opportunities for solving real-world problems in healthcare and biomedical sciences. Acta Inform Med. 2019;27:284–91. https://doi.org/10.5455/aim.2019.27.284-291.
55. Office for Civil Rights. How do HIPAA authorizations apply to an electronic health information exchange environment? 2008. https://www.hhs.gov/hipaa/for-professionals/faq/554/how-do-hipaa-authorizations-apply-to-electronic-health-information/index.html. Accessed 29 June 2019.
56. General Data Protection Regulation (GDPR), European Parliament and the Council of the European Union 2016.
57. Orel A, Bernik I. GDPR and health personal data; tricks and traps of compliance. In: Mantas J, Sonicki Z, Crişan-Vida M, Fišter K, Hägglund M, Kolokathi A, et al., editors. Special topic conference of the european federation for medical informatics (EFMI STC); 15–16 Oct 2018. Zagreb, Croatia. Amsterdam: IOS Press BV; 2018. p. 155–9.
58. Dagher GG, Mohler J, Milojkovic M, Marella PB. Privacy-preserving framework for access control and interoperability of electronic health records using blockchain technology. Sustain Cities Soc. 2018;39:283–97. https://doi.org/10.1016/j.scs.2018.02.014.
59. Karame G, Capkun S. Blockchain security and privacy. IEEE Secur Priv. 2018;16:11–2. https://doi.org/10.1109/MSP.2018.3111241.
60. Badr S, Gomaa I, Abd-Elrahman E. Multi-tier blockchain framework for IoT-EHRs systems. In: Shakshuki E, Yasar A, editors. The 9th international conference on emerging ubiquitous systems and pervasive networks. Leuven, Belgium; Oxford: Elsevier B.V; 2018. p. 159–66.
61. Hughes L, Dwivedi YK, Misra SK, Rana NP, Raghavan V, Akella V. Blockchain research, practice and policy: applications, benefits, limitations, emerging research themes and research agenda. Int J Inf Manag. 2019;49:114–29. https://doi.org/10.1016/j.ijinfomgt.2019.02.005.
62. Manion ST. Advancing health research with blockchain. In: Metcalf D, Bass J, Hooper M, Cahana A, Dhillon V, editors. Blockchain in healthcare: innovations that empower patients, connect professionals and improve care. Orlando: Merging Traffic; 2019. p. 465–76.
63. Fortuna KL, Walker R, Fisher DB, Mois G, Allan S, Deegan PE. Enhancing standards and principles in digital mental health with recovery-focused guidelines for mobile, online, and remote monitoring technologies. Psychiatr Serv. 2019;70 https://doi.org/10.1176/appi.ps.201900166.

Chapter 4
Cloud Computing and Cloud Biology

Mussaad Al-Razouki

Abstract As hybrid healthcare systems lean into the digital revolution, increased attention to the way data is accessed and stored is paramount. The revolution of cloud computing is now coming back full circle into biology with remote research labs and digital trials a growing trend. As hybrid healthcare systems generate higher quantities of big data, both novel techniques of data processing and storage are required to ensure both HIPAA compliance as well as quality based care.

Keywords Cloud computing · Cloud biology · Big data · SaaS · Edge computing Biodata · DNA storage · Singularity

What Is the Cloud?

The cloud has catalyzed the digitization of almost every sector of our global economy. This was especially true during the COVID era where companies that were able to quickly shift away from on-premise data processing and storage during the pandemic to a cloud centric model, rapidly capitalized on the important competitive advantage of higher quality computing power at a lower cost [1]. Unfortunately, this tectonic shift to all-things-cloud was not very common in healthcare. Many insurance companies, health systems, hospitals, medical centers and even a few large clinics still opt for costly on premise servers and data storage, feigning the excuse of draconic state laws on patient data or an archaic legacy system that hide behind the faux labyrinth of the Health Insurance Portability and Accountability Act (HIPAA) of 1996. Instead of 'plugging in' to the utility of data storage on the cloud, many healthcare stakeholders still choose to build their own (computing) power station. This is supported by the significantly slower growth of the public cloud

M. Al-Razouki (✉)
Business Development, Kuwait Life Sciences Company, Kuwait City, Kuwait
e-mail: mussaad@klsc.com.kw

© The Author(s), under exclusive license to Springer Nature Switzerland AG 2022
M. Al-Razouki, S. Smith (eds.), *Hybrid Healthcare*, Health Informatics, https://doi.org/10.1007/978-3-031-04836-4_4

Fig. 4.1 Healthcare lags behind the cloud-computing market during COVID-19

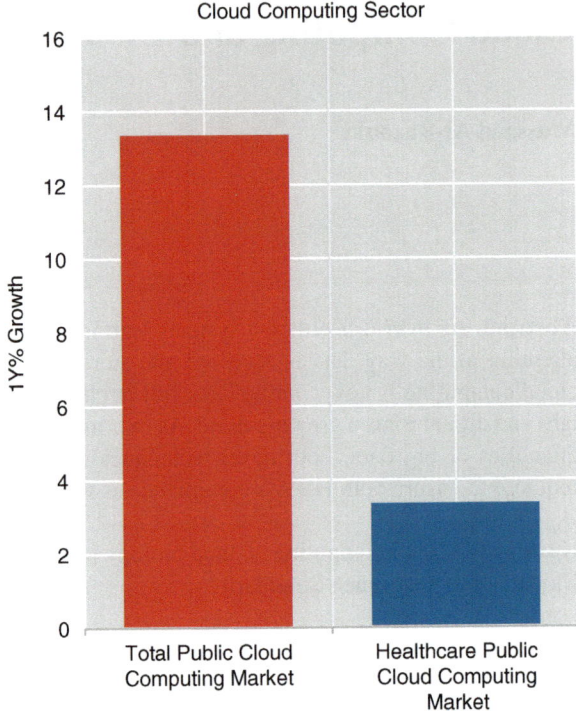

2019–2020 1Y Market Size Growth in Cloud Computing Sector

computing market in the healthcare industry compared to the total cloud computing market from 2019 to 2020 as shown in the diagram below (Fig. 4.1).[1,2]

Before we dive deep into the technical parts of this chapter, it is important to note that the subject of cloud computing goes beyond simple data storage or computer processing needs. Yes, there are concerns on patient privacy and data security, but those concerns are far outweighed by the rapid development of the data analytics required to process the ever growing quantities of data produced by patients and their access to the healthcare system.

Indeed, when it comes to simple data storage, there are three major choices for healthcare stakeholders: on-premise, cloud, or hybrid. Frankly speaking, a pure on-premise option will unlikely be sustainable in the near future leaving the options of cloud or hybrid. Even though this is a book on hybrid healthcare, the future will leave very little room for any on-premise storage of patient or health data. The cloud is the only true (and scalable) panacea.

A hybrid healthcare system requires on-demand availability of computing power to churn through the millions of patient data points generated by the provider or

[1] Markets and Markets, "Healthcare Cloud Computing Market."
[2] Fortune Business Insights, "Cloud Computing Market to Soar at 17.9% CAGR till 2028."

payor. Another key benefit of cloud computing is that it provides computer system resources without direct active management by the user. With patient data stored in remote data centers, hybrid healthcare payors and providers are able to decrease their information technology (IT) headcount and reallocate these full time equivalents (FTEs) to other more meaningful tasks. The redundancy of these large clouds, which often have core functions distributed over multiple locations from central servers, adds an extra layer of security when it comes to patient data and information processing.

Cloud computing cuts costs further by allowing different end users to share common IT resources thereby achieving coherence and economies of scale. Hospital and clinical real estate is expensive and therefore every inch of land or built-up-area should be leveraged to enhance patient care and the patient's experience. Wasting valuable space on servers is so late twentieth century. Payors and providers can also either avoid or minimize costly upfront capital expenditure thereby lightening the load on company balance sheets. The argument can even be made around the speed of implementation, where cloud computing allows enterprises to get their applications up and running faster, with improved manageability and maintenance, especially with respect to burst computing capability where above normal high computing power is required at certain periods of peak demand, as was the case during the height of the COVID19 pandemic.

The typical "pay-as-you-go" model of cloud computing aligns well with the lean and accountable business models of hybrid healthcare organizations. The availability of high-capacity networks, low-cost computers and storage devices as well as the widespread adoption of hardware virtualization, service-oriented architecture and autonomic and utility computing becomes even more important as medical devices evolve into important nodes in the Internet of Things (IoT) and patients and physicians demand more real time measurement of their bodily functions via quantitative self-reporting wearables [2].

As a result of these cost saving features, data from Gartner.com suggests an up to 50% cost reduction 3 years after migrating to cloud computing despite an initial spike in cost due to migration cost (Fig. 4.2).[3]

Hybrid Healthcare Service Models

As the future end state of hybrid healthcare heavily leans on the intersection of soft and hard services it is important to note that cloud-computing companies offer their services according to three standard models [2, 3]:

1. Infrastructure as a Service (IaaS)
2. Platform as a Service (PaaS)
3. Software as a Service (SaaS)

---

[3] Meinardi, "Is Public Cloud Cheaper than Running Your Own Data Center?"

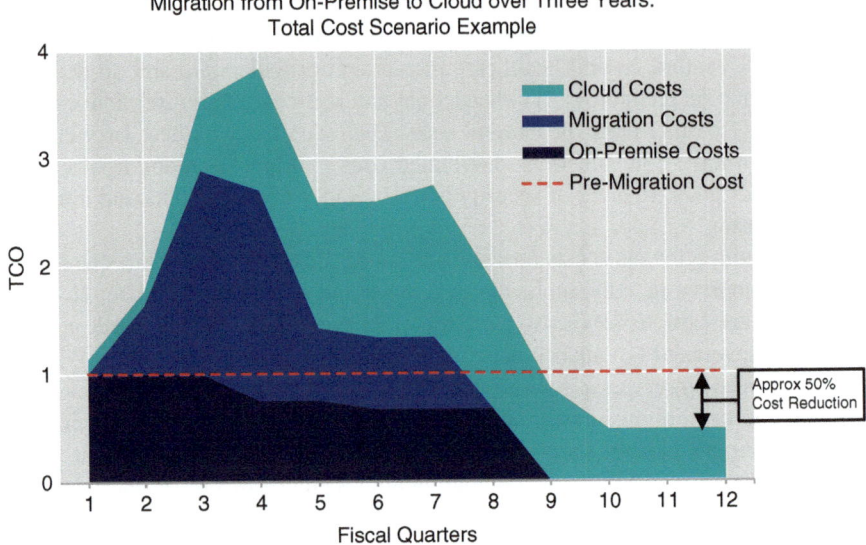

Fig. 4.2 Example of total cost of migration to cloud

Hybrid healthcare entrepreneurs and stakeholders need to be intimately familiar with these various cloud service models, keeping in mind that most service-oriented architecture actually advocates "Everything as a service" (with the more acronyms such EaaS or XaaS or simply aas added to the alphabet soup). These aforementioned models offer increasing abstraction; they are thus often portrayed as layers in a stack: infrastructure-, platform- and software-as-a-service, but these need not be related. For example, a digital health company can provide SaaS implemented on physical machines (bare metal) located in a hospital or insurance company, without using underlying PaaS or IaaS layers, and conversely a physician end user can run a program on IaaS and access it directly, without wrapping it as SaaS.

Indeed, the biggest difference between IaaS, sometimes called Hardware-as-a-Service (HaaS) and the two other cloud computing service models, PaaS and SaaS, is how much control the hybrid healthcare organization has over the cloud environment compared to how much the vendor (cloud service provider) controls.

With SaaS deployments, a health system's applications, data runtime, middleware, operating system, virtualization, servers, storage, and network are all delivered as a service by a third party provider. PaaS deployments only require the organization to develop new applications and provide data—the rest of the infrastructure is delivered as a service, giving said health system more control over its environment than SaaS.

With IaaS, hybrid healthcare stakeholders have the most options. They are able to implement applications, data, runtime, middleware, and their operating system. The virtualization, servers, storage, and network are all provided as a service for IaaS [4].

With IaaS comes access to user interfaces (UIs) and application programming interfaces (APIs). This gives local IT administrators the ability to modify how applications handle and store data as well as how hardware is used.

Some integration and data management providers also use specialized applications of PaaS as delivery models for data. Examples include iPaaS (Integration Platform as a Service) and dPaaS (Data Platform as a Service). iPaaS enables the end user to develop, execute and govern integration flows. Under an iPaaS integration model, the hospital system for example would drive the development and deployment of integrations without installing or managing any hardware or middleware. dPaaS, on the other hand, delivers both integration and data-management products as a fully managed service. Under the dPaaS model, the PaaS provider, not the end user, manages the development and execution of programs by building data applications for the end user.

Furthermore, mobility (more specifically mobile phones) has become an increasingly larger part of how we collect data and access the power of the cloud. This has led us to a mobile "backend" as a service (m) model (MBaaS), also known simply as a Backend as a Service (BaaS) where hybrid healthcare entrepreneurs developing web and/or mobile based apps are provided with a way to link their applications to cloud storage and cloud computing services with application programming interfaces (APIs) exposed to their applications and custom software development kits (SDKs). Services include user management, push notifications, integration with social networking services and more. This relatively recent model in cloud computing is rapidly gaining significant mainstream traction with traditional enterprise healthcare players and can be assumed to play an important role in the future, more mobile, hybrid healthcare system.

Choosing Cloud Computing Deployment Models: Private vs. Public vs. Hybrid

Healthcare stakeholders must eventually choose between either a public, private or hybrid deployment when it comes to their cloud infrastructure. Indeed, the major differences between public and private cloud is where the data is physically stored and how much on-site maintenance will eventually be required. The diagram below shows a glimpse of the differences between private cloud, hybrid cloud, and public cloud such as accessibility and data storage methods (Fig. 4.3).

Private Cloud

A private cloud is a closed infrastructure operated solely for a single healthcare system, hospital, insurance company, or digital health business that can be managed internally or by a third party, and hosted either internally or externally [2, 3]. As previously mentioned, self-run data centers are generally capital intensive. They have a significant physical footprint, requiring allocations of space, hardware, and environmental controls. These assets have to be refreshed periodically, resulting in additional capital expenditures. So when favoring a private cloud solution, hybrid

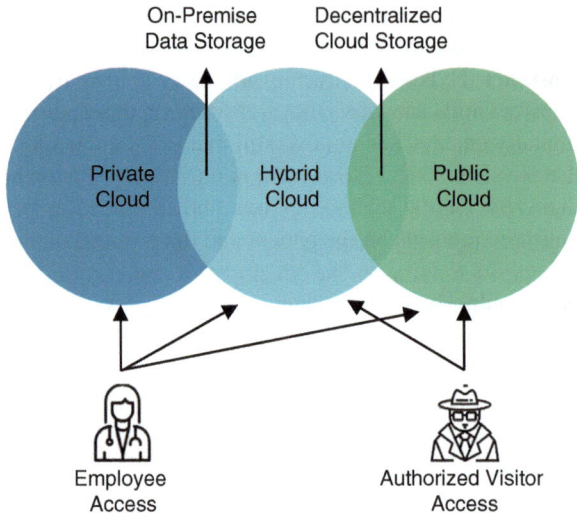

Fig. 4.3 Schematic of public, hybrid, and private

healthcare companies have to essentially spend costs upfront and therefore do not leverage the proper pay-as-you-go potential of cloud computing.

Public Cloud

A public cloud can be considered a more open infrastructure that is usually shared by multiple companies as services are delivered over the public internet [2, 3]. Obviously, security concerns increase substantially when services (applications, storage, and other resources) are shared by multiple customers, however most public-cloud providers offer direct-connection services that would allow hybrid healthcare organizations to securely link their legacy data centers to their cloud-resident applications.

Hybrid Cloud

As this is a book on hybrid healthcare, it seems obvious that combining the benefits of both private and public cloud computing into a hybrid cloud would be ideal. A hybrid cloud solution is a composition of a public cloud and a private environment, such as a private cloud or on-premises resources, that remain distinct entities but are bound together, offering the benefits of multiple deployment models. Hybrid cloud can also mean the ability to connect collocation, managed and/or dedicated services with cloud resources. A hybrid cloud service crosses isolation and provider boundaries so that it can't be simply put in one category of private, public, or community cloud service [2, 3]. It allows one to extend either the capacity or the capability of a cloud service, by aggregation, integration or customization with another cloud service.

Varied use cases for hybrid cloud composition exist. For example, a hospital may store sensitive patient data in house on a private cloud application, but interconnect that application to an appointment booking application provided on a public cloud as a software service.

Another benefit of a hybrid cloud is the ability to rapidly ramp up computing capacity in surge times that typically cannot be met by the private cloud. This capability enables hybrid clouds to employ cloud bursting for scaling across clouds and streamlines costs as end users pay for extra compute resources only when they are needed [4].

Hybrid Healthcare's Cutting Edge

Moving outwards from the clouEdge Computing is defined as a "mesh network of micro data centers that process or store critical data locally and push all received data to a central data center or cloud storage repository, in a footprint of less than 100 square feet."

Localizing data processing and storage puts less of a strain on computing networks. When less data is sent to the cloud, the likelihood of latency—the delay in data processing that results from the interaction between the cloud and IoT (Internet of Things) devices—decreases. This also places more responsibility on the hardware underlying edge computing technology, which consists of sensors for collecting data and CPUs or GPUs for processing data within connected devices.

As edge computing takes off, it is important to understand another technology that edge devices are involved with: fog computing. While edge computing refers more specifically to the computational processes being done at or near the "edge" of a network, fog computing refers to the network connections between the edge devices and the cloud [5].

In other words, fog computing extends the cloud closer to the edge of a network; therefore, "fog computing always uses edge computing, but not the other way around," according to the OpenFog Consortium. Data processing uses the edge, but it is not always immediate. Using fog computing, short-term analytics can be assessed at a given point in time and do not require full travel back to a centralized cloud.

The diagram below provides a visual illustration of the network between edge computing, fog computing, and cloud computing. Local devices collect and analyze data that is connected to the cloud through fog computing to reduce the amount of data sent to the cloud and hence latency. A network connection between edge devices and the cloud, fog computing provides short-term analysis without traveling back to the centralized cloud. Ultimately, cloud computing stores and analyzes long-term data for a variety of uses (Fig. 4.4).

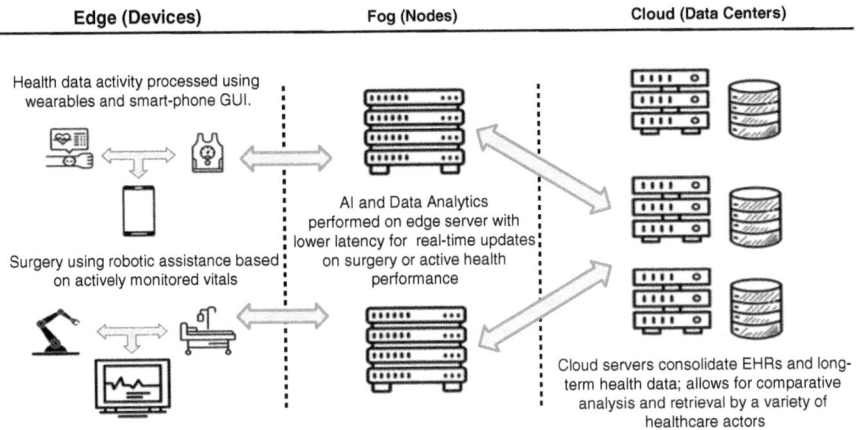

Fig. 4.4 Edge, fog, and cloud in a healthcare setting

So where is the Edge in Hybrid Healthcare? Traditionally there are three different edges in any industry, but considering the future of healthcare is nearing the singularity, I will add an extra special fourth dimension specific to Hybrid Healthcare at the end.

1. OT Edges—Operational Technology

OT is the hardware and software that detects or causes a change through the direct monitoring and/or control of physical devices, processes and events in the enterprise i.e. the suppliers subsector of healthcare. Think the Big Pharma pill production plants in New Jersey or the medical device mills of the Midwest. As we continue to develop the healthcare industry of the future known as precision medicine, these factories will have to increasingly compete with personalized 3D pill printers either at local pharmacy chains or within the home.

2. IoT Edges—Internet of Things

IoT is yet another buzzword that is taking the world by storm. In healthcare, IoT is applicable to both large medical equipment i.e. Imaging systems such as MRI's, CT scanners, etc., smaller personalized wearables e.g. smartwatches as well as a growing number of invasive medical devices e.g. pacemakers.

It is estimated that some 50 billion devices are connected to the Internet today, generating 50 zetabytes, or 50 trillion gigabytes of data annually. Today, people have become increasingly comfortable wearing fitness trackers, glucose monitors, smartwatches, and other health-monitoring wearables. But to truly capture the benefit of the massive amounts of data being collected, real-time analysis may be necessary—and while many wearable devices connect to the cloud directly, others can operate offline. Some wearable health monitors can locally analyze pulse data or sleep patterns without connecting to the cloud. Doctors can then evaluate patients on the spot and provide on-demand feedback about their health.

But the potential for edge computing in healthcare goes far beyond wearables. Consider the benefits of speedy data processing for remote patient monitoring, inpatient care, and healthcare management for hospitals and clinics. Doctors and clinicians would be able to offer faster, better care to patients while also adding an additional layer of security to the patient-generated health data (PDHD). The average hospital bed has upwards of 20 connected devices, generating a considerable amount of data. Instead of sending confidential data to the cloud where it could be improperly accessed, it would happen closer to the edge.

As previously mentioned, localized data processing means a widespread cloud or network failure will not impact the process. Even if cloud operations were disrupted, these hospital sensors operate independently, and could still function as intended.

In the not too distant future, medicinal nanobots such as cybernetic cytotoxic, cytokine secreting, killer T cells could also be connected to the World Wide Web by use of IoT Edges either worn by or implanted in the patient.

3. Enterprise IT Edges

Not to be confused with the above OT Edges, these EIT Edges as the white collar brothers of the blue collar OTE's. Think Electronic Health Record vendors and the big healthcare payors (or more specifically) InsureTech, who each 'manage' the healthcare of millions of patients. Buzzwords such as "Population Health" and "Predictive or 'Big Data' Analytics" also come to mind. Enterprise IT Edges need to also be consistently developed in line with HIPAA.

Cloud Biology

Moving away from purely technological systems and into the intersection of biology and computer science it is important to quickly cover the emerging field of Cloud Biology. What is the BioCloud and how is it important to hybrid healthcare?

So far, we have talked about the application of cloud computing on healthcare systems and their technology infrastructure. The BioCloud, involves applying the power of the cloud in biological, genomic/multiomic and even in pharmaceutical design. Simply put, Wet labs will be dried up and fully digitized via cloud biology, as software algorithms eventually replace the need for physical labs, biological specimens and chemical inputs with computer code. This would thereby enable drug discovery and other applications on the cloud the same way most of our day to day human interaction has moved out of the physical world and onto the digitized world of social media messaging.

The promise of the BioCloud is faster, cheaper and less ethically challenging medicine (no more animal or human trials). Hybrid healthcare will be able to take full advantage of the "virtualization" of biology in the way that Amazon, Microsoft and other big tech "cloud" providers have virtualized data centers or the way semiconductor "fabs" like Advanced Micro Devices (AMD) have virtualized the fabrication of new computer chip designs. But can Moore's Law on microchip size be applied to our own biological design?

The Biocloud involves far more than simply storing patient data on off-site servers. Clouding biology is far more encompassing and involves essentially the digitization of the contract research organization (CRO) space of healthcare and to eventually develop a hybrid system whereby a physical lab can either be managed remotely by the principal investigators or be completely replicated in a virtual system that could be labeled as a web-based wet lab. This will essentially allow smaller and less well-funded labs and biotech ventures access to the same "research power" found in Big Pharma. This long-tail approach to lab research will leverage the focus of researchers from around the globe that will simply 'plug into' these pooled resources and perhaps even allow for the cross-fertilization of scientific thought beyond our current reliance on peer-review publications and conference presentations.

However, as part of a hybrid healthcare system, it is important to note that we believe that biology and drug discovery should never really be completely decoupled from the old-fashioned, high-touch, physical lab environment. Even the most rigorous scientific process, much like most medical treatment, involves a delicate balance between art and science. Trial and error is the hallmark of scientific innovation. Without introducing the all-important and fallible human element, we may not have enough errors in our trials to spur on the innovation. Indeed, the hubris of breaking down a physical and/or biological problem into virtual components that can be modeled and prodded with digital data on the cloud is inherently risky and has not been successfully achieved yet. Therefore, as with other components of the healthcare system, a hybrid approach to scientific laboratory discovery is recommended.

These hybrid labs of the future will need to leverage bioinformatic tools to make sense of large biodatasets via adaptive algorithms and holistic hardware required for large-scale biodata analysis. Further research and development is needed to eventually upload biological tools on the cloud, build biodatabases on the cloud, and encourage cloud-based biocomputing.

Even today, our rate of accumulating biomolecular data is increasing exponentially. This bioinformatic explosion is being driven by the development of low-cost, high-throughput experimental technologies in genomics, proteomics, molecular imaging, amongst others. Our success in the life sciences will depend on our ability to rationally interpret these large-scale, high-dimensional data sets into clinically understandable and useful information, which in turn requires us to adopt advances in informatics. Indeed, the translational of biomedical informatics into the biocloud demonstrates the utility and promise of cloud computing for tackling the challenge imposed by this 'big data.' Cloud computing could be an enabling tool to facilitate translational bioinformatics research where the biomedical cloud, given the proper architecture, could integrate all the big data in one place and automatically process said data on a continuous basis. In this way, hybrid labs could continuously (and in real-time) observe the connections between genotypic profiles and phenotypic data. These cloud-supported translational bioinformatics experiments will promote faster breakthroughs in the diagnosis, prognosis, and treatment of human disease. Once again, based on the cloud centric concepts of resources on demand and pay as you go, scientists from across the globe with no or limited infrastructure can have access to scalable and cost-effective computational and laboratory resources [2].

Genetics IT Edges: From Selfie to Singularity

Taking a selfie typically involves spending 5–10 s taking, filtering and uploading a 30–50 MB photo or video (or several versions). So far, most of our data is either stored on our handheld devices or on our personal cloud accounts, both of which are rapidly running out of space.

Surprisingly our DNA is quite ideal as a medium for data storage. The data density of DNA is orders of magnitude higher than conventional computer storage systems, with 1 g of DNA able to represent close to 1 zettabyte or 1 billion terabytes or 1 trillion gigabytes of data. That's enough smart phones to fill an entire football stadium. DNA is also remarkably robust; DNA fragments that are thousands of years old have been successfully sequenced, essentially meaning that the information stored on DNA could itself last for thousands of years.

So, assuming an average human body of 65 kg houses about 60 g of DNA, each person on earth could store as much as 60 zettabytes or 60,000 exabytes of data. Just for comparisons sake IBM back in 2012 estimated that the entire world generates a total 2.5 exabytes of data per day. So not to worry, there will be plenty of space to store your selfies. Thankfully, the rapid adoption of DNA as a data storage medium should easily allow us to squirrel away these vast quantities of future digital data as we approach the singularity; where our biology becomes seamlessly integrated with our technology.

Another interesting consideration is that all the words ever spoken by humankind prior to the digital revolution is estimated to command a total storage of a mere 5 exabytes—meaning that in the future you could store the entire compendium of human knowledge pre-Internet, on your small finger nail.

The current limitations however with DNA storage, is the abysmally long time it takes to retrieve said stored data. This is where the power of the Genetic IT Edge could come in and help speed up the transliteration of all those analog C-Gs and A-Ts into 1 s and 0 s, thus allowing data to freely flow from nitrogenous nucleobases to digital databases.

Nevertheless, we can imagine a future hybrid end state to our health data storage and data processing needs whereby a patient (perhaps via their sensors) accesses the hospital's cloud based network (before or after their visit, which in turn could be either in person or virtual) and uploads the data to be processed on the cloud with the results downloaded back down into the patient's own DNA to be accessed at a later date. This cycle can be repeated across the entire patient population creating a deep data lake whereby anonymized data sets can be aggregated to come up with an immediate pulse of the entire population's health status thus providing important guidance to the future direction of an accountable healthcare system.

References

1. Bommadevara N, et al. Cloud adoption to accelerate it modernization. McKinsey & Company; 2018. https://www.mckinsey.com/business-functions/mckinsey-digital/our-insights/cloud-adoption-to-accelerate-it-modernization
2. Wang. Enterprise cloud service architectures. Inf Technol Manag. 2012;13(4):445–54. https://doi.org/10.1007/s10799-012-0139-4.
3. Mell P, Grance T. The NIST definition of cloud computing. NIST; 2011.
4. Montazerolghaem A, Yaghmaee MH, Leon-Garcia A. Green cloud multimedia networking: NFV/SDN based energy-efficient resource allocation. IEEE Trans Green Commun Netw. 2020;4(3):873–89. https://doi.org/10.1109/TGCN.2020.2982821.
5. Ray PP. An introduction to dew computing: definition, concept and implications. IEEE J Mag. 2017;6:723–37. https://doi.org/10.1109/ACCESS.2017.2775042.

Chapter 5
Wearables and Remote Monitoring

Raza Ali

Abstract Sensors have become embedded in modern life—powering our personal electronics devices and environments. In this chapter, we examine how hybrid healthcare can leverage these sensors for a wide range of applications. We outline the trends and opportunities for these devices in healthcare and also the particular challenges imposed by the domain. We then review two key areas for healthcare using wearable and remote monitoring: activity recognition and profiling and apps for personalised medicine and lifestyle monitoring.

Keywords Wearable sensors · Ambient sensors · Hybrid healthcare · Activity recognition · Behaviour profiling · Machine learning

The Growing Prevalence of Sensing Technology

Sensing technology has been driven by advances in the semi-conductor industry and has become a mainstay of modern life. Modern sensors are small, affordable and have powerful computing built-in. This allows development of devices that are not simply for data collection but can process data onboard. It opens up options for sensors transforming data before transmission for example to enhance privacy and improve context. Figure 5.1 illustrates a well-established and steadily growing market for personal, wearable devices with sensors built-in, colloquially termed wearables—driven in particular by smart watches and specialist devices for health and fitness.

Another trend enabling the hybrid healthcare environment is the rise of spaces and devices with sensing built-in. Ambient or environmental sensors such as

R. Ali (✉)
Nabta Health, London, UK
e-mail: raza@nabtahealth.com

© The Author(s), under exclusive license to Springer Nature
Switzerland AG 2022
M. Al-Razouki, S. Smith (eds.), *Hybrid Healthcare*, Health Informatics,
https://doi.org/10.1007/978-3-031-04836-4_5

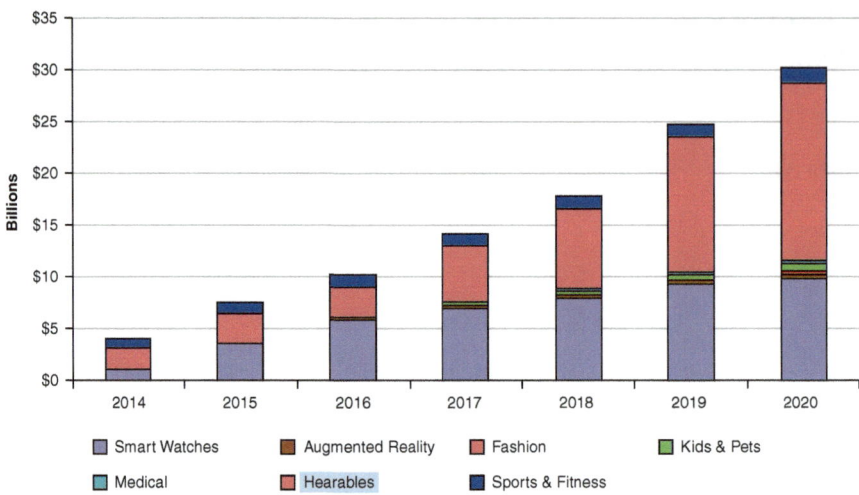

Fig. 5.1 Wearables market over the last 5 years [4]

location and cameras can combine with sensors residing in objects such as smart speakers, lightbulbs, thermostats, robot vacuums and more to both enable data collection and provision of contextual, personalised environments. Smart-homes [1] have long been studied in research environments with healthcare as a target application. This includes projects such as MavHome [2] and MIT's PlaceLab [3]. The home may also facilitate the operation of devices in the house based on sensed information. The sensors utilised in these projects include temperature, water flow and utility usage sensors as well as pressure sensors on furniture, proximity sensors for tracking user position in rooms as well as devices for monitoring vital signs. These technologies are now available through commercial technology providers including Google Nest™, Amazon Alexa™ and Samsung SmartThings™, which have created eco-systems for smart devices.

Wearable and ambient sensing can provide detailed pictures of many aspects of human life. Table 5.1 lists some of the commonly used sensors in commercial and research settings, along with an indication of their frequency of use.

Unsurprisingly, the potential of these technologies is maximised when leveraging more of them [5]. Ambient sensors impose the least burden on users once in-place—whereas wearables often offer the highest fidelity information. Multiple, independent sources of information increase not just the quantity of information but also the reliability of it, the resilience in the face of device failure and the ability of intelligent algorithms to make inferences from the data. An enabling technology for connecting multiple sensors is extensible, open-standards for connectivity setting up the potential for the 'Internet-of-Things' (IoT). These can emphasise low-power, local networking as in the ZigBee standard [6] or can allow ubiquitous wearable and ambient devices access to high-speed internet with the emerging 5G standard [7].

Table 5.1 Commonly used sensors with potential for use in hybrid healthcare

Sensor	Type	Information	Applications	Usage
Accelerometer, Gyroscope	Wearable	Movement, Activity, Posture	Behaviour profiling, Activity tracking, Fitness applications	High
GPS	Wearable	Location	Fitness applications, Behaviour Profiling	High
Passive Infrared (PIR), Contact	Ambient	Location	Indoor location tracking, Object usage tracking	High
Image/Camera	Ambient	Audio-visual	Location, activity	Medium
Flow	Ambient	Ambient	Water usage, leaks	Low
Temperature	Wearable	Core body temperature, Skin Temperature	Physiology, Fertility	Medium
Blood Oxygenation	Wearable	Blood oxygen	Respiratory health	Medium
Pulse	Wearable	Heart rate	Physiology, Fitness	High
Pressure	Ambient	Location, body posture and orientation	Sleep quality, posture	Low
Sweat	Wearable	Analytes from sweat e.g. electrolytes	Physiology, Fitness	Low

Challenges for Sensing in the Healthcare Domain

One of the most important areas for sensing is healthcare and as a result it has been an area of significant research focus. Chapter 7 outlines in more detail the factors driving this—including the growing healthcare needs of ageing demographics, reducing hospital admissions and the potential for patient centered care and the opportunity to provide better quality care with lower cost. Successful interventions in healthcare leveraging sensors must however overcome serious challenges.

A primary challenge for wearables and remote monitoring is incorporating privacy. The nature of the data imposes a significant cost if privacy is not taken seriously. In conventional healthcare there are stringent standards for storing and transmitting patient data—these must be adhered to [8]. Extensive meta-data about users can be valuable for analytical purposes—however each data source imposes regulatory constraints varying by region. Healthcare frameworks leveraging sensing [9, 10] have proposed addressing this through high security data transmission, leveraging anonymisation when possible, customising software architectures to regional and national regulations, adopting analysis that preserves privacy, and letting users control what information is collected and for what purpose—with conservative defaults.

To move hybrid healthcare into the mainstream it must cater for a wide range of healthcare needs and lifestyles. Individuals with chronic, non-communicable diseases (NCDs) such as heart disease will require different sensing modality and device type compared to women seeking fertility treatment. Lifestyle context—in addition to the underlying data requirements need to be factored into the system design and analysis [11]. The varied contexts for sensors pose challenges to algorithm development as well—it is often difficult to capture these in lab environments where sensors are calibrated and algorithms developed. Adaptive learning algorithms, along with the ability to re-calibrate sensors based on environment are key to overcoming this challenge [12].

Hybrid healthcare must also economically scale to potentially millions of users to deliver on its potential. Systems for hybrid healthcare must be designed with scalability in mind—from how data is transmitted and stored, to how it is visualised [9]. The rapid gains in computing power for small devices offers the potential of processing data on-board. A useful idea here is incremental processing: a substantial gain in performance can be achieved by processing the data as it arrives on devices and transmitting the information derived [13]. This is typically lower in volume and the data would otherwise require server-side computation. This can also be a privacy preserving strategy—for example in the case of vision sensors [14]. Avoiding the transmission, server-side computation and storage of data also has an unexpected environmental benefit—the internet is responsible for an estimated 3.7% of global carbon emissions [15] partially through the need to transmit and store huge amounts of data.

The rapidly standardised technology stack for cloud computing serves as a good foundation for flexible software architectures that can handle information from sensing devices scalably. Services for streaming data [16] for example can process data as it arrives and minimise the need to process at query time. Responsiveness can be enabled in these systems by leveraging events—allowing sensor devices to publish and subscribe to events that influence their behaviour [17]. Commercial standards such as SmartThings™ and IFTT™ make available these technologies for processing sensor data to consumers without requiring deep technical knowledge. To make sensing further accessible it must be available to end-users on personal devices such as smartphones and TVs—where powerful user interfaces leveraging chatbots and augmented reality can accessibly offer users context and explanation about their information [18].

Hybrid healthcare systems must not become the repositories of unutilised and uninformative personal information. Many sources of data will not offer useful information most of the time. This can be filtered at source—for example in naturally event-based sensors such as PIR. Alternatively, when information is fused, algorithms may analyse which dimensions of data offer the most information and choose to keep this at the highest resolution while discarding or archiving useless data. Dimensionality reduction techniques [19] such as Principal Components analysis (PCA) and Manifold embedding can represent information from very many sources in just a few dimensions. Alternatively—feature selection [20] can be used to identify the information most relevant to the context of the user's activity and only transmit and store this [21]. A further tool available to reduce storage and compute costs is compression and synopsis data structures [22]. Strategies can include downsampling, representation of statistical summaries and leveraging more advanced techniques like wavelet filtering [23] to preserve only the signal relevant to healthcare—not the noise of everyday life.

Applications Enabled by Wearable and Remote Monitoring in Healthcare

Analysing Activity and Behaviour to Improve Care Provision

Activity and behaviour are important clinical indicators of well-being. Activities of Daily Living (ADL) [24] can be used to infer the functional ability of people to live independently. Changes in frequency and performance of ADL may also signal the onset of disease, worsening of a condition [25] or be used to track recovery from surgery [26]. Recognising activities automatically is therefore an important and wide-ranging problem in the field of sensing [27]. A large range of sensors have been used for detecting and classifying activity—including cameras [28], wearables leveraging accelerometers and gyroscopes [29], activity information derived from smartphones [30] and combining ambient and wearable sensing [14].

The varied range of sensing technology offers the ability to customise applications to lifestyles, privacy priorities and health needs. For example, wearable sensors are very effective at differentiating between activities of different physical intensity. Sensors placed on objects can offer location and contextual information without the privacy issues attendant on more powerful, but potentially intrusive sensors like cameras. For example—sensors placed in drug dispensing boxes [31] can help track medication compliance. Cameras can offer the deepest degree of information about the user state—and depending on placement context and how information is extracted can be made palatable to end-users [32]. Infrared sensors offer an intermediate degree of information—these can track the movement of users across rooms. This can be used to generate a picture of an individual's room occupancy over the day, recognise activities from context (e.g. kitchen or toilet activity) and identify anomalous behaviour [9].

Activity analysis can be divided into two broad tasks—the first, termed 'activity recognition' deals with detecting the current user state in a typically small-time horizon. Building on this by incorporating temporal elements or sequencing is referred to as 'activity modelling'. To some extent, the latter can also be used for modelling complex activities from simpler, 'atomic' activities e.g., inferring 'food preparation' from a sequence of movement activities and location events. Whereas activity detection typically relies on discriminative machine learning algorithms, activity modelling often leverages sequence modelling algorithms such as Hidden Markov Models [33] and Long-Short Memory Neural Networks [34].

The effectiveness of wearables to identify ADL, as well as the potential to minimise the information extracted from the wearables is demonstrated in [35]. Figure 5.2 shows the data for several activities visualised in 2-D space using the

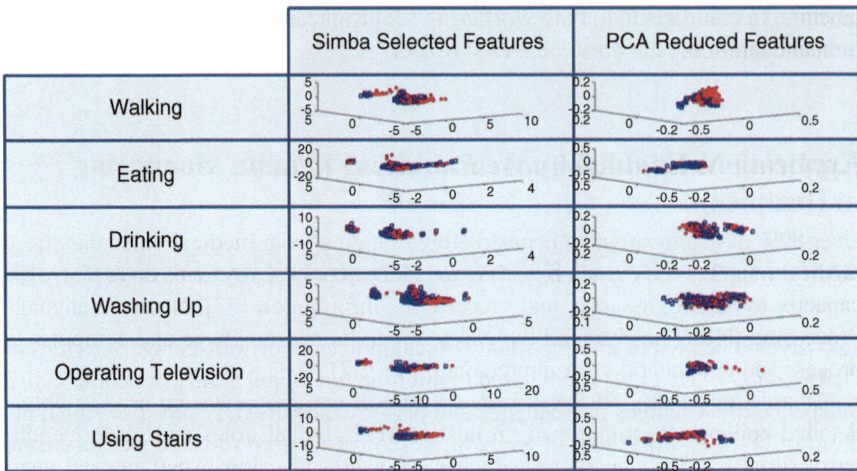

Fig. 5.2 Activities classified from sensor data in low-dimensional representation—blue points are from normal subjects, while red points are from impaired subjects [35]

feature selection algorithm Simba [36] and PCA. Both algorithms compress a large number of features extracted from the data in two dimensions, while still allowing the discrimination between impaired subjects (red) from normal subjects (blue).

ADLs and how they are performed can also offer insights around recovery from surgery. Current medical practice to assess recovery from surgery relies on patient questionnaires—for example the KOOS questionnaire for knee and mobility [37] and the CHAMPS physical activity questionnaire [38]. These questionnaires impose a compliance burden on patients, are difficult to control for subjectivity and there can be a significant delay between the onset of complications to the filling of questionnaires and subsequent analysis of it. Using sensors and remote monitoring allows for objective measures of recovery and timely interventions based on events automatically extracted from the data. Figure 5.3, taken from [35], shows the discrimination between subjects in early recovery (1–6 weeks after surgery) from subjects in late recovery (12–24 weeks after surgery) using accelerometer data collected while performing Step-up transitions (e.g. stepping onto stairs) and Stand-to-Sit transition (e.g. sitting into a chair). These activities are automatically identified in a continuous stream of sensor data by noting changes in data transformed into reduced dimensions using manifold embedding. The potential for this is to identify patients who do not follow the normal trajectory of recovery and direct care providers to them.

When wearable and ambient sensors are used to provide care to patients with chronic illnesses and requiring long-term care, an important aspect of behaviour to analyse is routine. Deviation from circadian rhythms in people can indicate a change in the state of health [39]. Furthermore, key indicators of wellbeing can be observed in daily routines for example sleeping habits, regular eating, exercise levels, routine social interactions. Typically, for this the sensors detecting movement and location both indoors and outdoors are important. As data accumulates rapidly over the

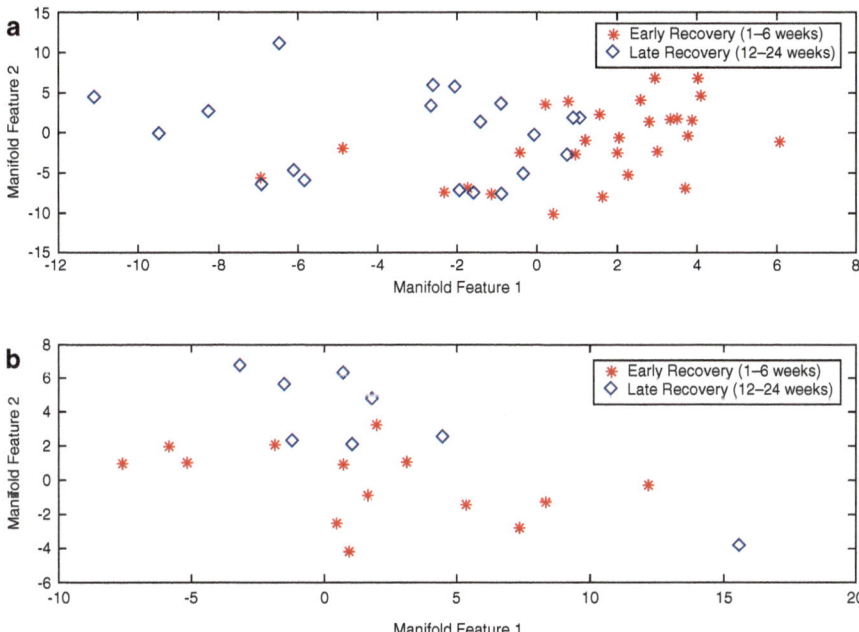

Fig. 5.3 Transitions from patients recovering from knee replacement surgery. Figures show embedding of accelerometer data while patients performed Step-up transition (**a**) and Stand-to-Sit transition (**b**) [35]

longer-term, abstracted pictures of an individual's routine allow the concise representation of their typical behaviour and allow care-providers to more easily see deviations. An example for this comes from the SAPHE project [40]—which deployed smart-home technology in partnership with Liverpool Primary Care Trust. A range of sensors were used—including wearable sensors such as accelerometers, ambient sensors including PIRs and connected devices such as smart weight scales. The patient cohort was typically elderly and requiring long-term care from community care providers who would otherwise prioritise their work using ad hoc means. Figure 5.4 shows the data abstracted about the individual's routine behaviour and showing a change in their routine resulting from an intervention from the healthcare worker, taken from [35]. These changes in routine behaviour derived from accelerometer and location sensors can allow timely interventions from care providers.

Personalised and Preventative Medicine Through Sensing and Smartphones

Widely adopted consumer devices such as smartphones and smartwatches carry a wide range of sensors. Accelerometers, GPS and gyroscopes are almost universal, and physiological sensors such as heart rate and skin temperature are also not

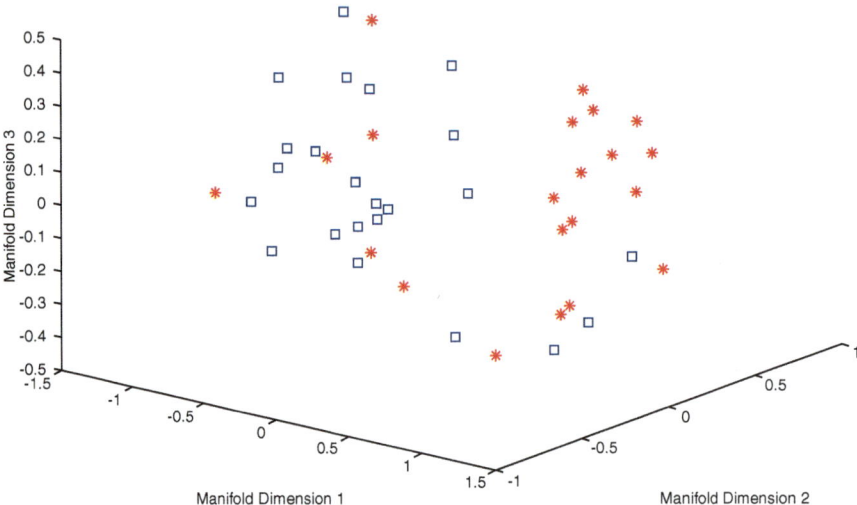

Fig. 5.4 Changes in routine behaviour (in red) compared to normal behaviour (blue) observed in a patient in a smart-home environment. Routine information is extracted from sensor data and visualised in a reduced manifold space [35]

uncommon. These devices therefore offer immense potential for enabling personalised and preventative healthcare.

Relatively soon after sensors became crucial for powering smartphone features like managing the screen orientation researchers were interested in studying the potential for use for activity and routine behaviour analysis [30]. Smartphones pose particular challenges however—they may not always be on the user's person and orientation and placement of the phone is often inconsistent. These factors are addressed—to an extent—in the ActiveMiles project, where rotation invariant features are derived and then clustered to get a basic indication of the user's activity levels. Combining with location data from GPS can give a rich picture of the user's activities and behaviour over time. Alternatively, the app can be calibrated with the phones placement at fixed locations e.g. belt buckles or pockets and machine learning models can discriminate between different activities using the sensor data (Fig. 5.5).

Wearables such as smart-watches and fitness trackers do not have the same challenges as with data collected from smartphones. Furthermore, a wide range of sensors are available as wearables—activity measures being the most common. These are widely used in the fitness tracking and sports markets and have extensive app eco-systems. More specialised sensors can be integrated into wearable and minimally invasive sensors. An example of this are sensors designed to track period cycles in women. Devices such as the OvuSense sensor [41] measure Core Body Temperature (CBT), changes in which are strongly associated with the phases of the reproductive cycle. OvuSense can characterise typical and atypical fertility cycles in addition to helping predict period and ovulation days [42]. OvuSense is one of the

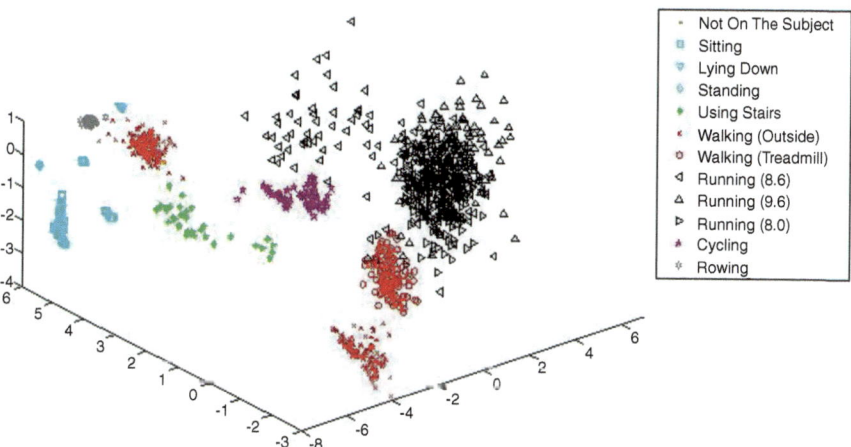

Fig. 5.5 Features from sensor data visualised in low-dimensional manifold space. Data is collected from a belt worn phone and activities can be clearly separated [35]

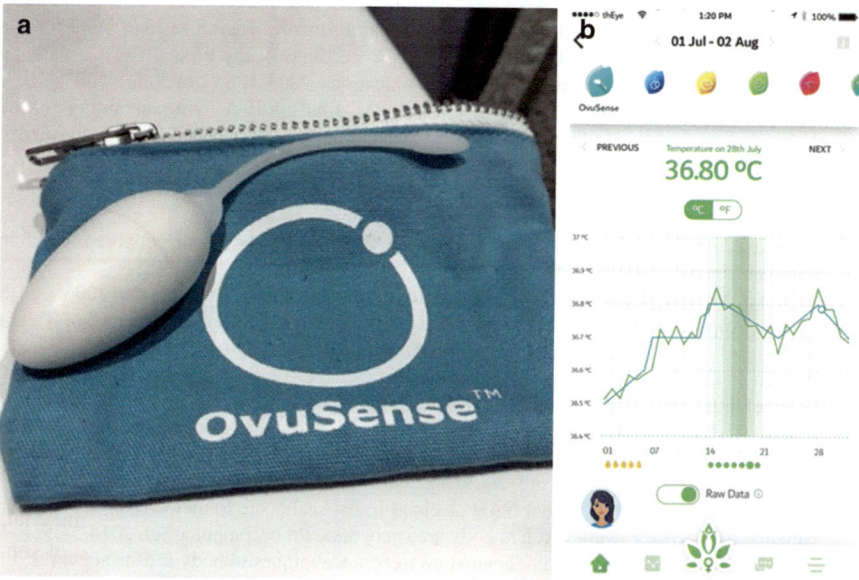

Fig. 5.6 The OvuSense sensor designed to track menstrual cycle using Core Body Temperature (**a**) and a screen designed to convey information extracted from the sensor in the Nabta app (**b**)

sensors supported by the Nabta app and will be a part of an ecosystem of sensors that Nabta app can draw information from, in addition to logs added by users themselves that give context to sensor data including mood, medications taken, food and water intake and more (Fig. 5.6).

Conclusion

Wearable and ambient sensors are inexpensive, ubiquitous and increasingly power-ful and easier to connect. A diverse set of healthcare and lifestyle monitoring use-cases are enabled by these devices ranging from care of chronically ill patients and post-operative recovery to delivering personalised medicine and helping patients take control of their health through insights derived from their data. Challenges remain—the need for privacy, catering for lifestyle differences, increasing regula-tory burdens and dealing with scale of data and more. Flexible, cloud-base software architectures, judicious data processing and use of compression and leveraging AI and machine learning can help address these challenges and deliver on the promise of sensing in healthcare.

References

1. Alam MR, Reaz MBI, Ali MAM. A review of smart homespast, present, and future. IEEE Trans Syst Man Cybern Part C Appl Rev. 2012;42:1190–203.
2. Cook DJ, Youngblood M, Heierman EO, Gopalratnam K, Rao S, Litvin A, Khawaja F. MavHome: an agent-based smart home. In: Proceedings of the First IEEE international conference on pervasive computing and communications, 2003. (PerCom 2003); 2003.
3. Intille S, Larson K, Beaudin J, Nawyn J, Tapia EM, Kaushik P. A living laboratory for the design and evaluation of ubiquitous computing technologies. In: CHI '05 extended abstracts on human factors in computing systems; 2005.
4. Hunn N. Global revenue from smart Wearables and hearables, *The market for smart wearable technology - WiFore Consulting.*
5. Yang G-Z, Hu X. Multi-sensor fusion. In: Yang G, editor. Body sensor networks. London: Springer London; 2006. p. 239–85.
6. Safaric S, Malaric K. ZigBee wireless standard. In: Proceedings ELMAR 2006; 2006.
7. Ejaz W, Anpalagan A, Imran MA, Jo M, Naeem M, Qaisar SB, Wang W. Internet of Things (IoT) in 5G wireless communications. IEEE Access. 2016;4:10310–4.
8. Aspden P, Corrigan J, Wolcott J, Patient safety: achieving a new standard for care. 2004. [Online]. https://www.ncbi.nlm.nih.gov/books/NBK216088/.
9. Elhelw M, Pansiot J, McIlwraith D, Ali R, Lo B, Atallah L. An integrated multi-sensing frame-work for pervasive healthcare monitoring. In: 3rd international conference on pervasive com-puting technologies for healthcare. 2009. pp. 1–7.
10. Khan FA, Ali A, Abbas H, Haldar NAH. A cloud-based healthcare framework for security and patients' data privacy using wireless body area networks. Proc Computer Sci. 2014;34:511–7.
11. Korel BT, Koo SGM. Addressing context awareness techniques in body sensor networks. In: 21st international conference on advanced information networking and applications work-shops (AINAW'07); 2007.
12. Hoey J, Boutilier C, Poupart P, Olivier P, Monk A, Mihailidis A. People, sensors, decisions: customizable and adaptive technologies for assistance in healthcare. ACM Trans Interact Intell Syst. 2013;2:1–36.
13. Talukder A, Ali S-M, Panangadan A, Jadhav C, Pidva R, Bhatt R, Chandramouli L, Monacos S. Optimal sensor scheduling and power management in sensor networks, Proc SPIE, vol. 5816; 2005.
14. Atallah L, Elhelw M, Pansiot J, Stoyanov D, Wang L, Lo B, Yang G. Behaviour profiling with ambient and wearable sensing, vol. 13; 2007. p. 133–8.

15. ClimateCare. Infographic: the carbon footprint of the internet. 22 April 2021. [Online]. https://www.climatecare.org/resources/news/infographic-carbon-footprint-internet/.
16. Samosir J, Indrawan-Santiago M, Haghighi PD. An evaluation of data stream processing systems for data driven applications. Proc Computer Sci. 2016;80:439–49.
17. Khriji S, Benbelgacem Y, Chéour R, Houssaini DE, Kanoun O Design and implementation of a cloud-based event-driven architecture for real-time data processing in wireless sensor networks, J Supercomput, 2021;1:651–59.
18. Jo D, Kim GJ. AR enabled IoT for a smart and interactive environment: a survey and future directions. Sensors (Basel, Switzerland). 2019;19(19):4330.
19. van der Maaten L, Postma E, Herik H. Dimensionality reduction: a comparative review. J Machine Learn Res JMLR. 2007;10:66–71.
20. Bachu V, Anuradha J. A review of feature selection and its methods. Cybern Inf Technol. 2019;19:3.
21. King R, Atallah L, Darzi A, Yang G-Z. An HMM framework for optimal sensor selection with applications to BSN sensor glove design. In: Proceedings of the 4th workshop on Embedded networked sensors (EmNets '07). Association for Computing Machinery, New York; 2007. pp. 58–62.
22. Gibbons PB. Synopsis structure. In: Ling LIU, Tamer ÖZSUM, editors. Encyclopedia of database systems. Boston, MA: Springer US; 2009. p. 2898–9.
23. Narasimhan SV, Basumallick N, Veena S. Introduction to wavelet transform: a signal processing approach. 1st ed. Alpha Science International Ltd; 2011.
24. Lin Z, Hanson AR, Osterweil LJ, Wise A. Precise process definitions for activities of daily living: a basis for real-time monitoring and hazard detection. In: Proceedings of the 3rd workshop on software engineering in health care, New York, NY, USA; 2011.
25. Paffenbarger RSJ, Hyde RT, Wing AL, Lee IM, Jung DL, Kampert JB. The association of changes in physical-activity level and other lifestyle characteristics with mortality among men. N Engl J Med. 1993;328(8):538–45.
26. Kwasnicki RM, Ali R, Jordan SJ, Atallah L, Leong JJH, Jones GG, Cobb J, Yang GZ, Darzi A. A wearable mobility assessment device for total knee replacement: a longitudinal feasibility study. Int J Surgery (London, England). 2015;18:14–20.
27. Chen L, Nugent CD. Sensor-based activity recognition review. In: Human activity recognition and behaviour analysis: for cyber-physical systems in smart environments. Cham: Springer International Publishing; 2019. p. 23–47.
28. Park DS, Zhang S, Wei Z, Nie J, Huang L, Wang S, Li Z. A review on human activity recognition using vision-based method. J Healthc Eng. 2017;2017:3090343.
29. Yu H, Cang S, Wang Y. A review of sensor selection, sensor devices and sensor deployment for wearable sensor-based human activity recognition systems. In: 2016 10th international conference on software, knowledge, information management applications (SKIMA); 2016.
30. Ali R, Lo B, Yang G-Z. Unsupervised routine profiling in free-living conditions — Can smartphone apps provide insights? In: 2013 IEEE international conference on body sensor networks; 2013.
31. Aldeer M, Javanmard M, Martin RP. A review of medication adherence monitoring technologies. Appl Syst Innov. 2018;1:1–27.
32. Apthorpe N, Shvartzshnaider Y, Mathur A, Reisman D, Feamster N. Discovering smart home internet of things privacy norms using contextual integrity. In: Proc. ACM Interact. Mob. Wearable Ubiquitous Technol., vol. 2; 2018.
33. Atallah L, Yang G-Z. Review: the use of pervasive sensing for behaviour profiling - a survey. Pervasive Mob Comput. 2009;5:447–64.
34. Uddin MZ, Soylu A. Human activity recognition using wearable sensors, discriminant analysis, and long short-term memory-based neural structured learning. Sci Rep. 2021;11:16455.
35. Ali R. Behaviour profiling using wearable sensors for pervasive healthcare. London: Imperial College London; 2012.

36. Gilad-Bachrach R, Navot A, Tishby N. Margin based feature selection - theory and algorithms. In: Proc of the 21th int conf on machine learning; 2004.
37. Roos EM, Toksvig-Larsen S. Knee injury and Osteoarthritis Outcome Score (KOOS) - validation and comparison to the WOMAC in total knee replacement. Health Qual Life Outcomes. 2003;1:17.
38. Stewart AL, Mills KM, King AC, Haskell WL, Gillis D, Ritter PL. CHAMPS physical activity questionnaire for older adults: outcomes for interventions. Med Sci Sports Exerc. 2001;33(7):1126–41.
39. Musiek ES, Bhimasani M, Zangrilli MA, Morris JC, Holtzman DM, Ju Y-ES. Circadian rest-activity pattern changes in aging and preclinical Alzheimer disease. JAMA Neurol. 2018;75:582–90.
40. Churcher GE, Bilchev G, Foley J, Gedge R, Mizutani T. Experiences applying Sensor Web Enablement to a practical telecare application. In: 2008 3rd international symposium on wireless pervasive computing; 2008.
41. Papaioannou S, Aslam M, Wattar BHA, Milnes RC, Knowles TG. User's acceptability of OvuSense: a novel vaginal temperature sensor for prediction of the fertile period. J Obstet Gynaecol. 2013;33:705–9.
42. Hurst B, Pirrie A, Milnes RC, Knowles T. Atypical vaginal temperature patterns may identify subtle, not yet recognised, causes of infertility. Fertil Steril. 2019;112(3):e244–5.

Part II
The Hybridization of Traditional Healthcare

Chapter 6
Disrupting the Delivery Mechanisms of Traditional Healthcare

Sophie Smith and Charles Newman-Sanders

Abstract With the increasingly rapid adoption of digital technologies by medical professionals across the globe, we are witnessing the first truly radical transformation of healthcare since the *Houses of Life* were established in Ancient Egypt in 2200 BCE (*Museum: House of Life*, 2017). In this chapter, we examine how hybrid healthcare seeks to reinvent the delivery mechanisms of traditional healthcare through the application of digital technologies, such as artificial intelligence (AI), the Internet of Things (IoT), and blockchain. We explore the effects of the Covid-19 pandemic on the willingness of healthcare providers and patients to adopt digital technologies, and we examine the dramatic overhaul of some of the key tenets of traditional healthcare such as the central nature of the provider. Finally, we evaluate various integrated care models against the theoretical efficacy of a truly hybrid healthcare ecosystem; one based around hybrid clinical pathways with the patient at the core.

Keywords Delivery mechanisms · Traditional healthcare · Hybrid healthcare Virtual care · Remote monitoring · Artificial intelligence · Patient-centricity

Introduction to Traditional Healthcare

Healthcare Defined

Healthcare, defined in the Oxford English Dictionary as "the organised provision of medical care to individuals or a community"—where "organised" implies adherence to a defined set of quality measures and outcomes—is a relatively novel practice. This is perhaps surprising if we consider that some of the first attempts to 'organise'

S. Smith (✉)
Executive, Nabta Health, Dubai, United Arab Emirates
e-mail: sophie@nabtahealth.com

C. Newman-Sanders
Nabta Health, Dubai, United Arab Emirates

M. Al-Razouki, S. Smith (eds.), *Hybrid Healthcare*, Health Informatics, https://doi.org/10.1007/978-3-031-04836-4_6

healthcare around a knowledge base were made by the Ancient Egyptians in 2200 BCE [1]. The first quality improvement documents for medical care were released by Florence Nightingale in England in 1863 [2]. In these, Nightingale referred to specific improvements she had made during the Crimean War of 1854, such as the reduction of overcrowding, provision of ventilation, and clearing of sewers, that collectively resulted in the mortality rate from disease dropping from 42.7% to 2.2% [3].

Nightingale's quality improvements were the first of a series of "tipping points", so-called by Malcolm Gladwell, that culminated in the traditional healthcare system(s) we know today. Other key tipping points include the introduction of sterilisation by Chamberland in France in 1879, the formalisation of the pharmaceuticals industry between 1881 and 1955, and the application of principles of mass production (courtesy of Henry Ford) in the 1940s and '50s [2].

The Architects of Traditional Healthcare Delivery Mechanisms

Most of the "tipping points" that resulted in today's healthcare systems can be traced back to a handful of key individuals. The pharmaceutical industry, for example, was built off the back of discoveries by the likes of Louis Pasteur (vaccinations, microbial fermentation, pasteurisation) and Emil von Behring (diphtheria antitoxin), with some of the first commercially available vaccines developed by Jonas Salk (polio), Pierre Descombey (tetanus), and Grace Eldering (whooping cough) [2]. Medical education owes its uniformity to Abraham Flexner, who in 1910 proposed a series of reforms that resulted in a standardised 4-year medical school curriculum and set of entry requirements.

Healthcare systems in the twenty-first century are largely uniform in terms of their constituents—educational and research institutions, medical suppliers, insurers, payers, claims processors, independent standard organisations, and healthcare providers. They owe their precise articulation in terms of the various touchpoints, authorities, and (often competing) interests, to three key tipping points: Nightingale's quality improvements, the introduction of technology to medicine in 1895 (when Wilhelm Conrad Rontgen accidentally discovered X-rays), and the provision of healthcare financing, mostly in the form of state-run medical insurance programs, from 1883.

For the purposes of this chapter, each constituent can be considered an "architect" of the delivery mechanisms of traditional healthcare; the mechanisms themselves, the technology, tools, and processes (including clinical pathways) deployed by those constituents as part of the organised provision of medical care.

Why Hybrid Healthcare Now?

Since Sir Tim Berners-Lee invented the World Wide Web in 1989, men and women around the world have had access to an unprecedented amount of information. Where previously individuals could not easily become specialised in subject matters they had not encountered through formal education, suddenly anyone could become an expert in anything, from origami to the Orient. And although "self-taught, self-made" has always been a lynchpin of entrepreneurship, particularly in the U.S. where few of the great names in business—Madam C.J. Walker, Henry Ford, John D. Rockefeller—studied extensively before founding the companies that made them famous, it was the Internet that made "self-taught, self-governed" possible—at scale and in all fields; even highly technical fields such as healthcare.

Since the early 1990s, patients have been able to access increasingly well-presented, evidence-based information about their health. Lay people with no formal medical background or training have gained the knowledge and skills required to become "architects" in the same healthcare system that previously governed their access to medical care. This shift in the balance of power has been cemented in recent years by further technological advances, such as the rise of sophisticated algorithms in machine and deep learning, increases in storage capacity and computational power, and an appreciation for big data and how to manipulate it. Today, machine learning is used to predict everything from a patient's progression along clinical pathways to the likelihood of chronic illnesses developing and, what is more, to share these insights with patients directly [4–8].

The final piece in the "why now?" puzzle is the Covid-19 pandemic. Prior to 2019, the adoption of new, technology-enabled delivery mechanisms by traditional healthcare architects was slow. Providers saw no reason to introduce telehealth platforms when virtual consultations offered no real time or cost savings, and negatively impacted footfall. Then the pandemic hit, and the response was a global lockdown. Government measures to enforce social distancing reduced access to in-person care and forced the introduction of virtual and remote care options—by private healthcare providers if they wished to stay afloat, and by public healthcare providers to meet the needs of high risk individuals.

Fast forward 18 months, and using chat, audio or video consultations to connect with doctors has become standard practice across the globe. At the height of the pandemic, Middle Eastern healthcare provider, Altibbi, succeeded in attracting 650,000 new subscribers from the Kingdom of Saudi Arabia ("KSA") alone [4]. Telehealth use by surgeons—nonexistent prior to the pandemic—increased exponentially during March and April of 2020 before levelling off at up to 60% cumulative use in some specialties [5]. The number of active surgeons during 2020 for each specialty are as follows: urology (n = 288), neurosurgery (n = 168), thoracic (n = 124), colorectal (n = 60), general surgery (n = 892), orthopedics (n = 698), obstetrics and gynecology (n = 1152), plastic surgery (n = 147), ophthalmology/ear, nose, and throat (ENT) (n = 876). The overall number of surgeons was 4405 [5].

This willingness of populations to access care in a new way was, is, the essential—previously missing—element that hybrid healthcare systems need to thrive.

Current State of Healthcare: Limitations of Today's Delivery Mechanisms

In many ways, the Covid-19 pandemic couldn't have come at a better time. Since the industrial revolution and rapid urbanisation in the early nineteenth century—which corresponded with the emergence of healthcare systems as we know them today—increases in environmental pollution and stress-mitigating behaviours such as smoking and the consumption of alcohol have resulted in a corresponding rise in non-communicable diseases ("NCDs").

NCDs sit on the opposite end of the spectrum to communicable diseases such as Covid-19; chronic conditions that cannot be transmitted from one person to another. They encompass everything from cancer to cardiovascular disease, obesity, and Type 2 Diabetes ("T2D"). Today, NCDs are a growing epidemic, threatening the ambition of countries around the world to achieve sustainable, universal access to health and health coverage for their populations. By 2025, it is estimated that NCDs will kill 41 million people globally each year, equivalent to 71% of all deaths. 15 million of those people will be between the ages of 30 and 69 years, with over 85% of "premature" deaths occurring in low- and middle-income countries [6].

In recent years, NCDs have placed an increasing strain on healthcare systems and economies around the world. WHO estimates that for every 10% increase in NCD mortality, economic growth is reduced by 0.5% [7]. The adverse effects of NCDs on healthcare systems is especially pronounced in low- and middle-income countries, where minimal health budgets are unable to support the growing dependence of NCD populations on costly medical solutions, such as drugs, as the first line treatment to reduce morbidity and premature mortality [8]. Coronary heart diseases, for example, is associated with seventy percent of deaths in low resourced countries versus twenty percent in high resourced countries [8].

Increasingly, it seems that traditional healthcare delivery mechanisms are not designed to treat the "accidentally unwell"—otherwise healthy individuals whose health has been compromised due to poor dietary and lifestyle choices, and who today make up the majority of the adult population [9]. Nor are they designed to cope with these individuals falling prey to communicable diseases such as Covid-19. During the pandemic, individuals with NCDs accounted for 78% of all Covid-19 ICU admissions and 94% of all deaths in the United States [10].

> *Of all the major health threats to emerge, none has challenged the very foundations of public health so profoundly as the rise of chronic noncommunicable diseases. Heart disease, cancer, diabetes, and chronic respiratory diseases, once linked only to affluent societies, are now global, and the poor suffer the most. These diseases share four risk factors: tobacco use, the harmful use of alcohol, unhealthy diets, and physical inactivity. All four lie in non-health sectors, requiring collaboration across all of government and all of society to combat them* [11]. (Noncommunicable diseases: a major challenge to public health in the Region, WHO, 2017)

To shift the burden of NCD management from established healthcare systems to individuals demands the active participation of industries outside of healthcare along with the application of corrective public health policies. It requires us to reimagine healthcare's delivery mechanisms by casting aside traditional provider-led, provider-centric models in favour of those that are patient-centric and patient-led; to enroll individuals as the lead architects in the project of their own health.

Digital Health Disruptors

Although the uptake of digital health solutions by established healthcare systems continues to be impeded by a number of factors such as lack of trust among clinicians, the perceived limitations of Artificial Intelligence, lack of access to data, and lack of interoperability between technology systems, a small number of "healthcare disruptors" are working to change this using different models of integrated care.

Integrated care, also known as comprehensive care, coordinated care, and integrated health, is a worldwide trend that seeks to provide more seamless, efficient, and effective care targeting the whole person and their needs at various ages and stages of life. The main differentiating factor between integrated care providers is the extent to which they are provider—as opposed to patient-centric.

Examples of integrated care models include the smart hospital, Hospital at Home®, and IoT-enabled care.

The Smart Hospital

Smart hospitals improve the provision of medical care by optimising and automating processes through the implementation of digital technologies such as cloud-based Hospital Information Management Systems (HIMS) and artificial intelligence. The aim of a smart hospital is twofold: to maximise productivity while providing better, more personalised, and more flexible care.

In order to qualify as "smart", a hospital cannot merely be digitalised; it must be able to generate unique insights that were not previously available, through the complete alignment of clinical processes and management systems [12]. This smart framework consists of three essential layers—data, insight, and access—with system-generated data parsed through machine-learning algorithms to generate meaningful insights that are subsequently able to be accessed and interpreted by different players in each healthcare system.

Current hotspots for smart hospitals include Dubai, Canada, Finland, South Korea and Singapore.

Case Study: Fakeeh University Hospital

Fakeeh University Hospital ("FUH") opened in 2021 in Dubai Silicon Oasis. The hospital is part of the Fakeeh Care group based in KSA and constitutes a Dh1.5 billion investment; the UAE's first smart hospital.

FUH is built on an integrated care model and aims to be both patient-centric and technology-driven. It achieves its aims through a combination of precision diagnostics, data-assisted decision making, and automated medication management. FUH places a premium on disruptive technologies. These include: comprehensive, two-way data integrations, to enable the efficient flow and harmonisation of information between systems and departments within the hospital; a state-of-the-art robotic pharmacy to automate the dispensing of medications; and, a novel patient "infotainment" system that supports interactions through a mobile app.

The integrated care model at FUH is underpinned by core values of medical excellence and scientific validation. The hospital is academically-minded, differentiating itself from other players in the market by prioritising the need to remain up-to-date with the latest advancements in clinical research and digital health technologies.

Hospital at Home®

Hospital at Home® is an innovative care model developed by John Hopkins University in the 1990s to provide hospital-level care in a patient's home. Designed to be a full substitute for acute hospital care, it was one of the first programs to use telehealth—providing nurse-supported, two-way telemedicine consultations with physicians as early as 2010—and is perhaps the earliest example of integrated care.

The program has been implemented by numerous healthcare and homecare providers across the United States, and is now increasingly available in other parts of the world such as the Middle East.

Case Study: TruDoc

TruDoc is a 24/7 population health management provider offering telemedicine, telemonitoring and home health services in line with NHS International Guidelines. Remote consultations are provided by a combination of licensed doctors and wellness experts via voice or video calls and live chat. In addition to remote consultations, TruDoc offers other services such as referrals to specialists, appointment-booking, medication delivery, and lab services at home.

From a technological standpoint, TruDoc differentiates itself from other integrated care providers by providing four connected entry points into its health management system. These are: a mobile app, on-site remote clinics, a hospital-based program that focuses on earlier discharge for patients in hospital, and the Hospital at Home® program licensed from John Hopkins University.

As part of Hospital at Home®, TruDoc provides on-site doctor visits and clinics for healthy, acute and chronic condition management. The objective of the Hospital at Home® programme is to reduce the long waiting times associated with traditional clinical pathways. TruDoc's target market for Hospital at Home® is the high risk 20% of the population who consume 82% of the medical costs; a group not adequately served by telehealth alone.

Hospitalised users are transitioned to the Hospital at Home® program on discharge. The program manages patients from the comfort of their own home with a range of benefits and positive outcomes, including cost savings of 19–30% versus traditional in-patient care, higher patient and caregiver satisfaction, a reduction in unnecessary hospital readmissions, reduced average hospital length of stay, better clinical outcomes, fewer complications, and less stress for family members and other caregivers.

IoT-Enabled Care

The "Internet of Things" refers to any device or object that is able to collect and share information using the Internet. In terms of healthcare, IoT devices mostly consist of connected medical wearables that are prescribed by physicians or purchased independently by patients to enable them to monitor different aspects of their health remotely. Today, IoT devices include everything from blood glucose monitors to fetal heart-rate monitors to realtime fertility monitors.

IoT-enabled care is a model of care underpinned by the active use of one or more IoT devices. It has all of the hallmarks of a standard integrated care model but, rather than being provider-centric in the sense that it is based around a traditional healthcare "architect" (a hospital or clinic), it is patient-centric.

Case Study: GluCare Health

GluCare Health is hybrid digital therapeutics company focused on Metabolic disease based in the UAE. GluCare Health practises a novel methodology of diabetes management focused on a hyper-personalized, behavioural change approach. It is the first provider globally to be certified by the International Consortium for Health Outcome Measures (ICHOM) for its practice of value based healthcare and the first outside of the United States to receive accreditation from URAC - a leading independent accreditation organisation.

The GluCare Hybrid Digital Therapeutics (DTx) model aims to correct deficiencies in the existing episodic model of care by moving from episodic and therapeutic care to a continuous, behavioural change model using Remote Continuous Data Monitoring ("RCDM").

As part of its continuous care model, GluCare Health utilizes different connected devices such as wearables, continuous glucose monitors, smart therapeutic inject-ables, weight scales, insulin pumps and blood pressure cuffs. Data is continuously streamed back from patients and is further analyzed by algorithms to provide action-able insights to the care team, who are able to communicate with patients via the GluCare Health app. This data is also integrated into the patient's Electronic Medical Record ("EMR").

GluCare Health's outcomes are currently amongst the best globally in compari-son to traditional or digital-only care . On average, patients reduced their HbA1c by around 2% in just 90 days, with the majority of patients requiring less medications. A reduction of just 1% has corresponding reductions of 21% in deaths related to diabetes, 14% in heart attacks, and 37% in microvascular complications. After 1 year of management, GluCare Health's average patient HbA1c is 6.6 [13].

Case Study: Pear Therapeutics

Pear Therapeutics develops Prescription Digital Therapeutics ("PDTs") to treat patients suffering with a range of diseases and disorders. Its provision of organised medical care is enabled by the original IoT device—the mobile phone.

Pear Therapeutics' lead product, reSET®, treats Substance Use Disorder and was the first PDT to receive authorisation from the Food and Drug Authority ("FDA") to improve disease outcomes. Pear Therapeutics' second product, reSET-O®, treats Opioid Use Disorder. reSET-O® was the first PDT to receive Breakthrough Designation and was authorised for prescription in December 2018 [14].

Pear Therapeutics' third and final product to date, Somryst®, is for the treatment of chronic insomnia. It was submitted for clearance through the FDA's traditional 510(k) pathway and was also reviewed by the FDA's Software Precertification Pilot Program before being authorised in March 2020.

Like traditional medicines, PDTs are developed in a GMP-compliant environ-ment, tested in randomised controlled trials demonstrating safety and efficacy, eval-uated and authorised by regulators such as the FDA, and used under the supervision of a prescribing physician.

NextGen Healthcare Delivery

If the first two decades of the twenty-first century were characterised by digital health disruption in the form of integrated care models of varying degrees of sophis-tication, the next two decades will be dominated by new, hybrid healthcare models. These hybrid models will use NextGen digital technologies such as virtual reality, deep learning, and blockchain to enable the decentralisation of care, where patients are the primary architects of their own healthcare delivery.

Enabling True Patient Centricity

The absence of true patient centricity in healthcare has, to date, resulted in significant racial and gender biases in healthcare delivery mechanisms—from the prescription of drug-based therapeutics, to the performance of routine procedures such as C-sections—with noticeably worse health outcomes among emerging market populations.

Not until 1994 did the United States' National Institutes of Health (NIH) mandate that women and minorities were to be included as subjects in clinical research and trials. Until then, women were largely excluded from clinical research and trials on the basis that they were considered to be "small men", with the research community refusing to entertain the fact that gender differences might affect clinical outcomes.

Today, women are still 50–75% more likely than men to suffer adverse reactions to drugs because most drugs have not been designed for or tested on women [15]. Moreover, a significant portion of the global population continues to be excluded from clinical trials, with 92% of trials occurring in the US and Europe, and the vast majority of the remaining 8% occurring in the Far East.

Hybrid healthcare aims to address racial and gender biases in healthcare by allowing individuals to become the primary architects of their own care. Platforms powered by machine learning with multiple IoT interfaces will allow patients to make informed decisions about everything from their progression along clinical pathways to the time, place and mode of care delivery. Lifestyle recommendations will be personalised according to a patient's age, stage and health goals, and will be culturally relevant. Health data will be patient-owned, patient-held and protected, with federated learning platforms such as Bitfount used to deliver machine learning algorithms to data, and not the other way round. Hospitals and clinics, even specialised clinics will become secondary—spokes in a complex network of delivery systems where every patient is its own hub.

Developing an Augmented Intelligence

One of the pillars of hybrid healthcare is the concept of augmented intelligence—combining the best of human intellect with machine learning capabilities in order to optimise health outcomes, particularly in situations where best practice guidelines conflict, for example, in the management of more than one non-communicable diseases in parallel.

Today, a plethora of artificially-intelligent systems are used to provide health information to patients at home [16]. These include sensors to detect heart rate and rhythm, smartwatches to track blood pressure and oxygen saturation levels, and systems to measure everything from blood glucose levels to ovulation in real-time.

The rapid development and commercialisation of clinically validated Point-of-Care ("PoC") devices and tests means that healthcare providers already have access to far greater volumes of clinically-accurate, patient-generated data than they did previously, and are increasingly being asked to use this data to diagnose, treat and rehabilitate patients.

Approximately 30% of the world's data today is generated by the healthcare industry, and this will increase to 36% by 2025 [17]. Physicians *will* require the assistance of machine learning algorithms to harmonise, analyse, and contextualise health data made available to them, or otherwise risk being overwhelmed or left behind. The result will be an augmented collective intelligence—systems that combine the best of human and artificial intelligence in terms of data collection, data analytics, and the delivery of qualified data insights.

Instilling Principles of Immutability Through Decentralisation

The final, defining traits of NextGen healthcare delivery and of hybrid healthcare itself is the principle of immutability through decentralisation that will be realised through the implementation of ledger-based technologies such as blockchain.

The decentralisation of care is the only way that true patient centricity can be achieved. Blockchain has the potential to define new standards for patient health record access and management. In the near future, blockchain will be used to create compliance-based cost incentives for payers; to provide value-based reimbursements to healthcare providers; to adjust premium calculations according to dietary and lifestyle behaviours; to improve the quality of medical records by reducing the prevalence of fabricated claims; and to deploy decentralised, peer-to-peer networks for clinical research and best practice [18].

To conclude, the growing prevalence of NCDs and their associated economic burden means that a shift away from traditional, provider-led care provision to new, decentralised models of care is necessary if healthcare systems are to survive. The disruption of traditional delivery mechanisms by hybrid healthcare and its core principles of patient centricity, augmented intelligence, and decentralisation, has come not a moment too soon. Prior to the Covid-19 pandemic, it would have been impossible to imagine the architects of traditional healthcare adopting so readily and at such pace the digital health solutions that would make hybrid healthcare possible. But adopt they did. Today, digital health disruptors are increasingly present, increasingly established, and increasingly capable of delivering better health outcomes than traditional healthcare.

In this world of emergent hybrid healthcare ecosystems with rapidly evolving digital technologies at their core, there's all to play for.

References

1. *Museum: House of life*. www.ucl.ac.uk. Accessed 17 Feb 2017.
2. Sheingold BH, Hahn JA. The history of healthcare quality: the first 100 years 1860–1960. https://www.sciencedirect.com/science/article/pii/S2214139114000043
3. Nightingale F. Notes on hospitals. 3rd ed. Greene, Longman, Roberts and Green, London, England: Longman; 1863.
4. HBC Editors. Altibbi achieves 3,000,000 telemedicine consultation in MENA. Healthcare Business Club.
5. Chao GF, Li KY, Zhu Z, et al. Use of telehealth by surgical specialties during the COVID-19 pandemic. JAMA Surg. 2021;156(7):620–6. https://doi.org/10.1001/jamasurg.2021.0979.
6. World Health Organisation. Noncommunicable diseases. https://www.who.int/news-room/fact-sheets/detail/noncommunicable-diseases
7. World Health Organisation. Health systems response to NCDs. https://www.euro.who.int/en/health-topics/Health-systems/health-systems-response-to-ncds/health-systems-response-to-ncds
8. Kassa M, Grace J. The global burden and perspectives on non-communicable diseases (NCDs) and the prevention, data availability and systems approach of NCDs in low-resource countries. IntechOpen. https://doi.org/10.5772/intechopen.89516.
9. Smith S, Alzabin S. The rise of the accidentally unwell, and its unforeseen impact. https://medium.com/hybrid-healthcare-is-the-future-of-healthcare/the-rise-of-the-accidentally-unwell-and-its-unforeseen-impact-f2308a933df2
10. Achenbach J, Wan W. New CDC data shows danger of coronavirus for those with diabetes, heart or lung disease, other chronic conditions. The Washington Post. 2020
11. Noncommunicable diseases: a major challenge to public health in the Region, WHO, 2017
12. Shah S. Understanding smart hospitals and why most aren't there yet. Healthcare IT News. https://www.healthcareitnews.com/blog/understanding-smart-hospitals-and-why-most-arent-there-yet
13. Glucare 90 days outcome report. https://glucare.health/wp-content/uploads/2021/04/GluCare-90-Days-Outcome-Report.pdf
14. Murphy M. Pear therapeutics announces formulary availability for its three FDA authorized prescription digital therapeutics at OptumRx. Business Wire: https://www.businesswire.com/news/home/20210810005275/en/Pear-Therapeutics-Announces-Formulary-Availability-for-its-Three-FDA-Authorized-Prescription-Digital-Therapeutics-at-OptumRx. 2021, Aug
15. Dusenbery M. The surprising reason we lack so much knowledge about women's health. Forbes (forbes.com). 2018 Aug
16. Topol EJ. A decade of digital medicine innovation. Sci Transl Med. 2019;11(498):eaaw7610.
17. Coughlin S, Roberts D, O'Neill K, Brooks P. Looking to tomorrow's healthcare today: a participatory health perspective. Inter Med J. 48(1):92–6. https://doi.org/10.1111/imj.13661.
18. Smith S, Pradhan M. Using blockchain to enable patient-centric care in the MENA region and to define new industry standards for personal health record access and management, Nabta Health. 2018 Jul

Chapter 7
Hybrid Home Healthcare

Mahiben Maruthappu and Paulina Cecula

Abstract Healthcare systems around the world are facing challenges related to population changes such as ageing and the complexity of long-term conditions. Hospital to home movement is already playing a crucial role in the delivery of care. The shift is driven by affordability, improved outcomes and convenience for patients. As home care will increase, the care of the elderly will become one of the fastest-growing sectors in the human labour market (Harari, 21 lessons for the 21st century, 2018). At the same time, technology is developing at an enormous pace, penetrating many industries, including medicine. Advances have been made in how healthcare is being delivered, how conditions are being monitored and how information is exchanged. As healthcare is looking for solutions, technology becomes critical in ensuring high quality of care and high independence for individuals (Maruthappu). From simple medical devices to artificial intelligence (AI), technology will play an important role in improving not only standards of care, but also the conditions of people working in the sector. It is likely that in the next few years, care will remain human-centred, with high-quality patient care at its core and technology being essential in supporting the whole hybrid healthcare system. This chapter will discuss the future of hybrid homecare and an example of a company that is already transforming the sector.

Keywords Homecare · Home nursing · Caregiving · Digital first · Marketplaces Eldercare · Silvercare · Telecare

M. Maruthappu
Cera Care, London, UK
e-mail: mahiben@ceracare.co.uk

P. Cecula (✉)
Imperial College London, London, UK
e-mail: pc2416@ic.ac.uk

M. Al-Razouki, S. Smith (eds.), *Hybrid Healthcare*, Health Informatics,
https://doi.org/10.1007/978-3-031-04836-4_7

The Need for Home Care

There are three main areas that can be identified as demand drivers for the care industry, especially home care, which are: demographic shift, the burden of long-term conditions and patients' preference to age at home.

The dramatic demographic shift is a major driver for the rising demand for home care. By 2025 there are going to be one billion more people in the world and 300 million of them will be over 65 years old [1]. It's been projected that the elderly in the US will double in number between 2018 and 2060 and become around a quarter of the country's population (U.S. Census Bureau, Population Projections). The situation is similar in the UK. In 2016, people over 65 accounted for 18% of the population, but in 2036 it will reach almost 24% (Fig. 7.1). The trend is likely to continue.

The demographic shift is not just numbers. Many other demographic factors can affect health perceptions, health seeking behaviours and healths needs of a population. For example, the geographical distribution of age groups is not equal across the countries with the elderly usually concentrated in more rural areas. It's also been observed that more elderly tend to live alone or are divorced than in previous generations. In the US, one-fourth of women aged 65–74 lived alone in 2018 [4].

Although life expectancy is increasing due to medical advancements and people are getting healthier in some aspects (higher cancer survival rates, less smoking), one can also observe increasing numbers of elderly living with chronic conditions, often multiple, such as dementia, diabetes, mobility impairments [5]. In the UK, more than every other person above 60 has a long-term condition and multiple long term conditions are on the rise [6]. Those illnesses have a huge impact on the NHS costs (Fig. 7.2). *Approximately 70% of the total health and care spending in England is attributed to caring for people with long-term conditions.* Moreover, societal inequality poses a challenge as long term conditions are 60% more prevalent and 30% more severe in the least privileged in British society compared with most privileged.

timeline	0–15 years old (%)	16–64 years old (%)	**Aged 65 and over (%)**	UK population
1976	24.5	61.2	**14.2**	56,216,121
1996	20.7	63.5	**15.9**	58,164,374
2016	18.9	63.1	**18**	65,648,054
2036	18	58.2	**23.9**	73,360,907
2046	17.7	57.7	**24.7**	76,342,235

Fig. 7.1 Table with projected age distribution in the UK population up to 2046 (based on data from the Office of National Statistics [2, 3])

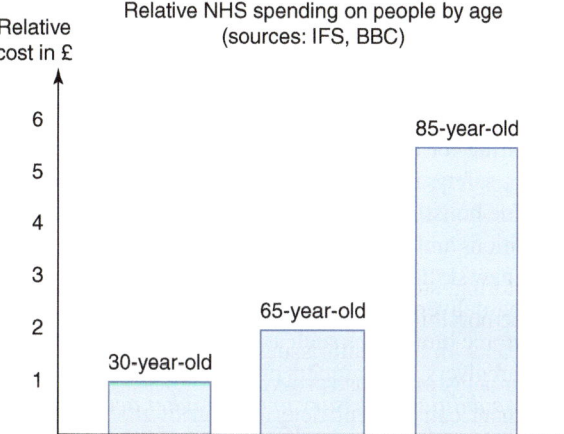

Fig. 7.2 NHS spending on people varies by age (adapted from BBC News [7, 8])

Although the demand for nursing and residential homes will also increase, it's been shown across surveys and studies that people prefer to age at home [9, 10].

Home healthcare market size is estimated to be worth $545.1 billion by 2028 [11]. Ageing populations, long-term conditions and people's hopes to age at home are not the only reasons for the increasing home care and retirement management market. Currently declining governmental support, cost-efficiency and increasing burden on family caregivers are also significant contributors. Home care is a cost-efficient alternative to expensive hospital stays. For instance, according to The Commonwealth Fund, "hospital at home" programs enable patients to receive care at home with fewer complications and over 30% reduction in the cost of care [12].

Let's now imagine an edlerly patient, Mary, age 75, living alone in a rural town in England. Her mobility is decreasing and she has diabetes, arthritis and depression. She is lonely, forgetful and cannot see her doctor often due to her frailty, GP practices being overstretched and living a significant distance away from the practice. The annual cost of her health and social care could be around £6000 per year. Despite, her health is declining. One day, she trips over and falls. She spends significant time on the floor before she gets admitted to the hospital. Following the accident, she becomes bed-bound and can no longer be independent. The social care is trying to find a residential home for her which makes Mary is very upset as she was hoping to stay at home.

This hypothetical scenario, is unfortunately a very common story for many elderly and frail patients.

The global trends and challenges explained may as well become opportunities for much-needed entrepreneurs and disruptors who aspire to transform the care system with the main objective being to ensure that ageing people can remain as independent as possible.

Challenges of Home Care

Social care is under a lot of pressure. The care industry has high stakes, limited resources and requires certain expertise.

Caring for a person is extremely complex. It involves looking after one's well-being, safety, health needs and activities of daily life. Home care is challenged to provide holistic care in increasingly complex situations. With the rise of long-term conditions and their various therapies and management, caregivers will increasingly need new skills. There's a certain level of difficulty in defining how much healthcare can be delivered at home with obstacles such as lack of medical equipment and workforce limitations such as lack of adaequate medical knowledge and training for the caregivers. Researchers pointed out that the home care industry needs to develop the *capabilities necessary to treat higher acuity patients with broader care needs in the home and community* [5]. On top of the complexity, home care is challenged by a lack of interoperability between systems in different parts of healthcare. Patients' health information is often dispersed between primare care doctors, hospitals, and care companies but only a comprehensive system can ensure comprehensive care. Lack of technology in-home care and care management is currently contributing to inefficiency and poorer quality of care provided. Other challenges include financing, reimbursements, regulatory constraints, measuring performance and shortage of care workers.

Future State of Home Care

The healthcare models will be shifting towards prevention, home care, patients' independence and collaboration between services. Home health and home care will play a crucial role in future healthcare models. Landers et al. proposed a transformation shifting delivery of care from hospitals to home while at the same time increasing patients' quality of life, timely delivery of medical interventions and reducing costs. One of the main reasons for the cost difference is that home care requiring less expertise and equiptment from the providers as compared to residential or acute care (hospitals). Given the potential to reduce costs for healthcare systems on a national level, reserachers advocated for policy makers to be involved in enabling the caregivers and home-care providers to best serve patients now and in the future.

Home Care Agency of the Future

American researchers looked into the competencies that a home care agency will need to have to cope with rising demands and constructed a model consisting of five core skills.

1. *Patient and person centred*—as patients are more engaged in their health and care, clinical decisions such as care plans need to reflect their values, preferences and needs [13]. With current healthcare trends, providing patient care is becoming closer to providing customer experience https://www.cerahq.com/. The success and performance measures will need to increasingly include patient satisfaction and preference [5].
2. *Well connected and coordinated*—in-house activities need to run smoothly to make sure that patients receive the right care at the right time. Cross-organisational integration will become crucial for comprehensive care. This means integration between community, primary and specialist care as well as mental health services to look at a patient's health holistically. Interoperability with other healthcare services needs to be established to ensure easy transitions of patients eg. between hospitals and homes.
3. *High quality*—provide reliable, responsive general and specialised care to patients. Care agencies will need to provide appropriate training for the carers, with continuous updates and opportunities to learn and grow. The care plans should be responsive and agile.
4. *Technology-enabled*—care homes will have to adopt technology to allow for improvements in efficiency, connectivity and care itself. Technology should be used to enable people, both patients and carers.
5. *Proactive*—in order to keep satisfying patients' needs, providing excellent care and taking home care to the next level, care homes will have to be reactive and proactive services. This means that the new approach will be to actively try spotting and preventing issues rather than waiting for an acute event to happen and treating it.

It is clear that the social care sector needs radical changes and more attention to keep up with the growing demands. One of the main reasons why social care currently lags 20 years behind healthcare in its provision of services is a failure to adopt the technology. From making existing care provision more effective to finding new ways of providing care, innovation will be crucial to ensuring we can meet the demands. While we are waiting for larger, slower reform against a backdrop of an ageing population and dwindling workforce, we need to embrace technology for immediate change. Although impossible to fix overnight, it doesn't have to be very difficult. Those shifts need to be acknowledged and embraced by institutions and healthcare professionals. Technology will be an inevitable part of delivering home care and to utilise it effectively we should aim to understand its benefits and limitations.

One of the main reasons why social care currently lags 20 years behind healthcare in its provision of services is a failure to adopt the technology. Although impossible to fix overnight, it doesn't have to be very difficult. While we're waiting for larger, slower reform against a backdrop of an ageing population and dwindling workforce, we need to embrace technology for immediate change. From making existing care provision more effective to finding new ways of providing care, innovation will be crucial to ensuring we can meet the demands. Technology will be an inevitable part of delivering home care and to utilise it effectively we should aim to understand its benefits and limitations.

Tech Applications in Care

Technology adoption in healthcare is much slower than across other industries due to reasons such as risk aversion, system fragmentation and lack of clear regulatory guidance. However, as research is proving more and more benefits of using technology in health and the patients' demands are rising, the technological transformation of healthcare becomes inevitable. To date, AI implementation has largely focused on younger, healthy smartphone users, dismissing those who attend A&E most frequently and use the most healthcare resources—the elderly [14]. *We talk about self-driving cars and all these great technologies, and yet we're regularly letting older people be left helpless on the bathroom floor for 48 hours because simple technology is not used (Parmentier, 2019).* As the system strives to make patients more independent and safe to live at home, it's crucial that innovations keep the patient, their consent, dignity and quality of their care in the centre of it.

In the UK, the government has set a clear vision for the use of technology, digital and data within health and social care, to enable the NHS and social care systems to improve outcomes [15]. Care Quality Commission groups, who regulate health and social care in England recognise that technology has the potential to bring plenty of benefits to the patients and the system [16].

1. Give people more control over their health, safety and wellbeing.
2. Support them to be more independent or feel less isolated.
3. Link them to services that are important for them.
4. Enhance the care or treatment providers offer.
5. Help them communicate with families, professionals and staff.
6. Help staff to prioritise and focus their attention on people who need it most.
7. Capture and compare data, and share good practice with peers.

Some of the biggest trends in homecare include: remote monitoring, automation and digitisation, prediction and prevention, and telemedicine.

Remote Monitoring

Being able to monitor a patient using sensors without the constant presence of carers is expected to revolutionize home care in the next few years. Internet of Things (IoT) devices can allow family members to monitor their loved ones and their environment remotely in real-time. IoT devices include smartphones, computers, smart speakers, smart homes, all connected to the web [17]. Part of the smart home technology could be voice recognition software, which allows vocalised commands to access lighting, household appliances, doors etc and could be helpful to the elderly's and those who struggle with mobility. Telecare includes personal alarms worn by the patients that can be activated to call for urgent help anytime. Telemonitoring refers to devices that can constantly monitor a patient's vital signs such as blood sugar level, temperature, blood pressure, heart rate and breathing. Some advanced technologies can even offer hospital-like standards [9]. The utilisation of devices and data analytics together offer promising results for the future of healthcare. Medical devices combined with information from sensors such as sleep and mobility patterns can offer comprehensive data about one's health. They can soon play a crucial role in disease detection, monitoring and treatment. According to doctor and CEO Meena Ganesh, medical devices could optimize both delivery and standard of care [9]. As devices are now able to do everything from monitoring a patient's heart rate to checking if they are performing their daily activities, more acute conditions and deterioration can be monitored and acted on quickly [14]. This means that even if an accident like a fall occurs, the alert systems can minimise the risk of severe consequences or death from being unable to receive immediate help. With the right data collection and analysis, very dangerous or even deadly accidents like falls could potentially be prevented. These will be particularly beneficial for high-risk populations and critically ill patients whose care plans need to be adjusted regularly and timely interventions can be determinant. Apart from the health benefits, technology can increase safety and security, which are crucial to ensuring the elderly's independence at home. Sensors can detect heat and floods and alarm the family or emergency services immediately [18]. Telecare and telemonitoring can also lead to cost savings as the carers aren't required to monitor the patient 24/7. In order to take advantage of those benefits, it's important to ensure that such devices are compatible and installed correctly. The devices will need to perfectly coexist together which again highlights the need for interoperability and integration. Successful utilisation will require both medical and technical skills. The long-term *benefit of smart home technology and wearables is that they enable users to become more autonomous and live in the comfort of their own homes for as long as possible* [14].

Automation and Digitization

Anyone with a relative who is receiving care at the moment will know how poor the communication can sometimes be with the carer or care team. Records are often handwritten on bits of paper and messages about the patient's health indicators can go awry [19]. Most care providers use pens, paper and whiteboards to manage their business, which means they're not as transparent, efficient or scalable as they could be if they harnessed technology [15]. As care companies need to focus on delivering the best quality care, automation has the potential to streamline processes and increase effectiveness. From providers perspectives, technologies like machine learning (ML) can be applied to a variety of operational tasks, from assigning caregivers to patients to scheduling appointments. Automation can also have a huge impact on the quality of care provided by caregivers. Traditionally, their responsibility was to fill in numerous paper files during their visit which reduces the time spent with the patient, often leads to information being lost or not captured and rarely reviewed. Digitization of the processes can ensure all crucial data is captured and saved in real-time. Thanks to voice recording technology, carers can even record their visit reports without typing. Tech can free up staff to focus on care rather than admin, to drive savings that push up carer wages, and ultimately deliver better care [15]. All combined, the technology can help with basic, operational or administrative tasks, freeing up the time to concentrate on the patient which will increase patient satisfaction and carers job fulfilment.

Prediction and Prevention

Across the world, prevention is one of the key objectives for healthcare systems and technology has a significant role to play in this [15]. One of the most exciting possibilities that can potentially revolutionise home care are ML and AI driven assessments and predictions. These technologies can be developed and trained to assess risk, predict illness and health deterioration. Such algorithms can be trained on the data collected from visit reports or constantly updated clinical data about the patient - such as they day-to-day needs, symptoms and level of independence. The technology can then quickly flag signs of deterioration which can be communicated to the care management team, the family or even automatically recommend a doctor appointment or a hospital visit. Such support system will also give carers more confidence in their decisions. Overall, preventitive technologies can lead to better healthcare outcomes by health issues being picked up faster and acted upon to prevent accidents and deterioration. As AI could also learn to understand what behaviours are normal for a particular patient, we could avoid unnecessary appointments which are a burden to the system. Aside from the technology offered by home care companies, there are plenty of lifestyle applications that can be used for preventive medicine. In the NHS, where 10% of the entire system budget is currently spent on type 2 diabetes—a largely preventable condition—the NHS Diabetes Prevention Programme is tackling this challenge by making use of apps that support healthier lifestyles and behaviour change. AI and social networking are being used to tailor solutions to specific needs and provide support for people as they embark on lifestyle changes [15].

Telemedicine

Elderly with complex illnesses who struggle with few-long term conditions and take a lot of different medications often require more frequent appointments with their primary care doctor. Some of those appointments do not necessarily need the patient to physically visit the clinic. Moreover, as the elderly also often experience mobility issues, the journey to the clinic may cause a lot of stress. That's why telemedicine, meaning the possibility to see a doctor via a video call, can be revolutionary for those patients. Telehealth can range from telephone calls, obtaining information from tools online to joining an online support group, bridging the geographic distances and providing access to healthcare for all [18]. It's important to highlight that the waiting time for a video call GP consultation is much shorter than for the actual visit. Combined with the data from medical wearables, doctors may still have the possibility to check a patient's blood pressure, heart rate, blood glucose levels at so on, all in real-time. Similarly to previous examples, when adopted correctly, telemedicine can lead to a decrease in negative healthcare outcomes and costs by preventing events such as hospital re/admissions and emergency department visits.

Apart from these four big trends, there are many other issues that are being addressed by new innovative technologies. One way technology is already helping is by making people stay on top of their medications. Going to see a GP just to repeat a prescription is a huge burden for the system as well as the patient. Very often the prescribed medications are not even taken in the way they should be. Now, a patient's repeated prescriptions can be delivered to their home (eg. *Lloyds Direct*).Mobile apps can also send patients reminders when it's time to take their medication. Other companies, like *KOMP* from Norway, believe that devices could help fight the elderly's loneliness and isolation. Their product is an elderly-friendly alternative to a tablet with a primary role to easily connect the patient with their family and loved ones. Others, like *Accenture Interactive* believe that AI voice assistants can also help isolated elderly to share their stories and save them for future generations. Many companies are trying to use chatboxes and AI to tackle the elderly's loneliness [9]. However, as a robot can never replicate the enormous benefits of human contact from a carer [15], it's important to emphasise that these technologies can be useful for the time when the patient cannot see their carers or family members. Another interesting trend is to use virtual reality (VR) to tackle various issues from loneliness to memory loss and dementia. *Revender* offers customized reminiscence therapy by showing personalised content to the patient that could even be a reconstruction of their wedding day. *Memory Co* develops personalised games and activities that aim to help patients recall certain events and facts which could prevent deterioration and keep them independent for longer. There are also more specialised services that use tech and devices to deliver physical and neuro-rehabilitation, such as after a stroke (eg. *Flint, Immersive Rehab, MindMaze*). This is particularly interesting as combined with the regular physiotherapy received by the patients in the hospitals, it can increase the effects and speed up the process of recovery.

As one can notice, there's some degree of overlap between the utility of those various care tech trends. Telecare, telemonitoring alongside apps and AI all combined have the best chance of success in preventative medicine. These won't work without early digitization and adoption of technology amongst carers, patients and healthcare professionals. Aspiring to produce a hybrid healthcare system the challenge will be to align people, services and technology. The usability and interface of those technological designs will need to be tested with those groups before implementation, especially the elderly with functional, hearing, visual and cognitive limitations. The teamwork between medics, engineers, entrepreneurs and patients will be crucial in order to truly utilise those possibilities. Both users and healthcare professionals will be able to give insights into the amount of information and features desired from a product. Just like a multidisciplinary teams (MDT) made of nurses, therapists and doctors work together in a hospital, home care medicine may require its own MDT team too. The costs savings, better outcomes and overall satisfaction will be a result of technology working in synergy with human healthcare services.

The Cera Care Case Study

The Current State of Care in the UK

In the UK, social care is under fire. Looking at the trends in demand, the need for care workers will be increasing drastically, in the UK and internationally. Just like healthcare systems are struggling with having fewer doctors than needed, the social care sector is challenged by a chronic shortage of care workers, estimated to be around 350,000 workers short by 2028 [20]. Coupled with the potential loss of talent because of Brexit, it is clear that the sector needs to work hard to maintain and expand the number of carers [15]. How should we respond to the challenges and growing demand?.

At Cera Care, the struggling state of social care motivated the company to find a solution. Cera's vision is to empower people to live their best lives in their own homes. The company specialises in helping people select the right care for their loved ones and offering continued support for as long as it is required [21]. Cera helps clients achieve high quality of life, satisfaction and independence by offering a wide range of care services to patients, both live-in and hourly, such as palliative, respite, post-discharge, dementia and elderly. Cera also hopes to reduce their needs for emergency care and hospitalisation thus reducing the cost burdens of care. For Cera, there are three key opportunities for using technology: digitisation, data, and the use of devices [15].

Digitization

Digitization can help tackle several issues that social care is currently facing. According to research as well as proven track record at Cera Care, digitalisation has helped streamline processes, reduce the burden of paperwork and improve quality of care. For Cera, digitization is about having all services in one, easily-accessible place so that a range of individuals, including general practitioners (GPs), families and carers can access up to date information on the individual being cared for. Cera is implementing an AI-driven "Dynamic Tasks" list for carers, personalised to patients needs and information from previous visits. The tasks depend on the patient's condition, mood, recommendations from healthcare professionals and patients' individual needs and preferences. Carers can access up to date information about the patient and reply to the highest priority tasks. The platform also allows for real-time updates about completed tasks and ensures vital information about developments in an individual's care are taken into account. This is particularly important where a person is unable to communicate for themselves or may be living with a condition like dementia. It gives carers the vital knowledge they need and is particularly helpful when they are on the move. The technology is effective—Dynamic Tasks have been proven to be 93% accurate at correctly identifying the 'next best action' for a visit, which can drastically reduce the risk of key tasks being missed and makes care more consistent [15].

Data

Just like banks use data to identify unusual activities in an account, Cera uses data to detect unusual changes in a person's health [22].

Cera has developed algorithms that can analyse carers' reports and predict if there's anything concerning happening to the patient. Using AI, Cera's Concern Predictor alerts caregivers to any possible deterioration in a person's physical and psychological health. The technology was built by analysing 68,000 care records—the digital paperwork for people receiving care. These were the reports created by carers that summarise each visit with a patient. Medical professionals reviewed the records to highlight key information and the annotated data was then run through machine learning models. The end result is a trained algorithm able to make accurate predictions and apply a score to indicate levels of concern [22]. It improves the quality of care on a few levels. Firstly, thanks to the analysis by medical professionals, the system can spot things that the carers wouldn't due to their limited medical knowledge. Secondly, thanks to AI, the system could even spot things that medical professionals wouldn't. The ability of technology to identify subtle patterns in data that would probably pass under the radar of humans enables Cera carers to identify undetected risks and the worsening of existing conditions. As with any predictive maintenance system, this information can then be used to intervene and implement strategies to help those in care much sooner. A great example of a hybrid approach to data analytics.

Using the technology developed at Cera, the operational staff now have the information they need to manage the health of clients in a way that was not previously possible—through actually predicting and hopefully preventing issues before they occur [15]. This not only increases the quality of care provided but also increases carers' job satisfaction as they can now feel more confident and supported. The overall aim is to create preventative care—avoiding health issues before they happen. Which is an aspiration that we should always try to prioritise for every aspect of healthcare. Cera can measure the success of preventative actions by looking at numbers of hospital admissions and patient deterioration. Cera hopes that this will reduce pressures on Acute and Emergency (A&E) units and NHS hospitals, which would otherwise cause significant strain on an older or vulnerable person, as well as drawing unnecessarily on strapped NHS budgets [15]. So far Cera has already achieved an accuracy of 82% and has identified 715 cases of increased concern. They are constantly working to improve the accuracy even further. It's a perfect example of how the collaboration of expertise between medical professionals and data scientists lead to the creation of a technology that is safe, effective and beneficial for patients and the system. It's also an example of how technology can enhance and help humans with providing the best quality of hybrid healthcare.

Devices

As discussed above, digital devices can monitor patients' health thus help us with providing continuous care. As the availability of such devices is increasing, health monitoring could be possible from wherever we are, including at home. Cera is utilizing devices such as lidar laser sensors to help with continuous monitoring of movement of the older patients they care for importantly, such devices allow the team to provide care even when a carer isn't there, with 24/7 monitoring and support. Cera is also currently working with IBM to pilot the use of these sensors in the homes of the elderly, with the aim of using the device to alert caregivers to possible deteriorations in a person's physical health, such as changes in gait, or emergency situations such as a fall [15].

Recruitment of Carers

Thoughtful recruitment of caregivers is at the core of the company's vision. Cera emphasizes that carers are absolutely crucial and that they need to be aware of the importance of their role and rewarded accordingly. The introduction of new technology in the care sector will be adopted only when carers understand the benefits of it and their feedback is included in the solution development process. Thus, Cera provides training sessions for all the carers that teach manual, care and medical but also technological skills. Moreover, the Cera operational staff often shadow carers during their work and observe how they interact with patients and technology, which allows the team to understand what is helpful or what is not working. With fears about AI replacing healthcare professionals, it's important to acknowledge possible concerns both current and potential care workers may have. As any hybrid healthcare pioneer will attest, there is a need to allay their concerns about how tech may impact the work they do and empower them to work with tech—showing how tech can actually improve their working lives. After all, technology can be a powerful tool to empower both carers and those they care for, one that can ultimately attract more people to the profession. Helping people understand that care can in fact be an innovative, forward-looking sector (contrary to some misconceptions) could help destigmatize it as a profession and attract both human capital and investment [15].

In 2019, the UK Minister of Care, Caroline Dinenage, backed a campaign by Home Instead Senior Care inspiring more people to work in care. The campaign is centred on the hashtag #YouCanCare to drive conversations on social media about the benefits of working in care and dispelling myths [15]. Social media is an untapped opportunity when it comes to recruiting carers and can be a really engaging method of communication, which is why care providers should consider running campaigns via the likes of Snapchat and Instagram Stories. Cera is already planning to implement this innovative recruitment model, whereby prospective employees can quiz real-life carers on all aspects of the job and apply directly from the app, streamlining the process and making it feel more personal [14].

Conclusions: The Collaboration of Humans and Technology

Let's go back to our patient, Mary, age 75, living alone in a rural town in England. As her health was deteriorating, her family decided to install sensors in the house to pick up any deterioration or potential issues to her mobility. She's also got used to wearing a wearable device that monitors her blood pressure and sugar levels. It also has an alarm that can immediately call help. Mary's GP has access to the data from the wearable and knows exactly when to alter her therapy, if needed arrange a phone or video call. Her family installed a smart home device in the kitchen that uses a friendly voice to remind Mary to take her medications. Her carer only needs to come in two times a day for short visits to help her with showering and healthy food preparation, which saves a lot of money for the relatives. They can see constant reports from carer's visits and suggest topics of discussion for them. Over time, sensors in Mary's house picked up that she takes more time to get up and her blood pressure seems to be lower than usual. Care management teams get an alert that it may be worth checking on her to prevent any falls. The field care coordinator visits her and performs a fall assessment. After consulting with the GP and therpaists, they conclude that she may need some home adjustements and some exercises which are then added to the care plan. Mary is now going for more walks with her carer and 1 day she manages to walk all the way to her old friend's house. Mary's mood and confidence improve.

This story doesn't have to be a futuristic story at all. Anticipated, hybrid health is closer than ever and technology is already revolutionising home care. There are several challenges before a widespread implementation such as ensuring that technologies are safe, and effective and promoting equality and access to care. We will have to all remember that there's a delicate balance between tech that empowers elderly people and those who care for them and the tech that distances vital carers from the profession [15]. We may also need a mindset shift as a society and a higher appreciation of the importance of caring as a profession [15]. It's vital to ensure that all stakeholders involved in the creation of the future of home care remember that the single most important relationship we want to nourish is the interaction between a caregiver and the patient. As we are developing new technologies.

References

1. PwC. Demographic change. [online]. 2020. https://www.pwc.com/gx/en/industries/financial-services/projectblue/demographic-change.html. Accessed 7 Feb 2020.
2. Ons.gov.uk. Population estimates - Office for National Statistics. [online]. 2021. https://www.ons.gov.uk/peoplepopulationandcommunity/populationandmigration/populationestimates. Accessed 6 Nov 2021.
3. Hayter C. Overview of the UK population – Office for National Statistics. [online]. 2020. Ons.gov.uk. https://www.ons.gov.uk/peoplepopulationandcommunity/populationandmigration/populationestimates/articles/overviewoftheukpopulation/july2017. Accessed 7 Feb 2020.
4. Prb.org. Fact sheet: aging in the United States – Population Reference Bureau. [online]. 2019. https://www.prb.org/aging-unitedstates-fact-sheet/. Accessed 7 Feb 2020.
5. Landers S, Madigan E, Leff B, Rosati R, McCann B, Hornbake R, MacMillan R, Jones K, Bowles K, Dowding D, Lee T, Moorhead T, Rodriguez S, Breese E. The future of home health care. Home Health Care Management & Practice. 2016;28(4):262–78.
6. NICE. Social care guideline scope. [online] NICE. 2014. https://www.nice.org.uk/guidance/ng22/documents/social-care-of-older-people-with-multiple-longterm-conditions-final-scope3. Accessed 7 Feb 2020.
7. BBC News. 10 charts that show why the NHS is in trouble. [online]. 2018. https://www.bbc.co.uk/news/health-42572110. Accessed 7 Feb 2020.
8. BBC News. 11 charts on the problems facing the NHS. [online]. 2021. https://www.bbc.co.uk/news/health-50290033. Accessed 6 Nov 2021.
9. Ganesh M. Home healthcare all set to transform lives in future. [online] Entrepreneur. 2019. https://www.entrepreneur.com/article/344116. Accessed 11 Feb 2020.
10. Bynum J, Meara E, Chang C, Rhoads J. A Report of the Dartmouth Atlas Project. Our Parents, Ourselves: Health Care for an Aging Population [Internet]. Dartmouthatlas.org. 2016 [cited 11 May 2020]. Available from: http://www.dartmouthatlas.org/downloads/reports/Our_Parents_Ourselves_021716_embargoed.pdf
11. Bloomberg.com. Home healthcare market size worth $545.1 billion by 2028: grand view research, Inc. [online]. 2021. https://www.bloomberg.com/press-releases/2021-09-28/home-healthcare-market-size-worth-545-1-billion-by-2028-grand-view-research-inc. Accessed 6 Nov 2021.
12. Home Healthcare Market Size, Share & Trends. Grand View Research. 2021 [online]. https://www.grandviewresearch.com/industry-analysis/home-healthcare-industry. Accessed 6 Nov 2021.
13. Market H. Home healthcare market worth $353.5 billion by 2022. [online]. 2020. Marketsandmarkets.com. https://www.marketsandmarkets.com/PressReleases/home-health-care.asp. Accessed 7 Feb 2020.
14. Forbes.com. How can we revolutionise social care in 2019? [online]. 2018. https://www.forbes.com/sites/benmaruthappu/2018/12/20/how-can-we-revolutionise-social-care-in-2019/#2b242ada4a22. Accessed 11 Feb 2020.
15. Maruthappu D. Why the UK's National Health Service is moving towards 'digital-first' | GovInsider. [online] GovInsider. 2019. https://govinsider.asia/health/digital-first-healthcare-uk-nhs-dr-ben-maruthappu-nhs-innovation-accelerator/. Accessed 7 Feb 2020.
16. Cqc.org.uk. How technology can support high-quality care | Care Quality Commission. [online]. 2020. https://www.cqc.org.uk/guidance-providers/all-services/how-technology-can-support-high-quality-care. Accessed 11 Feb 2020.
17. Tariq A. 4 hot tech trends in senior care. [online] Entrepreneur. 2020. https://www.entrepreneur.com/article/343986. Accessed 11 Feb 2020.
18. Demiris G, Kaushal R, Nilsen W. The future of home health care: workshop summary. National Academic Press. [online]. 2015. https://www.ncbi.nlm.nih.gov/books/NBK315926/. Accessed 11 Feb 2020.

19. Agetech could transform the care industry [Internet]. Ft.com. 2019 [cited 11 May 2020]. Available from: https://www.ft.com/content/ba4d0376-a7be-11e9-90e9-fc4b9d9528b4
20. Beattie J. Britain faces a social care catastrophe with 400,000 workers set to quit. [online] mirror. 2018. https://www.mirror.co.uk/news/politics/britain-faces-social-care-catastrophe-13643490. Accessed 11 Feb 2020.
21. Carecare.co.uk. Care & Care Limited. [online]. 2020. http://www.carecare.co.uk/. Accessed 11 Feb 2020.
22. Finch S, Prevett R, Cox L, Prevett R, Finch S, Finch S, Finch S, Cox L. Transforming social care: digitization and data – DisruptionHub. [online] DisruptionHub. 2019. https://disruptionhub.com/Digitization-data-devices-transforming-social-care/. Accessed 11 Feb 2020.

Chapter 8
Maternal Hybrid Healthcare

Yasmin AbuAyed and Katie Wainwright

Abstract Pregnancy, childbirth, and raising a child are in the main a normal event, encompassing the physical, emotional, mental, social, and cultural elements of the mother and family (International Confederation of Midwives [Internet], 2017). Women receive normal routine care if it is available to them. Care if it is available is often fragmented and increasingly obstetrically led. Care provision is centred around the organisation delivering the care rather than the women and babies accessing the care. All of this adds to the increasingly institutionalised medicalisation of pregnancy and birth and lack of appropriate training and exposure to normal birth leading to deskilling the birth professionals.

The World Health Organization (WHO) states that skilled care before, during, and after childbirth can save lives—both of women and their babies (World Health Organisation [Internet], 2019). Recent research also concludes that investing in midwifery could prevent 66% or two thirds of maternal deaths, stillbirths and neonatal deaths (Nove et al., Lancet Glob Health 9:e24–e32, 2021).

There is a shortage of 900,000 midwives across the world (International Confederation of Midwives; World Health Organisation & United Nations Population Fund [Internet], 2021). The use of technology and the move to hybrid healthcare would ease this pressure and allow the knowledge, expertise and skill of midwives to be shared globally. This would assist women who may not be able to access even the most basic routine care to access the knowledge and expertise to support and guide them through their pregnancy and parenthood. It would also help to streamline and improve efficiency for women who are able to access care.

Keywords Midwife · Digital · Birth · Pregnancy · Antenatal · Continuity Technology · Medical · Telehealth

Y. AbuAyed (✉) · K. Wainwright
Rise Birth Center, Dubai, UAE

Epical Global Ltd, Shrewsbury, UK
e-mail: Yasmin@RiseBirthCenter.com; katie.wainwright@epicalglobal.co.uk

© The Author(s), under exclusive license to Springer Nature Switzerland AG 2022
M. Al-Razouki, S. Smith (eds.), *Hybrid Healthcare*, Health Informatics, https://doi.org/10.1007/978-3-031-04836-4_8

87

Overview of the Current Maternal Care Landscape

Approximately 4.4 babies are born every *second* [1, 2]. Maternal care is a very significant portion of healthcare and safety practices tend to vary widely around the world. Care may be provided by midwives, obstetricians, or general practitioner doctors in a village clinic, birth center, home setting, or hospital. This chapter will focus on the current landscape of maternal care, the impact of care, and a few suggested best practices for the future of maternal care in the context of hybrid healthcare.

There is room for improvement globally in maternal care. Some countries suffer from staff shortages, some have high infant death rates, some have racial disparities, some have incredibly high intervention rates, and some countries' health systems are restricted by limited access to both care and treatment options.

Maternal care has significantly improved over the last 200 years; as technology and new practices emerged, there was an increase in their use. While the advancements were certainly life-saving, there is currently a tendency to overuse some of these practices. A few of these non-evidence based practices are mentioned below.

Non-Evidence Based Maternal Care Practices

Induction

Induction involves starting labour artificially. There are instances where this may provide more benefits to mother or baby than risks. Medical indications for induction may include: HELLP syndrome [3]; intrauterine fetal death coupled with an infection, bleeding, or broken water [4]; and blood group isoimmunization (Rh incompatibility) with maternal titre ratio 1:40 or higher [5].

Induction without medical indication is not supported due to the increased risk of complications. The following clinical indications are commonly offered an induction however there is not sufficient evidence to support use of induction in these cases:

- Gestational diabetes [6, 7]
- Twin gestation [6]
- Fetal macrosomia (big baby) [6, 8]
- Oligohydramnios (low amount of amniotic fluid) [6]
- Cholestasis of pregnancy [6]
- Maternal cardiac disease [6]
- Fetal gastroschisis [6]
- Decreased fetal movements [9]
- Fetal growth restriction [4]
- Small for gestational age (SGA) [10]
- Suspected interuterine growth restriction (IUGR) [11]

- Preterm prelabour rupture of membranes (water breaks before 37 weeks gestation) [12]
- Post 40 weeks gestation [13]
- Intrauterine fetal death without infection [4]

There are complications with any method of induction. Depending on the type of induction, the complications include:

- Increased risk of caesarean birth [14–17]
- Increased risk for chorioamnionitis [18]
- Higher odds of developing autism in boys who were exposed to oxytocin for longer periods of time during labour and received higher total doses of oxytocin [19]
- Uterine fatigue [20]
- Increase likelihood of postpartum haemorrhage [14, 21]
- Increased use of epidural [14]
- Increased risk of instrumental birth [14]
- Increased risk of episiotomy [14]
- Decreased chance of spontaneous vaginal birth [14]
- Increased chance of instrumental birth [14]
- Risk of uterine rupture [22, 23]
- Uterine hyperstimulation [4]
- Increase risk of infection [4]
- Nausea [4]
- Vomiting [4]
- Diarrhoea [4]
- Fever [4]
- Hypotension (lowered blood pressure) [4]
- Abnormality of heart rate in baby [4]
- Change in mother's heart rate [4]
- Cord prolapse [24, 25]
- Potential long-term change to uterine receptors for future labors [4]
- Increase in pain [4]
- Increase in speed of contractions [4]
- Bleeding [4]
- Reduction in freedom of movement for the mother
- Vaginal tenderness [4]

Another consideration is the overdosage and misuse of IV administered uterine stimulators. A study out of Pakistan showed the largest contributing factor to mother's being admitted to the ICU was "misuse of oxytocin" (31% of patients), the next highest reason was 15% of patients [26]. This is particularly concerning when the fatalities of the patients in ICU was 27% [26]. Developed countries also misuse induction drugs. An example of this is in the UK with synthetic oxytocin; the licensed instructions set limits of how much to initially administer, the rate of increase, and a maximum dose. In contrast, the Royal College of Obstetricians and

Gynaecologists advises a higher starting dose, a quicker increase, and an over 50% higher maximum dose meaning if the RCOG regime is followed, the administration is an unlicensed use of the drug. Table 8.1 details the aforementioned contrast. Going outside of the licensed dosages legally requires consent from the patient and there is public concern over whether this conversation is happening and consent is being granted by the birthing mother [27].

No Support for Vaginal Birth after Cesarean (VBAC)

Evidence supports vaginal birth after cesarean [30] however it can be extremely difficult to find providers who will attend to VBAC births. In America for example, American College of Obstetricians and Gynecologists recommends facilities that support VBACs to have the ability to perform an emergency cesarean birth; many smaller hospitals in rural towns do not have this capability and as a result do not offer support for VBAC mothers.

The main concern about attempting a VBAC is the increased likelihood of a uterine rupture. The irony is that induction of labor actually has a higher chance of uterine rupture than VBAC. A study looking at instances of uterine rupture for mothers with a prior cesarean birth concluded the incidence of rupture was 0.5% [31]. Depending on the type of medication used for induction, the instance of uterine rupture for induced birth is 1.1%–6% [22].

There may also be trauma from the first birth that needs to be emotionally worked through and finding providers and systems that facilitate this healing, whether it be through recognition, assessment, or accessibility, is hard. Mental health workers are not always covered by insurance and maternal care providers may not assess or recognize the need for further trauma work to help the preparation for a vaginal birth after cesarean.

Risks continue to increase for the birth giver every subsequent cesarean received. Table 8.2 shows the risk of 'major complications' [32]:

Table 8.1 Manufacturer's dosage recommendations vs. RCOG regime for induction

	Drug licensed limits [28]	RCOG regime [29]
Maximum initial dose limit	4 mU/min	1 mU/min
Maximum rate of increase	2 mU/min every 20 min	4 mU/min every 30 min
Maximum dose limit	20 mU/min	32 mU/min

Table 8.2 Risk of maternal major complications with every cesarean birth

2nd Cesarean	3rd Cesarean	4th Cesarean
4.3%, 1 in 23	7.5%, 1 in 13	12.5%, 1 in 8

No Support for Vaginal Birth of Breech Presentation

The risk of neonatal morbidity for a breech vaginal birth is .9/1000 [33]. The risk of neonatal morbidity for a cesarean breech birth is .8/1000 [33]. The absolute risk for some birth givers would be considered quite low and a worthwhile trade-off to having a cesarean birth. However, it can be quite challenging to find providers willing to attend a vaginal breech birth. The ones who do may also be scrutinized by their own community of fellow maternal care providers. The art of attending breech births is not always part of the education a midwife or obstetrician would receive, further impacting the ability to find suitable and confident providers for breech vaginal birth.

Electronic Fetal Monitoring

Electronic Fetal Monitoring was introduced and marketed as a way to reduce cerebral palsy. In reality, it has led to more birth interventions and cesarean births [34]. In contrast to the original purpose, emergency cesarean birth has been found to increase the risk of cerebral palsy [35]. Electronic Fetal Monitoring persists as a way to have 'proof' and justification for birth related injuries and litigation [36]. The monitoring is subject to interpretation and not particularly accurate. A study reviewing 155,636 children found a false positive rate of 99.8% for multiple late decelerations or decreased variability in fetal heart rate; only .19% of the babies with these decelerations showing from the monitoring actually had cerebral palsy [37].

As shown above, many routine practices are not following evidence-based care. Examples of the same overuse of interventions can be found globally. The countries who have lower rates of intervention and better outcomes for mothers and babies share the following: midwifery-led care, and choices of birthing location including hospitals, birth centers, and home. Table 8.3 indicates the top countries in four different categories.

More digital platforms are arising which help families understand the benefits and risks of interventions during labor and birth. Having access to the evidence is getting easier and more comprehensive as the years go by which will help to decrease some of the non-evidence based practices.

Cost of Maternal Care

Maternal care can be costly especially in countries that do not offer government funding for health care, for example the average out of pocket costs for families accessing maternity care in the USA with insurance is $4500 [42]. This is in addition to any insurance payments and care covered by that insurance.

Table 8.3 Best rated countries and their maternal care practices

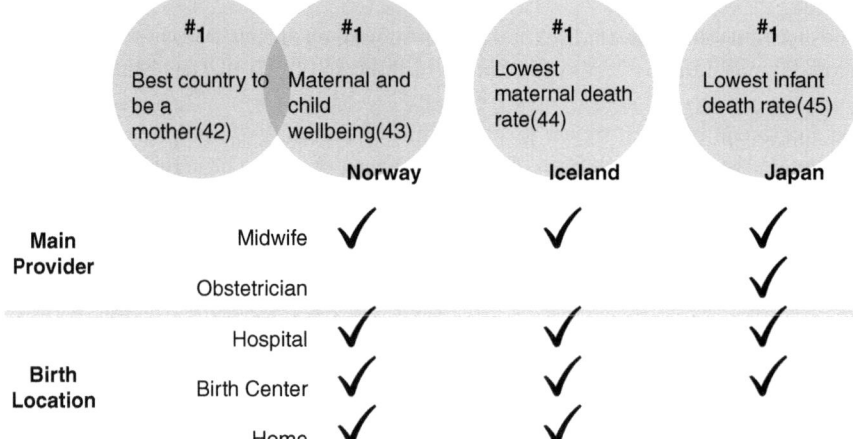

		Norway	Iceland	Japan
Main Provider	Midwife	✓	✓	✓
	Obstetrician			✓
Birth Location	Hospital	✓	✓	✓
	Birth Center	✓	✓	✓
	Home	✓	✓	

In contrast, even in countries where the cost is low, people often choose to pay for additional care to meet their individual needs. In the UK for example, maternity care is provided free at the point of delivery via the National Health Service (NHS). However, there are a proportion of women that will pay for additional care via independent midwives to ensure they receive the support and advocacy they feel may be lacking elsewhere. This may be due to requesting birth support outside of the NHS prescribed guidelines, or the desire for continuity throughout their pregnancy and birth journey that is not provided by their lead care provider.

This is in direct contrast with those countries and populations where no care is received at all.

Delivery of Maternal Care

There is a divide between how midwives are educated and how obstetricians are educated; the two practices are very different and quite complimentary. Table 8.4 is a summary of main differences between the midwifery and obstetrical models of care.

The World Health Organisation (WHO) reports that the poorest women have the least access to routine antenatal care. This can be detrimental for many reasons. An example is the absence of physical health monitoring for mother and baby; this lack of support can impact maternal mental health due to potential periods of worry and stress [43].

The WHO also recommends that all women should have access to maternity care within their first trimester of pregnancy. Whilst this is being achieved by over half

Table 8.4 Differences and impact between midwifery and obstetrical models of care

Midwifery model	Obstetrical model	Impact
Trained in physiological birth	Trained for complications and emergencies	Obstetricians are less equipped to support straight-forward natural birth
Body is trustworthy unless proven otherwise Reactive	Birth is dangerous until proven safe Preventative	Reactive care avoids unnecessary interventions
Woman-centered focus, philosophy of supporting the woman's informed choices	Hospital policy focus, concern over "allowing" for woman requests	A birthing person is more empowered to be a decision-maker with woman-centered care
Continuity of care providers	New staff attends during labor and birth	Unfamiliar people may hinder the birth process
Attend home birth and birth center births	Typically attend hospital births	Community settings foster a feeling of safety which physiologically assists the process

of the world's population, there is a massive gap where women receive little to no care at all. We know that the areas with the lowest rates of early antenatal care (before 12 weeks as defined by WHO) have the highest rates of maternal morbidity and mortality [43].

Access to care alone is not a total solution, the quality of care is important and the level at which the woman and her family are in control of their own decisions and care provision, including the information they have access to.

The gold standard of midwifery care is provided through continuity of carer models. Continuity of carer refers to the provision of care consistently by one named midwife, or a small team of midwives during pregnancy, labor and throughout the postnatal period. The midwife adopts the role of care navigator and ensures the right care is provided, at the right time, and by the right person [44].

There is a plethora of evidence to support continuity of carer models and the increase in improvements in clinical outcomes. Women who receive continuity of carer from a midwife consistently report a significant improvement of their care experience [45], and the following examples of clinical outcomes can be evidenced for midwifery led continuity of carer provision:

- Women are 16% less likely to lose their baby [45]
- Women are 19% less likely to lose their baby prior to 24 weeks gestation [45]
- Women are 24% less likely to experience preterm birth [45]

Not only are clinical outcomes improved, but there are also increased cost savings made across the service provision due to a reduced number of interventions, reduced number of epidurals, reduced number of instrumental births, reduced number of neonatal care cots required, and less ongoing costs due to poor outcomes at birth [46].

Impact of Maternal Care

Birth is the first encounter to see your child, the experience can greatly alter the early parenting days. There surely is a difference between parents who had an empowering and encouraging birth experience and those who struggled, felt bewildered and were not participating in the decision making. A positive experience can contribute to more confidence in parenting. When a birth experience is traumatic, that puts an additional strain on the parenting role. A difficult birth experience can contribute to postpartum depression and/or post traumatic stress disorder.

Benefits of Physiological Birth

Mothers who have a physiological birth enjoy a full range of hormones that provide a natural high and pain relief. Oxytocin, the love hormone, is abundant and creates the special bond between parent and child in the first hours of life. Mobility is greater when laboring and birthing without medication. Recovery is also quicker. Breastfeeding is generally established within the first hour of birth which is highly beneficial for the long term breastfeeding relationship.

Medication taken during labor is passed to the baby. Babies born to mothers who had a medication free birth tend to be more alert and have high initial health assessment scores. Babies act out a number of reflexes while being born vaginally. If they miss these vestibular stimulations, the balance and spatial orientation sequencing does not properly begin. If the reflexes are not expressed, the effect could be a life-long lack of coordination [47]. The microbiome in a vaginally born infant is also different from an infant born via cesarean section. The birth microbiome sets up the immunity for life. Asthma and allergies are more common among cesarean babies because of this microbiome difference [48]. There are also increased risks of childhood diabetes and autism with cesarean births [19, 49, 50]. A 2020 study showed an increase in autism for infant boys who were exposed to synthetic oxytocin for prolonged periods with high cumulative dosages [19].

If women are fully aware of these impacts, they may make different decisions for themselves. In the end, the birthing person should know what is happening to their body and the process for their baby during birth and have their informed decisions be supported by care providers.

Future of Maternal Care

One of the most effective ways to improve maternal care globally is to support midwifery-led care. Depending on the current practices in each area, this could mean (a) to increase the role of midwife in countries that are not yet recognizing their education and abilities, (b) introducing midwifery-led care models and structuring licensing models accordingly, (c) supporting existing midwifery-led models to reduce midwife burnout, and (d) increasing and promoting midwifery educational programs globally.

Part of supporting midwives is providing appropriate working locations and conditions. A midwife that is trained and capable of handling all care from prenatal through birth to postnatal should be given the autonomy to do so. Great options for providing this are home-birth models, birth center facilities, and multi-disciplinary hospital teams where the straightforward pregnancies first see a midwife and if required or desired, obtain obstetrical care. Ideally options would be available for midwives so they can choose a working location and model that suits them. Midwives could work in caseloading models or rotational team models; flexibility in governmental structuring would allow for preferred models to be available for all.

An overarching desire would be to see continuity of carer across all maternity provision—whether in person or through digital means. As noted above, the impact of continuity alone can have far reaching positive implications for women and their families throughout pregnancy and childbirth and growing strong families.

All women should have a choice of birthing location, not everyone is well suited for a community birth, nor are all comfortable with a hospital birth. Better outcomes will be achieved when mothers are informed of their options, informed of what birth looks like in reality, and in turn empowered to make their own decisions. This is how birth trauma is reduced and higher satisfaction with the birth experience is gained.

All care providers for maternal care should also have appropriate working conditions. Things to be considered for any unit should be the patient/provider ratio, fostering work/life balance, and accounting for shift work by providing adequate time to catch up on sleep/recover. Adopting appropriately sized caseloads to be able to provide safe, effective midwifery-led continuity of care will have a direct impact on outcomes and satisfaction rates for both mother and midwife.

Another way of assisting care provision is the use of hybrid health systems, namely telehealth. Incorporating telehealth appointments into routine care can make care more efficient and free up clinicians for face to face care when it is really needed. In the last 12 months, Microsoft has launched a new health-centric cloud. This combines some of Microsoft's existing platforms such as MS Teams to enhance medical telehealth, inter-clinician collaborations and transcription of patient consultations into organised medical notes using speech recognition [51]. These intelligent platforms will enhance patient care and also clinician to clinician collaboration and multi agency working.

Digital Influences on Maternal Care

Covid 19 has accelerated the use of digital platforms and consumer demand for more remote and virtual services across healthcare, including maternity care. This surge resulted in the use of telehealth being 78 times higher in April 2020 than it was in February of the same year [52].

The global telehealth market is now expected to reach $460 billion by 2030, with the largest telehealth market within the USA and remote patient monitoring being the most frequently used mode of telemedicine in the USA [53].

The World Health Organization (WHO) recognises the value of digital interventions to health care services, including recommending telehealth as a complimentary addition to in-person health care and other benefits including [54]:

- Digital records management
- Client to provider telehealth
- Provider to provider telehealth
- Education for clients
- Decision making toolkits for providers and clinicians

Opportunities for Digital Healthcare in Maternal Care

Current Use of Technology in Maternity care

Maternity care across the globe has been static at best, and detrimental at worst. In order to move maternity care into the twenty-first Century, the use of virtual care that is midwife-led, and preferably inclusive of continuity is an imperative first step.

The rapid advances in technology and telehealth leave us in no doubt that the combination of knowledge and technology can combine perfectly with the potential to make a lasting impact for pregnant women and their families.

To be able to ensure that all women, from anywhere in the world, can access safe and effective midwifery knowledge on demand, the use of innovative technologies can create sustainable behaviour change and long-term impact on the physical and mental health of families.

This is already happening within the healthcare field with a 17% increase in telehealth within the healthcare sectors overall, including a massive 50% increase within the psychiatric sector. However, despite a 7% increase in telehealth use in the gynaecology speciality (non pregnancy related), maternity care does **not** feature in the statistics at all [56]. Although some use of digitalization is present within maternity services, these statistics confirm the overall static nature of maternity care and indicate this sector has some way to go in order to embrace the value and initiation of telehealth and digital resources within maternal care provision.

An interesting hybrid healthcare approach would be to provide maternal health services using similar hybrid health models as mental health (see Chap. 10 for more on hybrid neuroscience and mental health). Increasingly, people are accessing online therapy. This is an opportunity to access specialized care for unique situations such as VBAC preparation, working through traumatic births, or general anxiety over pregnancy and birth.

There will always be a need for the touch and physical presence of a midwife, for that there is no question. What is likely though, is the potential that technology has to enhance and complement the care that is received in person, through hybrid systems. This can include telehealth appointments—with or without remote monitoring devices to measure physical health and wellbeing. This can also include the enhancement of clinician-to-clinician liaison, digital records and data flow and systems [54]. Education and preparation for birth and parenting is imperative to clinical outcomes and patient satisfaction. Digital resources and support forums for pregnant women can foster a sense of community and allow them control over their learning journey, and a support system for their families long after their pregnancy has ended.

We already know the power of information, coupled with continuity of carer within the field of maternity care. To align and merge the strength of continuity of carer with the power of technology should be our aspiration for not only the future, but for today. The technologies are there already, and our fellow healthcare sectors are flying ahead with integration. Amazon is already working on telehealth solutions and is planning to revolutionise healthcare with AI driven chatbot health care services [51]. Through a continuity model of care, the move to incorporating digitalization into maternity care is supported and would reduce the risk of fragmenting care. If the woman and the midwife know each other and have a relationship, the injection of digital elements of care can be done with confidence and maintain the level of continuity for seamless care provision, whether in person or not.

Virtual reality (VR) is increasingly being used in medicine [55]. For example, it has been studied for the potential reduction of pain in labour and childbirth with positive results [56] and also specifically for reduction in pain and anxiety of women experiencing episiotomy during their first pregnancies [57]. The use of VR has been shown in these studies to reduce anxiety scores during and after perineal repair in the intervention with VR groups [57], and is an effective non-medical method to reduce pain during episiotomy [58]. The studies conclude that simulation via VR is another way that technology can be used to prepare pregnant women and is generally accepted as a useful method. Further research is required but the potential is high for a variety of uses including reduction in anxiety and pain [56, 59].

Other uses of technology to improve services could include VR training for those care providers to gain confidence and competence with scenarios such as VBAC or vaginal breech births and to fully support women with all their choices and options for care.

Hybrid healthcare using technology is more than just telehealth. Access to information and support networks digitally can ensure women and their families get the support and information they need to make informed choices and become confident parents.

Some advances have been made within the maternity field. For example, Ethiopia has one of the highest maternal and child mortality rates in the world, contributed to by lack of access to education and nutrition information. Field studies have shown great promise for the developing world with a serious game 'easycare' which has been designed to provide education on wellbeing and nutrition and has been designed for both illiterate users and those with little to no experience of digital resources [60].

There is an appetite for health care to be received digitally [56], and so now is the time to seize the opportunity for change, capitalize on this and move maternity care forward globally.

Our Childbearing Generations

The world we live in is perfectly poised to become completely digitized. With many areas of change there is normally a degree of resistance, but there has never been a better time to embrace digital advances in maternal care with our childbearing generations as they are already our digital warriors.

Generation Y (millennials) who make up 1.8 billion or 23% of the population worldwide [56], are tech savvy and keen to make a positive impact on the world they inhabit. 93% of this generation own a smartphone [61], and 59% use the internet as their main source of accessing information.

Generation Z are referred to as digital natives and spend an average of 15.5 h a week on their smartphones. They are constantly learning and over 60% of this generation say that technology makes them feel that anything is possible. This is a tech savvy generation because [62]:

- 95% own a smartphone
- 82% own a laptop
- 78% own a gaming console
- 29% use their smartphone after midnight every night
- 69% use the internet as their primary source of accessing information

These generations, due to their ages, are likely to be using maternity care across the world. Therefore, as it is clear technology plays an integral part of their lives already, hybrid healthcare would be a natural progression for these generations. Apple owns almost 50% of the market share of smart watches, and with plans ahead for their health app to link directly to patient medical records, the potential to change the delivery of maternity care forever is right here, right now [51].

Barriers to Digital Healthcare in Maternity

Due to the rise in the use of telehealth borne out of necessity during the COVID 19 pandemic, there has been an increased acceptance and confidence with people using such methods to access elements of healthcare [56]. This should go some way to overcome the barriers associated with change and ease the transition to a hybrid model of healthcare. This is further supported as 40% of people have indicated that they would want to continue with telehealth in their lives moving forward past the pandemic, and 57% of physicians who offered telehealth have indicated that they wish to continue to do so [56].

The culture within maternity care needs to be addressed in order to fully embrace this hybrid system of care. Change management has always been difficult and can take a long time to embed new ways of working and ensure systemic change within an organization or health care service. Due to the blended nature of in-person and digital care required for the provision of maternity care, there may be a tendency to retain more and more 'essential' in person care, thus stalling the move forward to engaging the benefits of digital platforms and resources. For example, not moving antenatal appointments to virtual appointments and embracing the support of technology to do so with remote monitoring due to a reticence to 'let it go' from in-person care. This could be due to a resistance to change and a fear of losing in-person care. It should be remembered that in-person care will always be required in maternity care provision, and therefore the addition of technology to complement the service provision should be seen as an asset and not a threat.

In addition, hospital and maternity care providers will encounter the challenge of data flow and integration across existing systems—both internally for example in the case of electronic health records and externally with other providers where care may be shared.

Visions for Digital Healthcare in Maternity

Technology and digital platforms have the capacity to be able to change and transform the way that global health services are delivered and accessed [63]. It is inevitable and required that this digitalization of maternity care continues to grow and develop to enable maternal care to be provided within a hybrid system.

The vision for a hybrid healthcare system for maternity care would range from the most basic services for those communities in digital poverty, to fully integrated digitalization of care for those with access to more sophisticated and advanced technologies.

Examples of this vision include:

- Basic text messaging service to sophisticated AI enabled live chat to facilitate women being able to connect to a midwife for support and information/advice.
- Fetal monitoring remotely, coupled with monitoring of maternal health in the form of blood pressure and urinalysis, combined with virtual appointments and virtual education.
- Artificial Intelligence (AI) employed to support machine learning that can monitor remote working and other digital interventions and diverts them suitably for in person support when appropriate.
- Enhanced education for women and clinical training for midwives using gamification, VR and other immersive learning methods.

All these elements of the vision are based upon technologies already in use in other sectors of healthcare, or those that are in development.

Artificial Intelligence (AI), for example, is already fairly mainstream, with smart watches and voice activated digital assistants. AI within healthcare can help to organise patient routing and pathways, whilst supporting clinicians decision making [64].

AI is already in use within health consultations, such as those provided by Babylon Health—the user adds their symptoms to the AI powered APP and an appropriate course of action is recommended for the APP user—powered by AI. There are other APPS available with AI powered virtual assistants/doctors/nurses who help people manage chronic health conditions [64]. This could easily be adapted to pregnancy specific conditions and powered by AI Midwives. AI has already been shown to help radiologists accuracy in detecting cancer [64], so the potential to assist midwives and obstetricians to detect pregnancy abnormalities or fetal anomalies with the use of AI to increase accuracy and efficiency is phenomenal. The possibilities using AI and other intelligent technologies within maternity care services across the globe are exponential.

There is a global shortage of midwives, and care providers, so therefore hybrid maternity care is not a nice-to-have, but in fact an essential way forward for women across the globe to have access to care and information/education in a meaningful way, resulting in a real impact for women, babies and families.

References

1. The World Counts [Internet]. Theworldcounts.com. 2021 [cited 12 August 2021]. https://www.theworldcounts.com/stories/how-many-babies-are-born-each-day.
2. Birth rate, crude (per 1,000 people) | Data [Internet]. Data.worldbank.org. 2021 [cited 12 August 2021]. https://data.worldbank.org/indicator/SP.DYN.CBRT.IN?end=2019&start=2019.
3. Haram K, Svendsen E, Abildgaard U. The HELLP syndrome: clinical issues and management. A review. BMC Pregnancy Childbirth. 2009;9(1):8.
4. Wickham S. Inducing labour: making informed decisions. 2nd ed. Birthmoon Creations; 2018.
5. Goluboff N, Mckenzie JW, Brown AB. Induction of labour for prevention of stillbirth from Rh hemolytic disease. Can Med Assoc J. 1963;89:1313–9. https://www.ncbi.nlm.nih.gov/pmc/articles/PMC1922301/
6. Mozurkewich E, Chilimigras J, Koepke E, Keeton K, King V. Indications for induction of labour: a best-evidence review. BJOG Int J Obstet Gynaecol. 2009;116(5):626–36.
7. Berger H, Melamed N. Timing of delivery in women with diabetes in pregnancy. Obstetric Med [Internet]. 2014;7(1):8–16. https://www.ncbi.nlm.nih.gov/pmc/articles/PMC4934937/
8. Recommendations | Inducing labour | Guidance | NICE. [cited 2021 Nov 12]. https://www.nice.org.uk/guidance/ng207/chapter/Recommendations
9. Hofmeyr G, Novikova N. Management of reported decreased fetal movements for improving pregnancy outcomes. Cochrane Database Syst Rev [Internet]. 2012 [cited 19 August 2021], 4(4) https://www.ncbi.nlm.nih.gov/pmc/articles/PMC4058897/
10. Ofir K, Lerner-Geva L, Boyko V, Zilberberg E, Schiff E, Simchen M. Induction of labor for term small-for-gestational-age fetuses: what are the consequences? Eur J Obstetrics Gynecol Reprod Biol [Internet]. 2013;171(2):257–61. https://www.ejog.org/article/S0301-2115(13)00466-1/fulltext
11. Boers K, Vijgen S, Bijlenga D, van der Post J, Bekedam D, Kwee A, et al. Induction versus expectant monitoring for intrauterine growth restriction at term: randomised equivalence trial (DIGITAT). BMJ [Internet]. 2010;341(dec21 1):c7087. https://www.bmj.com/content/341/bmj.c7087
12. Bond D, Middleton P, Levett K, van der Ham D, Crowther C, Buchanan S, et al. Planned early birth versus expectant management for women with preterm prelabour rupture of membranes prior to 37 weeks' gestation for improving pregnancy outcome. Cochrane Database Syst Rev [Internet]. 2017 [cited 15 August 2021];2017(3) https://pubmed.ncbi.nlm.nih.gov/28257562/
13. Rydahl E, Declercq E, Juhl M, Maimburg RD. Routine induction in late-term pregnancies: follow-up of a Danish induction of labour paradigm. BMJ Open. 2019;9(12):e032815. https://bmjopen.bmj.com/content/9/12/e032815
14. Dahlen HG, Thornton C, Downe S, de Jonge A, Seijmonsbergen-Schermers A, Tracy S, et al. Intrapartum interventions and outcomes for women and children following induction of labour

at term in uncomplicated pregnancies: a 16-year population-based linked data study. BMJ Open. 2021;11(6):e047040. https://bmjopen.bmj.com/content/11/6/e047040.long

15. Davey M-A, King J. Caesarean section following induction of labour in uncomplicated first births- a population-based cross-sectional analysis of 42,950 births. BMC Pregnancy Childbirth. 2016;16(1):92.

16. Zhao Y, Flatley C, Kumar S. Intrapartum intervention rates and perinatal outcomes following induction of labour compared to expectant management at term from an Australian perinatal centre. Aust N Z J Obstet Gynaecol. 2017;57(1):40–8.

17. Kjerulff KH, Attanasio LB, Edmonds JK, Kozhimannil KB, Repke JT. Labor induction and cesarean delivery: A prospective cohort study of first births in Pennsylvania, USA. Birth. 2017;44(3):252–61.

18. Erekson EA, Myles TD. Risks for chorioamnionitis with both induction and augmentation of labor. Obstet Gynecol. 2006;107(Supplement):32S–3S. https://journals.lww.com/greenjournal/Fulltext/2006/04001/Risks_for_Chorioamnionitis_With_Both_Induction_and.75.aspx

19. Soltys S, Scherbel J, Kurian J, Diebold T, Wilson T, Hedden L, et al. An association of intrapartum synthetic oxytocin dosing and the odds of developing autism. Autism. 2020;24(6):1400–10.

20. Grotegut CA, Paglia MJ, Johnson LNC, Thames B, James AH. Oxytocin exposure during labor among women with postpartum hemorrhage secondary to uterine atony. Am J Obstet Gynecol. 2011;204(1):56.e1–6. https://pubmed.ncbi.nlm.nih.gov/21047614/

21. Khireddine I, Le Ray C, Dupont C, Rudigoz R-C, Bouvier-Colle M-H, Deneux-Tharaux C. Induction of labor and risk of postpartum hemorrhage in low risk parturients. PLoS One. 2013;8(1):e54858. https://www.ncbi.nlm.nih.gov/pmc/articles/PMC3555986/

22. Dekker R. EBB 113 - the evidence on VBAC - evidence based birth® [Internet]. Evidencebasedbirth.com. 2020 [cited 2021 August 19]. https://evidencebasedbirth.com/ebb-113-the-evidence-on-vbac/.

23. Fitzpatrick KE, Kurinczuk JJ, Alfirevic Z, Spark P, Brocklehurst P, Knight M. Uterine rupture by intended mode of delivery in the UK: a national case-control study. PLoS Med. 2012;9(3):e1001184. https://journals.plos.org/plosmedicine/article/figure?id=10.1371/journal.pmed.1001184.t001

24. Yamada T, Cho K, Yamada T, Morikawa M, Minakami H. Labor induction by transcervical balloon catheter and cerebral palsy associated with umbilical cord prolapse: cerebral palsy and cord prolapse. J Obstet Gynaecol Res. 2013;39(6):1159–64. https://pubmed.ncbi.nlm.nih.gov/23551955/

25. Huang C-C, Landy H, Kawakita T. Risk factors for umbilical cord prolapse at the time of artificial rupture of membranes. AJP Rep. 2018;08(02):e89–94. https://www.ncbi.nlm.nih.gov/pmc/articles/PMC5945286/

26. Khaskheli M. Iatrogenic risks and maternal health: issues and outcomes. Pakistan J Med Sci. 1969;30(1):111–5.

27. Shepherd L. Induction with synthetic oxytocin: less is more [Internet]. AIMS. 2019 [cited 15 August 2021]. https://www.aims.org.uk/journal/item/unlicensed-oxytocin-doses.

28. Oxytocin 5 IU/ml Concentrate for Solution for Infusion - Summary of Product Characteristics (SmPC) - (emc) [Internet]. Medicines.org.uk. 2018 [cited 14 Aug 2021]. https://www.medicines.org.uk/emc/product/9457/smpc

29. Royal College of Obstetricians and Gynaecologists. Induction of labour [Internet]. London: RCOG Press, 2001. p 24. http://www.perinatal.sld.cu/docs/guiasclinicas/inductionoflabour.pdf.

30. Guise J-M, Eden K, Emeis C, Denman MA, Marshall N, Fu RR, et al. Vaginal birth after cesarean: new insights. Evid Rep Technol Assess (Full Rep). 2010;191:1–397. https://europepmc.org/article/nbk/nbk44571

31. Motomura K, Ganchimeg T, Nagata C, Ota E, Vogel JP, Betran AP, et al. Incidence and outcomes of uterine rupture among women with prior caesarean section: WHO Multicountry Survey on Maternal and Newborn Health. Sci Rep. 2017;7(1):44093. https://www.ncbi.nlm.nih.gov/pmc/articles/PMC5345021/

32. Nisenblat V, Barak S, Griness OB, Degani S, Ohel G, Gonen R. Maternal complications associated with multiple cesarean deliveries. Obstet Gynecol. 2006;108(1):21–6. https://pubmed.ncbi.nlm.nih.gov/16816051/

33. Bjellmo S, Andersen GL, Martinussen MP, Romundstad PR, Hjelle S, Moster D, et al. Is vaginal breech delivery associated with higher risk for perinatal death and cerebral palsy compared with vaginal cephalic birth? Registry-based cohort study in Norway. BMJ Open. 2017;7(4):e014979. https://www.ncbi.nlm.nih.gov/pmc/articles/PMC5566597/

34. Alfirevic Z, Devane D, Gyte GM, Cuthbert A. Continuous cardiotocography (CTG) as a form of electronic fetal monitoring (EFM) for fetal assessment during labour. Cochrane Database Syst Rev. 2017;2(5):CD006066. https://pubmed.ncbi.nlm.nih.gov/28157275/

35. O'Callaghan M, MacLennan A. Cesarean delivery and cerebral palsy: a systematic review and meta-analysis. Obstet Gynecol. 2013;122(6):1169–75. https://pubmed.ncbi.nlm.nih.gov/24201683/

36. Sartwelle TP, Johnston JC. Cerebral palsy litigation: change course or abandon ship: change course or abandon ship. J Child Neurol. 2015;30(7):828–41. https://journals.sagepub.com/doi/10.1177/0883073814543306

37. Nelson KB, Dambrosia JM, Ting TY, Grether JK. Uncertain value of electronic fetal monitoring in predicting cerebral palsy. N Engl J Med. 1996;334(10):613–8. https://pubmed.ncbi.nlm.nih.gov/8592523/

38. A deep dive into the best countries in the world to be a mother [Internet]. Com.au. [cited 2021 Nov 12]. https://www.insureandgo.com.au/travel-hub/best-countries-to-be-mother.jsp.

39. Save the Children. State of the World's Mothers Report 2015 [Internet]. https://www.savethechildren.org/content/dam/usa/reports/advocacy/sowm/sowm-2015.pdf.

40. Roser M, Ritchie H. Maternal mortality. Our world in data [Internet]. 2013 [cited 2021 Nov 12]. https://ourworldindata.org/maternal-mortality.

41. Junior VL. Countries with the lowest infant mortality rates [Internet]. Worldatlas.com. 2018 [cited 2021 Nov 12]. https://www.worldatlas.com/articles/countries-with-the-lowest-infant-mortality-rates.html.

42. Institute for Healthcare Policy & Innovation, University of Michigan [Internet]. ihpi.umich.edu. 2020 [cited 13 Nov 2021]. https://ihpi.umich.edu/news/having-baby-may-cost-some-families-4500-out-pocket-study-finds.

43. WHO | More women worldwide receive early antenatal care, but great inequalities remain. 2017. https://www.who.int/reproductivehealth/early-anc-worldwide/en/?fbclid=IwAR15T64XGJ2UAWk-f97p-fIq2ZA6iYR9Q1ds6kNRkK0VqAxpCrlI6Kxitxc.

44. National Health Services. Implementing Better Births: Continuity of Carer [Internet]. 2017 Dec. https://www.england.nhs.uk/wp-content/uploads/2017/12/implementing-better-births.pdf.

45. Sandall J, Soltani H, Gates S, Shennan A, Devane D. Midwife-led continuity models versus other models of care for childbearing women. Cochrane Database Syst Rev. 2016;4:CD004667. https://www.cochrane.org/CD004667/PREG_midwife-led-continuity-models-care-compared-other-models-care-women-during-pregnancy-birth-and-early

46. NHS England [Internet]. england.nhs.uk. 2017 [cited 13 Nov 2021]. https://www.england.nhs.uk/ltphimenu/maternity/targeted-and-enhanced-midwifery-led-continuity-of-carer/.

47. Harper B. Waterbirth certification course for providers. 2020 June.

48. Sevelsted A, Stokholm J, Bønnelykke K, Bisgaard H. Cesarean section and chronic immune disorders. Pediatrics. 2015;135(1):e92–8.

49. Al-Zalabani AH, Al-Jabree AH, Zeidan ZA. Is cesarean section delivery associated with autism spectrum disorder? Neurosciences (Riyadh). 2019;24(1):11–5.

50. Chavarro JE, Martín-Calvo N, Yuan C, Arvizu M, Rich-Edwards JW, Michels KB, et al. Association of birth by cesarean delivery with obesity and type 2 diabetes among adult women. JAMA Netw Open. 2020;3(4):e202605.

51. Mesko, Bertalan [Internet]. 2021 [cited 13 Nov 2021]. https://www.linkedin.com/pulse/big-tech-medicine-how-amazon-apple-microsoft-google-mesk%25C3%25B3-md-phd/?trackingI d=P6AHxPDjQxKTp893QMA5GA%3D%3D.
52. Mckinsey & Company [Internet]. 2021 [cited 13 Nov 2021]. https://www.mckinsey.com/indus-tries/healthcare-systems-and-services/our-insights/telehealth-a-quarter-trillion-dollar-post-covid-19-reality.
53. Statistica [Internet]. statistica.com. 2021 [cited 13 Nov 2021]. https://www.statista.com/statistics/671374/global-telemedicine-market-size/.
54. WHO. Recommendations on digital interventions for health system strengthening. 2019.
55. Ministry of Defence. Human Augmentation – The Dawn of a New Paradigm. A strategic impli-cations project. 2021 May.
56. MSCI [Internet]. MSCI.com. 2020 [cited 13 Nov 2021]. https://www.msci.com/docu-ments/1296102/17292317/ThematicIndex-Millenials-cbr-en.pdf/44668168-67fd-88cd-c5f7-855993dce7c4.
57. Shourab NJ, Zagami SE, Golmakhani N, et al. Virtual reality and anxiety in primiparous women during episiotomy repair. Iran J Nurs Midwifery Res. 2016;21(5):521.
58. JahaniShoorab N, Ebrahimzadeh Zagami S, Nahvi A, Mazluom SR, Golmakani N, Talebi M, Pabarja F. The effect of virtual reality on pain in primiparity women during episiotomy repair: a randomize clinical trial. Ira J Med Sci. 2015;40(3):219–24.
59. Hajesmaeel-Gohari S, Sarpourian F, Shafiei E. Virtual reality applications to assist pregnant women: a scoping review. BMC Pregnancy Childbirth. 2021;21(1):249.
60. Font JM, Hedvall A, Svensson E. (eds.) Towards teaching maternal healthcare and nutri-tion in rural Ethiopia through a serious game. Extended Abstracts Publication of the Annual Symposium on Computer-Human Interaction in Play 2017:ACM.
61. PEW Research Centre [Internet]. pewresearch.org. 2019 [cited 13 Nov 2021]. https://www.pewresearch.org/fact-tank/2019/09/09/us-generations-technology-use/.
62. Jason Dorsey [Internet]. jasondorsey.com [cited 13 Nov 2021]. https://jasondorsey.com/blog/gen-z-and-tech-dependency-how-the-youngest-generation-interacts-differently-with-the-digital-world/.
63. Hagan D, Uggowitzer S. Information and communication technologies for women's and chil-dren's health - a planning workbook. Geneva; 2014.
64. The Medical Futurist [Internet]. medicalfuturist.com. 2021 [cited 13 Nov 2021]. https://medi-calfuturist.com/artificial-intelligence-will-redesign-healthcare/.

Suggested Reading

International Confederation of Midwives [Internet]. 2017 [cited 13 Nov 2021]. https://internation-almidwives.org/assets/files/statement-files/2018/04/eng-appropriate-maternity-services-for-normal-pregnancy.pdf.pdf
World Health Organisation [Internet]. 2019 [cited 13 Nov 2021]. https://www.who.int/news-room/fact-sheets/detail/maternal-mortality
Nove A, Friberg IK, de Bernis L, McConville F, Moran AC, Najjemba M, Ten Hoope-Bender P, Tracy S, Homer CSE. Potential impact of midwives in preventing and reducing maternal and neonatal mortality and stillbirths: a lives saved tool modelling study. Lancet Glob Health. 2021;9(1):e24–32.
International Confederation of Midwives; World Health Organisation & United Nations Population Fund [Internet]. 2021 [cited 13 Nov 2021]. https://www.unfpa.org/sites/default/files/pub-pdf/21-038-UNFPA-SoWMy2021-Report-ENv4302_0.pdf.

Chapter 9
Hybrid Neuroscience and Mental Health

Valentina M. Bos and Mussaad Al-Razouki

Abstract The nature of neuroscience has always been hybrid. The biological mechanisms of neurons work on a hybrid of chemical, physical and biological basis. Treatments for mental illnesses are becoming increasingly accepted as a hybrid between medical and behavioral approaches. Even diagnosing a patient with a major neurological disorder such as Alzheimer's disease consists of a behavioral assessment complemented by a brain scan. In analyzing how digital solutions are transforming the space of therapeutic neuroscience, we can safely say that hybrid solutions are here to stay. Three primary contributions are facilitating novel hybrid neural therapies, namely: advances of research on the brain, shifts in perspectives on mental illnesses and the rapid development of new technologies (both software and hardware). The combination of these factors welcomes a variety of different approaches to tackle mental illnesses and neurological diseases, from their screening and prevention to their detection and treatment.

Keywords: Neurons · Neurotransmitters · Central nervous system (CNS) Peripheral nervous system (PNS) · Neuromodulation · Neurodegeneration Alzheimer's disease (AD) · Parkinson's disease (PD)

Introduction

Due to the prevalence of mental illnesses and neurological disorders it is safe to assume that we all know someone who has suffered from one or both. Yet, traditional tools available to diagnose and treat the mind remain limited. Prior to the

V. M. Bos (✉)
Department of Biological Sciences, Columbia University, New York, NY, USA
e-mail: vmb2133@columbia.edu

M. Al-Razouki
Business Development, Kuwait Life Sciences Company, Kuwait City, Kuwait
e-mail: mussaad@klsc.com.kw

© The Author(s), under exclusive license to Springer Nature
Switzerland AG 2022
M. Al-Razouki, S. Smith (eds.), *Hybrid Healthcare*, Health Informatics,
https://doi.org/10.1007/978-3-031-04836-4_9

global Covid-19 pandemic, more than fifty percent of adults who lived with a mental disorder in the United States went without any treatment [1]. This is largely attributable to the persisting societal stigmatization around mental illnesses, even though there has been much improvement in the previous century where people with psychosis, or other mental illnesses were deemed dangerous and locked away into asylums with little to no support and estranged from society.

Thankfully, the way in which we conceptualize mental diseases has changed drastically since then, in the eyes of both the public and the traditional medical establishment. The advent of imaging techniques allowed us to visualize how psychological symptoms have a real biological basis. To take the instance of major depressive disorder (MDD), with imaging we can now see concrete chemical changes in sites of mood and emotional regulation in the brain. In addition, imaging technologies now can confirm MDD to be more than a mood disorder, as it also manifests in alterations in cognitive areas of the brain (versus emotional). Specifically, imaging studies [2] show a reduced size of the hippocampus—the principal site of episodic memory formation—as well as deficits in functions such as speech production [3]. These symptoms are coupled with chemical changes in sites of mood and emotional regulation of the brain. However, despite our better understanding of the illnesses the stigmatization around those who are affected persists.

A large reason for our current lack of physiological and neurological understanding of mental illness is the inherent complexity of the brain itself. Our most 'complex' organ is composed of a hundred billion brain cells, or neurons, passing seemingly infinite amounts of information to each other in very complex patterns and pathways. These nerve cells, together with the electrical impulses and chemical messengers they use to communicate together; generate the entire array of human behavior and cognition: thoughts, emotions, memories, intelligence, consciousness (and more). From faults within these same pathways, diseases can occur in incomprehensible ways. We understand many of the functional patterns in the brain of a person with MDD, however we still do not know what exactly causes them.

The previous decade of research has brought about the general consensus that genetic heritability does not exclusively determine psychiatric pathogenesis. The expression of our DNA, whereby the genetic code is transformed into "visible" characteristic, or a phenotype, is linked with multiple environmental influences. In fact, the accumulating evidence suggests [4] that key events in a person's lifetime are particularly telling of the manifestation of a mental disorder, particularly early life exposure such as prenatal exposures to maternal mood as well as early life trauma and neglect. Nevertheless, these sensitive periods are only one aspect that may influence the development of illnesses later in life. The brain must be analyzed as a holistic entity and treated via a hybrid approach that melds traditional in-person medicine with newer digital methods. To fully understand the root cause of a disease and develop new cures, we must look for both potential errors in our DNA sequence, together with a person's behavior, environment, and history.

Thankfully we are approaching a revolution in neuroscience. Mental illnesses are becoming destigmatized with the help of digital platforms and hybrid neuroscience technologies. Our collective Covid-19 experience has galvanized our approach to previously incurable neurological diseases which are now firmly under the research spotlight, attracting more funding than ever and laying the ground for future state-of-the-art hybrid technologies.

Alone in the first half of 2020 during the COVID-19 pandemic, the U.S. digital mental health platforms have raised $5.4B in venture funding, the largest funding year ever [5]. Depression is also increasing as we continue to learn about the brain, and hybrid technological solutions are opening new doors to solutions for screening, diagnosing, and treating these diseases. The Alzheimer's disease diagnostics and therapeutics market size was $6.6 Bn in 2020 with a CAGR of 5.36% forecasted until 2026 [6]. Therapeutic technologies that target ALS symptoms, such as Brain Computer Interfaces (BCI) was estimated to have a $179 Mn market size in 2019. In contrast, the market for neuromodulation devices was reported at a $4.5 Bn value in 2020, a figure that is expected to double by 2026 [7]. Perhaps the hybrid solution that will experience the highest growth in the coming years is the psychedelic industry; with a value of $2B in 2019, analysts predict a 16.3% CAGR , forecasted to reach a value of $6.9 Bn in 2027 [8].

Current Hybrid Neuroscience

The Rise of Self-Therapy

Mental health awareness has spread immensely with Covid-19, with a collective experience of isolation and socio psychological stress causing a surge in cases of anxiety and depression. By the end of 2019, 42% of adults in the United States reported symptoms of anxiety or depression, which increased by 30% from the start of the pandemic [1] Psychological distress can result in real, physical symptoms of mental illnesses, yet through self-therapy we also have considerable power over whether they manifest. One form of self-therapy is meditation, a term that can refer to different practices ranging from controlled breathing to an intense focus on a particular activity.

Meditation is a powerful tool for self-therapy and has long been used in (mostly Eastern) religious and spiritual practices. However, its integration into daily routines within Western society is only gaining popularity today. This is partly because it requires regular practice and patience to master the technique and see visible results within weeks, making it difficult for individuals to solely learn the technique and commit to it long enough to notice progress.

The demand for meditation-facilitating tools skyrocketed with the aforementioned isolation during the pandemic, considering that more than half of the U.S. counties didn't have a psychiatrist [1]. Meditation-guide software applications (apps) helped fill in this gap. Fast growing digital health startups such as Calm and Headspace provide digital first courses tailored towards different needs such as stress reduction, sleep quality, productivity, or patience in which the user is guided through each step by a specialized health coach. Both apps launched in 2012 by British entrepreneurs, Calm and Headspace gained momentum in 2018, coinciding with a vast growth in the entire industry (five thousand new meditation apps launching since 2015) [9]. As the first mental health app to reach unicorn status, Calm's success story boasts 100 million downloads, four million subscribers and a $2 billion valuation in its latest financing round in late 2020 [6]. In contrast, its rival, Headspace, tags behind with 65 million downloads, two million subscribers and a $320 million valuation as of June 2020. The effects of COVID-19 go unnoticed, with Calm doubling both its valuation, number of subscribers and total downloads from 2019 to 2020.

The different features of both digital platforms makes their success unsurprising. Courses of specific day limits, ranging from 10 day to 30 days on Headspace, create a sort of commitment that mimics therapy appointments and therefore adds accountability that independent meditation practice would not offer. Digital devices also allow users to track progress and therefore create a tangible way of tracking one's own mental health. Together, the digital ability to revive meditation practices are pivotal in helping individuals maximize their control over their health.

As meditation is a mental exercise where preferred results are often realized in a serene physical space amidst a group of like-minded individuals with similar mental health goals, it would be ideal for many of these meditation-guide platforms to cross over into the hybrid healthcare realm by offering coordination tools for their users to meet in the physical world—social distancing rules considered.

Tools of Detection and Treatment of Neurological Diseases

Alzheimer's Dementia is one of the most prevalent and problematic major neurological diseases in the United States today (Fig. 9.1) [10]. In a rapidly ageing population structure, we are increasingly conscious of the decline and slowing of cognitive skills. The thought of losing our memory, language skills and cognitive traits that define us is universally daunting, for the elderly and also for those who share the collective memory of the past.

The general cause of dementia is understood to be neurodegeneration, or the damage and death of neurons. The specific area of the brain damaged determines which cognitive functions are impaired and therefore the type of dementia. Alzheimer's, a disease that is responsible for 60–80% of cases of dementia, is less localized within the brain, with damage of the hippocampus, the site essential for memory formation, is often the first to deteriorate. We used to think of old age as inevitably causing memory loss, whereas we now understand it to only represent a risk factor. As the root cause of Alzheimer's is not yet universally accepted, and a definitive cure still hasn't been found, there is very high opportunity and urgency to tackle the diseases associated with dementia in all of its processes: prevention, early detection, diagnosis, progression and treatment.

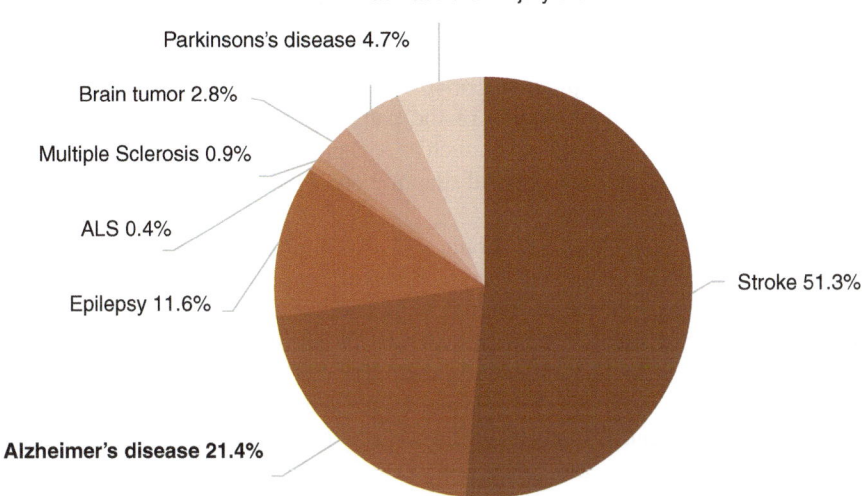

Fig. 9.1 Annual incidence of most common major neurological disorders in the U.S. Source: US Pharmacist [10]

Detecting symptoms of dementia requires being able to detect cognitive clues of decline, such as forgetfulness, disorientation, trouble with coordination, and in turn, directing the affected person to a clinician that can carry out different clinical tests to rule out other possible diagnoses and confirm with imaging techniques. Without people who look after you closely, detecting these clues can be challenging. Especially in old age where different medications can also mimic temporary memory loss, cases will often go unnoticed; an elderly person in a nursing home will often only be suspected of dementia and their condition will deteriorate significantly before a referral to a clinician. Furthermore, once in the hands of a practitioner, the diagnosis itself is not simple; it is made over a mix of subjective assessments over several consultations which may occur over many months. An MRI brain scan without behavioral analysis and repeated assessments will not show the nature of the disease at hand.

Digitalizing detection and treatment is a principal focus around the world in attempts to decrease the burden on all fronts affected by the $1 trillion Alzheimer's industry [11].

Brain+ is a leading hybrid health platform in implementing digital therapeutics that is currently used by 1.5 million people worldwide. Co-founded in 2013 by Kim - Baden-Kristensen and Ulrik Ditlev Erkisen, Brain+ is developing clinically proven digital therapies and detection technologies targeted especially towards dementia.

As the traditional path of diagnosis is obscure, lengthy and often too late down the dementia/Alzheimer's continuum, Brain+'s technology exemplified by their native app "Starry Night" has the advantage of tracking any early preclinical detection of Alzheimer's disease through memory tests. The availability of data monitoring, storing progress and deterioration results and high accessibility allows for the possibility to detect decline before noticeable behavioral symptoms surface. And, as with all health issues, the earlier the diagnosis, the greater the mitigation and or delay of disease progression. For 40% of dementia cases, early detection and treatment can prevent deterioration of the pathologies [12]. However even with incurable neurodegenerative diseases such as Alzheimer's, early diagnosis is crucial in prolonging one's independence and adapting one's lifestyle and avoiding unnecessary admission to a care home.

In addition to early detection, Brain + is also digitizing the evidenced- based therapy of Cognitive Stimulation Therapy. This therapy is traditionally an in-person therapy for patients suffering from mild to moderate forms of dementia that takes place in small groups with a therapist leading different stimulating social activities to improve different cognitive functions, including memory. Digitizing this therapy essentially consists of an app that provides a virtual audio coach to deliver therapy sessions to the patient. By making it digital, it is more accessible to patients and their progress can be tracked more systematically. Though delivered on a digital platform, Brain+'s CST app nevertheless remains hybrid in nature. Due to the social and interactive nature of the therapy, it is carried out by the patient affected as well as an accompanying family member or provided carer that partakes in the activities with the patient.

Pharmacological Treatments of depression

Platforms such as Brian+ highlight the power of early dementia diagnosis as a way to delay the disease and its associated decline in cognition, however the root cause of Alzheimer's dementia remains unknown with no definitive cure yet widely available. Thankfully, there has been a tremendous amount of funding directed to pharmaceutical and biotechnological research to provide a clinically acceptable therapeutic. The biological theories around Alzheimer's are mostly based on the biomarkers, or small molecules that help indicate the presence and location of the disease. For Alzheimer's, the two main biomarkers currently are beta-amyloid and tau proteins. One widely accepted hypothesis states that their presence in high amounts throughout the brain is a cause of the disease [13]. Amyloid proteins are believed to accumulate in a particularly toxic form; in the brain of an Alzheimer patient, this protein is present at abnormally high levels and tends to clump together in the synaptic spaces between neurons that is functionally crucial for two neurons to communicate. Tau proteins accumulate inside these neurons and block the functions necessary to keep them alive. Both beta-amyloid and tau build up leads to disruption of communication between neurons, ultimately leading to their death and a state of dementia in the patient.

These biomarkers are the key target of research in this field, however little progress has been made in terms of real world clinical application. There was a 20-year drought in the development of new drugs to treat Alzheimer until 2021 with the approval of Aducanumab, an amyloid targeting drug developed by Biogen. Aducanumab works by removing the accumulation of amyloid plaques, and in doing so prevents neuronal cell death. However, the recent FDA approval did not elicit a global response of relief and instead created quite the stir within the Alzheimer's community as the drug's clinical efficacy remains under a lot of scrutiny as 10/11 members of the FDA's independent Peripheral and Central Nervous System Drugs Advisory Committee voted to not approve the drug due to lack of definitive evidence of patient benefit—the 11th panelist voted "uncertain". Nevertheless, the drug was eventually approved through FDA's "accelerated approval" channel, as the interpretation of the clinical trials reports were revised several times (Fig. 9.2). With the approval of aducanumab, the spotlight is turning on other companies developing amyloid-targeting pharmaceuticals. For example, Eli Lilly's donanemab currently under development, received Breakthrough Therapy designation by the FDA a few weeks after aducanumab's approval, moving it to the fast-track drug approval process.

Furthermore, despite progress in detecting and possibly treating amyloid plaques, the crux of the research theory does not tell the entire story. A crucial caveat to Biogen and Eli Lilly's approach, is that PET imaging still shows the spread of these plaques in patients on aducanumab and donanemab. Furthermore, research also shows how healthy brains with amyloid deposits sometimes don't ever develop Alzheimer's and how some patients with Alzheimer's have very few amyloid deposits suggesting a correlation conundrum rather than a clinical causation [15] .

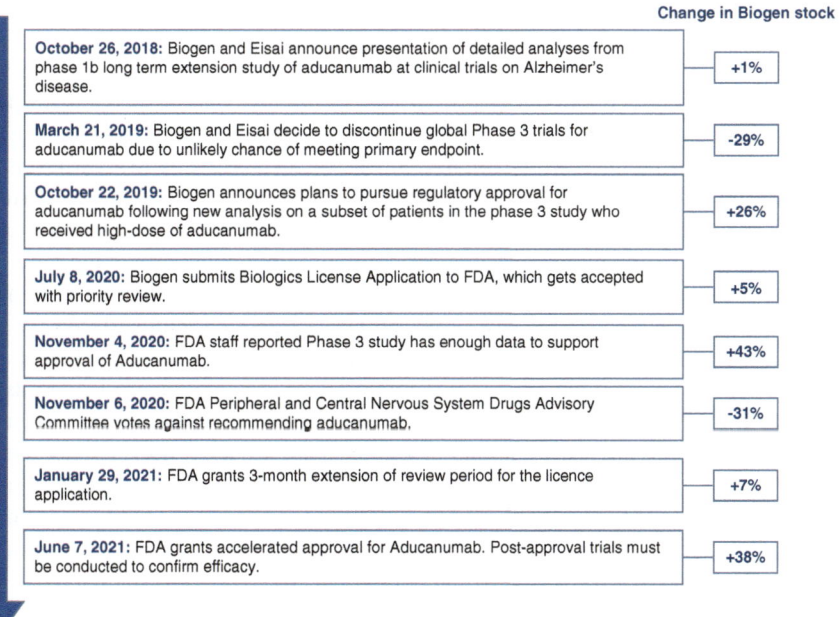

Fig. 9.2 Timeline of aducanumab approval. Source: [14]

Although amyloid plaques have been pivotal in helping us understand which areas of the brain are affected, their detection and treatment in Alzheimer's patients remains a challenge that is highly reliant on advances in digital technologies. For instance, the secret weapon used by Biogen to discover aducanumab is Neuroimmune's digital technology platform, Reverse Translational Medicine [16]. This platform essentially screens large amounts of immune responses to the beta-amyloid protein in both healthy elderly and Alzheimer patients, then conducts high-throughput analyses involving robotics, data processing software and liquid handling devices [17]. This digital approach allows the screening of millions of different tests, and ultimately helped Biogen identify an antibody that would bind to beta-amyloid deposits and remove them.

The success of pharmacological treatment of Alzheimer's is thought to be a function of the progression of the disease. Generally, the later the patient is diagnosed with the condition, the greater the amount of amyloid plaques and tau tangles in the brain, and the less effective the drug will be in treating them. Early diagnosis is therefore crucial in delaying the disease progression. However, diagnosis is a non-linear process that involves the physician testing for the behavioral symptoms as well as confirming the presence of biomarkers through brain imaging—currently, if there is no amyloid detection in the brain, the patient won't be diagnosed with Alzheimer's [18]. These amyloid-detecting brain scans are most commonly conducted by a PET scan, where radioactive tracers are sent to the brain and bind to amyloid deposits. Once bound, they are detected by the brain scan and the location of amyloid deposits can be visualized on a screen. However, this is an expensive process, considering one scan can cost more than $3000 in the U.S. and usually more than one screen is required.

Efforts to transform the biomarker-based Alzheimer diagnosis are widespread. Researchers are looking into revolutionizing imaging by creating technologies that can detect amyloid buildup in the retina of the eye, which would highly simplify the procedure in avoiding a costly brain scan that exposes patients to high levels of radiation [19]. Others are studying Alzheimer's to discover novel biomarkers. Much of the Alzheimer research is focused on beta-amyloid and tau proteins, however there could be several more molecules that are causal to or indicative of the presence of Alzheimer's. Yet, with only two significant biomarkers established, we can imagine the process of discovering new proxies for the disease difficult and slow.

We may see the future of Alzheimer screening and diagnosis to convert to the hybrid space. Digital biomarkers are being integrated as secondary endpoints in clinical trials for other major neurological disorders such as Parkinson's disease, multiple sclerosis and schizophrenia [20]. For example, Sage Bionetworks developed an app called mPower that can monitor the treatment response and predict disease severity in patients with Parkinson's Disease. This is done by recording a 20 second voice recording and analyzing features such as jitter, changes in prosody and fundamental frequency, before and after medication, and compared to measurements from traditional methods. Finding digital markers that can confirm the presence of Alzheimer's is a method that could be proposed to accelerate Alzheimer screening and diagnosis.

Advances in Research Techniques

Alzheimer's is not the only major neurodegenerative disorder without a definitive cure to date. With devastating neurodegenerative diseases such as Parkinson's and Amyotrophic Lateral Sclerosis (ALS), there is an increasing amount of research to find innovative hybrid tools to arrive at statistically significant clinical endpoints. Where pharmacological approaches have been disappointing not only in the case of Alzheimer's, but cross neurodegenerative diseases, different angles to heal are largely welcomed—including both gene editing and approaches to harness already existing biological mechanisms-Neurogenesis, or the growth of new neurons, is part of the latter.

Neurodegeneration is a problem unique to the central nervous system. All cells in our bodies continuously divide: they are born, give birth to new cells that will replace them, and die. It is the natural cycle of our internal biology. But not neurons. Most brain cells that are present throughout adulthood were created during embryonic development through a process known as neurogenesis. Stem cells, which are cells at their most unspecialized state, differentiate into specific types of neurons, at specific times and regions of the brain while we are still in our mother's womb. Once these neurons reach the mature state, they can no longer divide.

This is the reason why a cut in the skin can heal, while injury to the brain can be permanent - whether a concussion or a stroke, it is very difficult for damaged neurons to replenish themselves. This is also the primary issue of neurodegenerative diseases. For instance, Parkinson's disease results from damage to dopaminergic neurons (neurons that synthesize the neurotransmitter dopamine) in the substantia nigra region of the brain. Without these neurons, the pathway that mediates voluntary movement and inhibition is suppressed, resulting in impaired motor control such as the tremors and rigidity that typically characterize patients with Parkinson's. These lost dopaminergic neurons cannot be replenished, and therefore the disease cannot be definitively cured as of yet. Moreover, without treatment, the symptoms only get worse as more neurons of the substantia nigra die. Besides stimulation therapies (see *Neural Implants*), the primary pharmacological method of treatment currently is to provide L-dopa, a building block of dopamine, in attempts to increase supply of dopamine to restore to normal brain activity. This treatment helps with the symptoms of Parkinson's, such as the tremors, however it is not nearly enough to restore normal activity.

While mature neurons cannot divide to form new ones, a hallmark in neuroscience was achieved when it was discovered that neurons can be replenished through neural stem cells. First discovered in humans in 1998 by Dr. Peter Eriksson and colleagues, we now know of certain storage sites in the brain that contain these unspecialized nerve cells. Specifically, there are two prominent parts of the brain that store neural stem cells: the dentate gyrus of the hippocampus and the subventricular zone in the lateral ventricles. The hope and focus of our hybrid healthcare approach today is to be able to direct these cells to undergo neurogenesis in order to replace the lost cells in neurodegenerative diseases, like those of the substantia nigra in Parkinson's disease or of the hippocampus in Alzheimer's patients.

If scientists manage to successfully direct neurogenesis to cure neurodegenerative diseases, this would be a compensatory solution. That is, the root of the disease would not be cured, however normal functions would nonetheless be restored. In contrast, a different angle is to target the root cause of the disease, through gene editing. While many agree that there is an environmental component that determines if neurodegenerative diseases manifest, in diseases such as Alzheimer's, Parkinson's and ALS, scientists believe that there is also an important genetic contribution. The genetic component refers to having either a risk gene, a gene within your DNA that increases the chances of developing the gene but does not guarantee it, or a deterministic gene, a gene that directly causes the disease. In the case of Alzheimer's disease, scientists have identified both. The APOE-e4 is the first risk gene identified and the one with the strongest effect on the risk, with 40–65% of people diagnosed with Alzheimer's having it [19]. Specifically, APOE-e4 is linked to amyloid and tau pathological presence [21]. Certain deterministic genes have been found in a few hundred extended families worldwide, and are tied to causing early onset of the disease, usually starting in a person's early 40's and mid 50's. However, these genes account for 1% or less of all Alzheimer cases [21].

Gene therapy refers to manipulating the human genome at specific points in our DNA, such as at the site of risk and deterministic genes, to prevent a disease from manifesting. Specifically, it consists of delivering a copy of a therapeutic gene to the affected cells, and using the cell's own machinery to continuously express the "correct" genetic material—the promise of gene-editing is therefore a permanent solution from a one-time treatment. However, to target the correct genes in the pathway of disease expression requires a comprehensive understanding of the disease development as well as the correct tools to help precisely guide the therapeutic genes to the target cells without leaking into neighboring cells.

Until we arrive at a complete picture of major neurodegenerative diseases, where all genes involved in pathogenesis are discovered and we find the root cause, patients are relying on mechanisms that improve the symptoms. Besides pharmacological additives, a different neuromodulator mechanism is that of directly stimulating neurons with electrical activity.

Neural Implants

Neurons communicate with each other through electrical impulses and chemical messengers. When one end of a neuron senses a change in voltage, it sends an impulse down the length of the cell, causing the opposite end to release chemical messengers to activate the next neuron, which in turn also experiences a change in voltage. A hybrid functionality if you would that encompasses biology, chemistry and physics. There is also a hint of (biological) data science in the functionality of neurons as these impulses store detailed information within their specific timing and frequency —a pattern that creates a sort of neurological Morse code. While psychopharmaceuticals attempt to restore chemical balances and gene therapies attempt to fix the expression of all molecules in the ecosystem, a different approach to neuro-modulation comes from harnessing (or hacking) the electrical modality of communication to produce desired biological responses. The fact that there are hundreds of different types of neurons involved in thousands of different functions acting by the same mode of communication suggests how in theory, all functions of the nervous system could be helped and healed through electrical intervention—naturally, the question remains how.

This suggestion has been put to the test since the first electrical stimulation therapies 80 years ago. Introduced by Ugo Cerletti in 1938, the electroshock consisted of applying an electric current on the skull and inducing epilectic seizures in patients with severe psychosis. The resulting seizure was thought to more or less remodel neural connections in a way that was claimed to show clinical improvement [22]. Since then, innovation has taken the course of developing methods of stimulation by minimizing the invasiveness, making them a permanent solution to each patient, preventing any collateral effects on the brain and increasing accessibility as treatment options for everyone. The ultimate goal is to move beyond one-time therapies and develop cybernetic neurostimulation technologies that bridge our own biology with hybrid healthcare technology.

The most established form of neural implants available today is Deep Brain Stimulation (DBS), first approved by the FDA to treat essential tremor in 1997. This therapy consists of surgically inserting electrodes through the skull and into the brain, where they send electrical signals to specific regions that associate with the symptoms. The exact pattern of these signals is established by a neurostimulator, a pacemaker-like package implanted under the skin connected to the electrodes with wires. Today, DBS is considered the most common treatment for Parkinson's disease, while also treating obsessive compulsive disorder and epilepsy [23]. Similar applications of neurostimulation, such as Epidural stimulation, are also used to treat spinal cord injuries, where damage affects principal sites of information transfer from the central nervous system to the rest of the body. Here, microelectrodes powered by implantable devices can directly elicit electrical impulses in the neurons sending information to the targets of the peripheral nervous system. The effects are powerful, having the potential to allow paraplegics to stand up again and even walk.

The accuracy with which microelectrodes can target specific neural pathways makes them more reliable when compared to administering drugs, where the clinical effects are less clear with respect to the timing of action, spatial specificity of the affected neurons and the dosing needed. [24]

However, these technical innovations must still surpass biological obstacles. Finite battery life is one major setback of traditional implants; once a DBS neurostimulator battery runs out, it must be replaced through surgery. Battery replacements constrains the lifetime of implants while causing additional trauma for a patient to undergo repeated surgery [25]. Researchers around the world are therefore investigating alternative modes of powering the neural signals. One such approach is ultrasound powering where ultrasound waves sent from a site outside the body can travel in the form of sound waves to the implant site. Here, the pressure from these vibrational waves is then converted into electrical energy by a transducer.

Moore4Medical, a project combining efforts from diverse research institutions and companies, also highlights the possibility of using ultrasound waves to directly stimulate nerves in addition to powering the implant. Dr Vasiliki Giagka, a specialist in implantable devices and a part of the Moore4Medical project, explains that "in combining different acoustic waves, we can create very small focal points to target specific locations inside the body" [26]. This specificity might allow stimulation to reach the level of individual neurons rather than the bundles of neurons that make up nerves. Moore4Medical's aspiration in incorporating ultrasound technology in the nervous system reflects the hybrid direction that neuroscience is heading. To have rechargeable implantable devices means that stimulation devices can become a permanent part of a patient's body. In addition, new and more specific ways to stimulate nerves will make the experience of having a digital "supplement" in the body a less noticeable and more "normal" experience for the patient.

While invasive deep brain stimulation is pivotal in helping treat Parkinson's disease, other less invasive, while also less potent stimulation approaches are reaching the all-important commercialization stage for more invasive mental health issues. For example, there are studies that demonstrate how directing stimulation to certain areas of the brain can help alleviate symptoms of depression. Flow is a Swedish startup that commercializes this concept through a portable headset that noninvasively delivers constant low electrical impulses to the frontal lobe; a part of the brain that controls emotional expression. This approach aims to "redress imbalances in brain activity" [27]. Because the device does not require medical guidance or prescription and delivers stimulation from outside the skull rather than implanted electrodes, it is a less potent form of stimulation. The full hybrid healthcare therapy is complemented by a virtual AI therapist app that helps with behavioral treatment, a combination that is hoped would eventually maximize the chances of recovery from clinical depression.

The Brain Computer Interface/Brain Sensors

Amyotrophic lateral sclerosis (ALS) commonly known as Lou Gehrig's disease, used to strip people of their independence as well as their ability to connect and interact with the environment, depriving them of some of the basic tenets of basic human experience—their independence and their identity. As the disease exclusively degenerates neurons that control movement, paralysis can reach all muscles of the body– e.g. the legs thus impairing the ability to walk or stand, the face thus impairing the ability to laugh, communicate and create relations. The late Dr. Stephen Hawking was probably the best-known ALS case. We have witnessed firsthand how he was able to regain his ability to share his groundbreaking theories on black holes and origins of the universe through a customized PC developed by Intel. This PC, replaced and upgraded every 2 years, acted as an assistive computer technology that could pick up his eye movements, squeezes in the cheek and a thumb switch to help him dictate his thoughts onto a computer screen.

With the rate at which neural prostheses are advancing, technologies used by the late Stephen Hawking are today obsolete. The dawn of a new decade has brought with it neural implants that can be coupled with artificial intelligence to sense brain activity and translate it into tangible words, thoughts and even actions. This means that electrodes can not only send impulses to activate nerves (stimulation), but also pick up signals from the brain and relay them to a computer interface that uses algorithms to decode them (sensors). These sensors are called brain computer interface (BCI) and can either help the patient communicate, or in the case of amputees, relay the information back into a robotic limb to induce a desired action.

The promise of this sensor is powerful. When the electrodes of the sensor are inserted in the motor cortex of the brain that controls movement, a cursor on the computer screen can be induced to move depending on the brain signal commands it receives from the ALS patient. The mere thought of movement induces movement. While this technology has much promise, in reality it is not as simple as wearing a mind-controlling device that allows anyone to interact with a computer. Just like a baby learning to walk through trial and error, these patients must learn exactly which bodily sensations and intentions *will* the cursor on the screen to move. It takes extensive training and close medical supervision, not to mention immense willpower and grit, to create a new brain-digital extension connection. This hybridized approach is hardly accessible to anyone, as it must take into account the mental health of the patient, compatibility between the patient brain and computer interface, and the quality of the technology itself. Also, the invasiveness of having to first remove the skull to insert the electrodes complicates the treatment in its current state. The alternative would be to use a non-invasive technology to pick up signals, such as electrocephalography (EEG). However the clinical issue here is that these signals are so weak that it is difficult to locate where they are coming from. Overcoming these challenges requires advances in digital technologies and continued research on the brain. On the other hand, the patient's effort will always be necessary for them to function and for the hybrid solution to succeed. BCI companies must therefore take a page out of the digital mental health platform playbook and consider implementing programs to help train and provide mental support to patients attempting to achieve brain-digital symbiosis.

The downscaling of neural implants to grain sized pieces and the development of biocompatible materials has recently led neuroscientists from the Australian BCI company Synchron to discover a way to bypass the traditional open brain surgery procedure necessary to insert electrodes into the brain. In other words, they were able to insert electrodes without touching the skull and even brain tissue. This interesting hybrid neural health technology called Stentrode, involves an electrode the size of a match stick that is inserted directly into the blood vessels that travel to the brain [28]. These blood vessels naturally reach all areas of the brain, as they are the principal mode of importing nutrients and oxygen as well as exporting waste across all brain cells. The ingenuity of Stentrode was therefore to implant electrodes into the brain through a natural path—without the burden of surgery. A catheter-like tool helps direct the flexible electrodes into the blood vessels from the base of the neck, leaving the electrodes to lace the inside of the blood vessels in a fixed position to record brain activity. The recorded signals are relayed to a second implant in the chest, and wirelessly reported back to a computer interface for interpretation and action.

With this device, Synchron is a leader in the field of brain computer interfaces. In 2020 they conducted their first human trials on daily activity, testing out the Synchron technology on four patients with severe paralysis [29] The results were promising, showing they were able to carry out tasks such as texting, emailing, shopping and online-banking [24]. With FDA approval in 2021, Synchron will proceed to carry out trials for its commercialization.

The success of restoring a patient's ability to induce movement ignites the realm of possibilities and the potential of boosting other parts of our brain. Founded in 2016, Elon Musk's venture, Neuralink , aspires to expand brain computer interfaces to target more disorders than those related to the motor nervous system. It therefore differs from standard BCI approaches in that it collects information from 1024 electrodes in different areas of the brain: the visual cortex, auditory cortex, somatosensory cortex and motor cortex [30] . These electrodes are connected to a "chip" that is surgically implanted within the patient's skull, which wirelessly relays the signals to a computer interface. Although Neuralink has only been tested on rodents this far, the company aims to cure diverse neurological disorders including deafness, mental illness and blindness. Thus, compared to its competitor Synchron, Musk's brain chip takes a more holistic hybrid neuroscience approach, where one chip has the potential to integrate several different therapeutic functions.

Movement to Traditional Therapies

Amidst a large movement towards a digital approach to therapeutics, there is also a growing resurgence into the application of traditional naturalistic methods of healing. The psychedelic industry is one form of natural healing , currently at a $4.75Bn Market size and expected to reach $10.7 Bn by 2027 [31] . Several psychedelic, micro dosing, startups have made their way to the public markets and are on route to disrupt the mental health industry, in a movement that has even been baptized as the Psychedelic Renaissance. Favorite amongst the classes of natural therapeutics are classic hallucinogens, a sub-category of psychedelics that are derived from natural compounds (Table 9.1):

The biomedical industry's interest in psychedelic therapeutics has arrived, however a bit behind the curve. In fact, it was centuries ago when indigenous communities became knowledgeable about these drugs and started using them as part of their holistic healing practices consisting of spiritual practices, plant-based medicines and community involvement—essentially, part of an indigenous hybrid healthcare approach. Furthermore, biomedical research has been complicated and delayed due to the uncontrolled consumption of psychedelics during their mass rediscovery throughout the counter-cultural decades of the 1950s, 60s and 70s, when these substances were labelled as "drugs of abuse" and failed to gain recognition amongst the

Table 9.1 Classification of classic hallucinogens

Scientific name	Natural source	Illegal street name
Lysergic acid diethylamide (LSD)	Ergot (fungus)	Acid
Dimethyltryptamine (DMT)	Chacruna, Jurema, Yopo, and dozens of other plant species	The Spirit Molecule, Dimitri
Psilocybin	Psilocybin mushrooms	Magic Mushrooms, Shrooms

medical establishment. Today, leading research institutions such as John's Hopkins University are resuscitating biomedical knowledge in this field, with doctors and scientists keen to discover more about how psychedelics influence the mind and body, and how they can be practically used in the treatment of mental illness.

Current evidence shows the strong potential of psychedelics in treating anxiety, treatment-resistant depression, post-traumatic stress disorder (PTSD), and addictions. For example, patients suffering from major depression have experienced lasting improvement after treatment with psilocybin, with little to no adverse effects after the first day [32]. Notably, these findings also show that effects were reported with no hints of dependency, thus favoring this substance over traditional pharmacological treatments, such as the highly addictive benzodiazepines that are widely used for anxiety. There is also a rise in supplementing psychedelics and talk therapy into a hybrid healthcare approach known as psychedelic-assisted psychotherapy (PAP). This practice is thought to facilitate healing by allowing the patient to be introspective and to share their feelings, thoughts, and memories which come to mind [33].

Once a substance of abuse, the FDA has recently declared the professionally supervised use of psychedelics a "breakthrough therapy". However, passing clinical studies does not come without its own set of challenges as we have noted earlier during our discussion of Alzheimer's and aducanumab. In incorrect doses, psychedelics can cause adverse effects such as panic, nausea, and anxiety. There are also many other side effects such as hallucinations that we still know little about. We do know however that classic hallucinogens bind to certain types of serotonergic receptors—that is, due to their molecular 3D composition, where they can activate the same neurons that are activated by serotonin, a neurotransmitter that in the brain is involved in the entire body to regulate several factors such as mood, reward, cognition and memory. Serotonin (along with dopamine) are colloquially known as the happiness neurotransmitters. Although researchers are understanding the neural effects every day, much is still unknown. Careful regulation and several more clinical studies on their effect is therefore essential to integrate these natural substances into novel hybrid therapies targeting mental health.

Indeed, hybrid healthcare platforms are pivotal in facilitating this movement. A notable example is EntheogeniX Biosciences, a Delaware based company that created an AI-enabled computational biophysics platform that can essentially predict the potential side effects of different psychedelic-derived drugs before using them in a clinical trial. Similarly, MindCure, a Vancouver based company is aiming to enhance the safety of the process throughout treatment through a monitoring system where patients undergoing PAP can track their progress and report different aspects of their experience. This hybrid platform includes protocols, assessment tools, and a communication stream with practitioners. MindCure currently only operates in Canada, one of the few countries where psychedelic therapy is legal, however its local success provides us with insight into how other countries might also use similar platforms to create a safe space for users and transparency between patients and clinicians. Startups such as MindCure are crucial in hybridizing the digital and the natural to realistically and carefully execute psychedelic therapeutics.

A Hybrid Future for Neuroscience

One of medicine's holy grails is developing treatments targeting the trinity of (incurable) neurodegenerative diseases—ALS, Parkinson's and Alzheimer's. No significant progress on finding the root cause of these diseases has been made in the last three decades. However, we are coming to an unprecedented time for biotechnological tools as well as urgency from society. Breakthroughs in gene therapies and digital systems to map out neural networks in immensely greater capacity than humans ever could, give reason to believe that we are soon coming to a tipping point.

And while the interest in the brain is largely medical, many others see a futuristic, recreational potential of brain technologies. If a brain computer interfaces allow patients to control digital parameters just by thinking about it, why not allow anyone to access the digital world through the mind? This thought might reflect Elon Musk's longer-term aspirations for Neuralink. A platform where people can communicate without the burden of an external device. In a no-longer dystopian reality, we are at the beginning of a shift from telephony to telepathy.

In this point of view, thought control of digital devices is a desirable feature for healthy people insomuch as the disabled. Part of this has already become reality. Once a year, a Cybathlon is held at the Swiss Institute of Technology (ETH) where competitors gather from around the world to play videogames purely controlled by the mind.

The direction of this trend of invasiveness of digital platforms shouldn't come as a surprise. Less than 20 years ago, telephones were fixed lines; now, they are a permanent accessory on our bodies (and constantly *on our minds*). We now wear our social media and communication platforms on the wrist or within connected eyeglasses. As a society, we are no longer separated by distance or wires; the only remaining limitation is our use of technology through an external device. Whether direct access to the digital world without a physical intermediary is desirable is a question that people are starting to face themselves with. While there is a self-evident convenience to having immediate access to all digital aids, from communication to information, there is also the risk that spending time in a digital world connected through our minds will alienate us from the physical world. The COVID-19 period alone demonstrated adverse effects of isolation that came from digital communication without physical interaction, especially concerning mental health.

While the singularity of merging our brain's biology with the digital sounds like science fiction, many are quick to forget that digital neural aids are now commercialized at an extremely fast rate outside the realm of medicine. Within sports, more and more athletes are incorporating electromagnetic stimulation technologies (EMS) to optimize their training sessions and game day performance . To name a few of the best athletes in the world, Usain Bolt, Rafael Nadal and Cristiano Ronaldo all endorse EMS to boost their most intense training. In conventional training, muscle contractions are commanded from nerve impulses from the brain and spinal cord when performing specific movements. EMS can direct electrical impulses, generated by electrodes placed in a position directly above muscle to stimulate muscle groups at controlled times. Hybridizing conventional training with EMS brings significant advantages over solely training with one of the two methods. Traditional training typically requires a mental effort that equals the physical effort, whereas EMS training will not fatigue the brain of the athlete, as the simulations do not involve input from the central nervous system. At the same time, conventional training is still important as training the mind is an important element in training in each sport. Thus, not only does a hybrid EMS training structure allow athletes to boost their conventional training sessions and competitive performance by putting in less time to achieve the same (or even greater) effect on the muscles, but in professional athletes who experience high mental strain, this solution helps to prevent over-stimulating their nervous system and to maintain a healthy mind.

Other athletes are betting on the theory that very light, non-invasive stimulation achieved by transcranial direct current stimulation (tDCS) to certain brain parts during exercise will also make training more effective. To master a basketball shot, the player not only has to train his physical strength, but must also develop the technique on how to score—the exact movements needed under different scenarios (the precious final seconds of a game with the score tied), the order of actions, accuracy, how much force to use at each distance from the hoop etc. The brain is heavily involved in this learning process, where it wires and rewires the connections between neurons with each attempted shot. By stimulating the neurons involved in learning, it will speed the process up and create a better end result on game day.

This theory was integrated in the training technology developed by Halo Neuroscience, a startup founded in 2013 and acquired by Flow Neuroscience in early 2021. Worn as a headset, the device sends tCDS impulses to the primary motor cortex as the person is learning a specific motor skill, and is thought to develop muscle memory faster. Although Flow Neuroscience repurposed the stimulation technology to the scope of tackling mental illnesses, their muscle-memory biohacking device provides a glimpse into the hybrid future of cognition-performance technologies.

Beyond seeking digital extensions to transcend physical human limitations, it will be possible to change one's own biology . With increasing amounts of big data processing to map and interpret the entire human genome, we will be able to understand exactly which genes determine different cognitive traits. For instance, researchers from around the world are identifying genes that are involved with intelligence [34]. With gene therapy, it is already possible in theory to alter or upgrade the DNA sequence of a particular set of genes to enhance a persons' cognitive skills. However, a major obstacle from theoretical to practical is of course ethical. Undoubtedly, pushing the limits of our cognition has all sorts of benefits. The potential to transcend the boundaries of our DNA to become more intelligent, higher functioning humanoids merits curiosity, fascination and practicality. However, the break in natural selection, as well as the moral divisiveness it would implicate when gene editing is only available to a certain societal class, makes one question—is it worth it? Just because we know how to clone humans doesn't mean that it is ethically right to do so. And just because neural implants could allow any human to access the internet and make phone calls through thought, doesn't mean that we should.

References

1. https://www.forbes.com/sites/katiejennings/2021/06/07/venture-funding-for-mental-health-startups-hits-record-high-as-anxiety-depression-skyrocket/?sh=23975db01116.
2. https://www.theguardian.com/society/2015/jun/30/chronic-depression-shrinks-brains-memories-and-emotions.
3. https://www.health.harvard.edu/blog/sad-depression-affects-ability-think-201605069551.
4. https://ajp.psychiatryonline.org/doi/10.1176/appi.ajp.2019.19010020.
5. https://www.fiercehealthcare.com/tech/funding-for-digital-behavioral-health-startups-surged-amid-covid-19-pandemic.
6. https://www.mordorintelligence.com/industry-reports/alzheimers-diagnosis-and-drugs-market#:~:text=Market%20Overview,forecast%20period%2C%202021%2D2026.
7. https://www.fortunebusinessinsights.com/industry-reports/neuromodulation-devices-market-100561.
8. https://www.prnewswire.com/news-releases/psychedelic-drugs-market-size-is-projected-to-reach-10-75-billion-by-2027%2D%2D301273405.html.
9. https://www.businessofapps.com/data/calm-statistics/.
10. https://www.uspharmacist.com/article/incidence-and-prevalence-of-major-neurologic-disorders.
11. https://www.alzint.org/about/dementia-facts-figures/dementia-statistics/.
12. https://www.cdc.gov/aging/publications/features/dementia-not-normal-aging.html.
13. https://www.alz.org/national/documents/topicsheet_betaamyloid.pdf.
14. https://www.drugs.com/history/aduhelm.html.
15. https://www.alzforum.org/news/research-news/when-theres-no-amyloid-its-not-alzheimers.
16. https://www.neurimmune.com/news/neurimmune-welcomes-biogens-news-on-clinical-benefit-of-aducanumab.
17. https://www.neurimmune.com/technology/rtm-technology-platform#:~:text=Reverse%20Translational%20Medicine%E2%84%A2%20(RTM,healthy%20during%20the%20aging%20process.
18. https://www.nature.com/articles/d41586-018-05721-w.
19. https://link.springer.com/chapter/10.1007/978-3-030-26269-3_6.
20. https://alz-journals.onlinelibrary.wiley.com/doi/full/10.1016/j.trci.2018.04.003.

21. https://www.alz.org/alzheimers-dementia/what-is-alzheimers/causes-and-risk-factors/genetics.
22. https://www.ncbi.nlm.nih.gov/pmc/articles/PMC3157831/.
23. https://www.mayoclinic.org/tests-procedures/deep-brain-stimulation/about/pac-20384562.
24. Chari A, et al. Surgical neurostimulation for spinal cord injury. Brain Sci. 2017;7(2):18. https://doi.org/10.3390/brainsci7020018.
25. https://bioelecmed.biomedcentral.com/articles/10.1186/s42234-020-00052-6.
26. https://blog.izm.fraunhofer.de/we-could-be-treating-diabetes-asthma-and-parkinsons-tomorrow/.
27. https://www.nsmedicaldevices.com/analysis/brain-stimulation-headset/.
28. https://www.businesswire.com/news/home/20201028005613/en/Patients-with-Severe-Paralysis-Use-Stentrode-Brain-Computer-Interface-to-Text-Email-Shop-Bank-Online-First-in-human-Study-Reports.
29. https://jnis.bmj.com/content/13/2/102.
30. https://neuralink.com/approach/.
31. https://www.globenewswire.com/en/news-release/2021/03/18/2195240/28124/en/Global-Psychedelic-Drugs-Market-Report-2020-Market-Size-is-Projected-to-Reach-10-75-Billion-by-2027.html.
32. https://www.hopkinsmedicine.org/news/newsroom/news-releases/psychedelic-treatment-with-psilocybin-relieves-major-depression-study-shows.
33. Schenberg E. Psychedelic-assisted psychotherapy: a paradigm shift in psychiatric research and development. Front Pharmacol. 2018;9(733) https://doi.org/10.3389/fphar.2018.00733.
34. https://www.nature.com/articles/ng.3869.epdf.

Chapter 10
Combating the Compounding Effects of Chronic Disease

Christian Hense and Michael Schelper

Abstract Chronic diseases and conditions impact millions of people every day, across the globe. Caring for patients with chronic diseases creates both a medical and economic burden which is increasingly unsustainable. When physicians apply digital health technology tools and solutions as part of their prescribed medical care both time and costs can be saved. But what's even more important—patients outcomes increasingly improve when physicians and technology work together. In this chapter, we will focus on three main chronic diseases—heart disease, cancer, diabetes. Each face unique challenges that give birth to unique opportunities and innovative methods of chronic disease management in a hybrid healthcare era. Early detection and prevention are key to effectively manage these conditions, however when a disease has already developed there are many approaches on how to best care for the patients. Technological advances play a vital role, supporting clinical professionals with relevant digital tools that transform patient data into a very valuable resource, via Patient Reported Outcome Measures (PROMs), which will eventually lead to improved clinical outcomes. Patients with chronic conditions needs empathy, time and attention from their care givers, and hence the evergreen need for a hybrid approach to managing these complex and ongoing cases.

Chronic Diseases on the Rise

We've all been affected by chronic illness at some point in our lives. Whether it is a close family member, a friend, or navigating supportive care for a community member who needs a little extra help—chronic conditions have touched all of us. Chronic diseases and conditions lead to disability, decreased quality of life, and an enormous

C. Hense (✉) · M. Schelper
Universal DX, Madrid, Madrid, Spain

Anvano, Dubai, United Arab Emirates
e-mail: michael.schelper@anvano.com

© The Author(s), under exclusive license to Springer Nature Switzerland AG 2022
M. Al-Razouki, S. Smith (eds.), *Hybrid Healthcare*, Health Informatics,
https://doi.org/10.1007/978-3-031-04836-4_10

economic burden on both the patient and the healthcare system. Unfortunately, it does not appear to be an issue that is slowing down—especially with the average age of most populations increasing.

Chronic conditions greatly disrupt quality of life and provide several limitations for patients and their families. Factors including functional, physical, social, and cognitive limitations all contribute to a higher demand on caregivers and the healthcare system [1]. When the time spent by patients and physicians combine with the financial strain on both patients and the healthcare system as a whole, there is a dire need to find innovative solutions beyond the status quo. This is exactly where technology continues to step up and provide tools, systems, and pathways which enable patients and healthcare systems to deliver in their quest for quality chronic disease management and care.

Beyond technology creating pharmaceutical therapies and treatment protocols, technology is now bringing healthcare monitoring and solutions to the patient on a continuous basis and outside of the traditional healthcare infrastructure. Waiting to make an appointment with a physician, waiting to schedule a test, and waiting to review results is time that could be better spent by patients elsewhere, especially those suffering from chronic care conditions who need continuous follow up on a monthly or even weekly basis. With so many patients needing continuous care for their chronic conditions, this means physicians and staff must allocate an enormous amount of resources and time to see patients in person, as chronic conditions compound the time needed to provide optimal care to patients. Optimal care that's required to span multiple years and multiple comorbidities more times than not. Though, with technology, including artificial intelligence (AI) solutions (see Chap. 2), patients can use home-based healthcare monitoring devices (see Chap. 7) to share information in real-time with their healthcare teams. Their family members can have the peace of mind when their is monitored frequently and accurately, and healthcare workers can in turn focus on in-person patient care more closely by using these tools that allow them to leverage their time more efficiently.

The Centers for Disease Control and Prevention (CDC) defines a chronic disease as a condition that requires ongoing medical care or one that interferes with daily life for 1 year or longer [2]. Heart disease is the number one cause of death globally, accounting for 32% of all deaths worldwide [3]. Cancer is the second leading cause of death worldwide, accounting for one out of every six deaths [4]. These facts make chronic illness the number one cause of death on a global scale and one that affects many aspects of a country's health and economic status. Chronic conditions and diseases drive the $3.8 trillion spent every year on healthcare costs in the United States [2, 5]. They are a global issue and are often caused by preventable risk factors as outlined in Fig. 10.1 including tobacco use, less than ideal nutrition, lack of physical activity, and excessive alcohol use all contribute to the most common chronic diseases [2]. Obesity for example is a major risk factor for heart disease and diabetes and it has tripled on a global scale since the 1970s with nearly two billion people overweight in 2016 [6]. When someone has multiple chronic conditions, this further complicates their recovery as treatment plans and goals can vary for each disease, not to mention the ballooning of healthcare costs. It often results in one

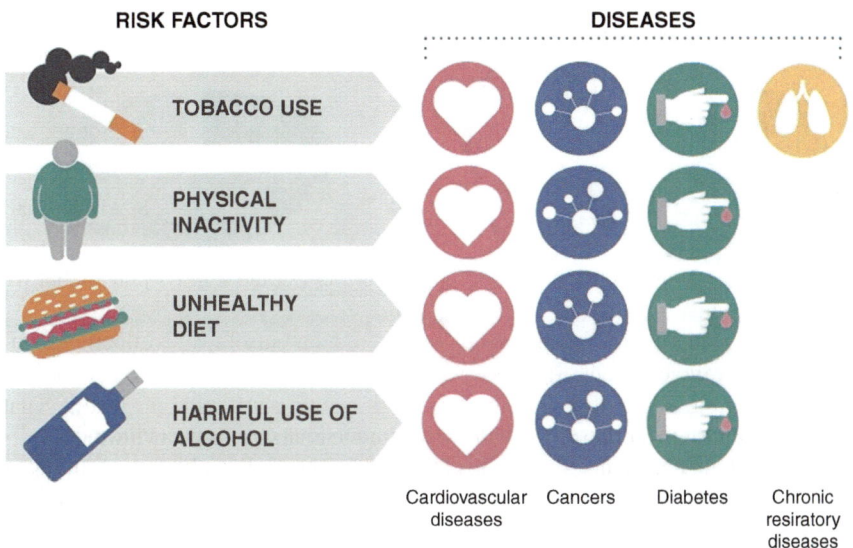

Fig. 10.1 Chronic disease risk factors—global alliance for chronic diseases [7]

chronic disease being the primary condition and becomes better managed than the others [1].

Age continues to be the largest corollary factor for developing chronic disease. Over 80% of Americans that are 65 years of age or older have multiple chronic conditions compared to only 18% of Americans who are between the ages of 1–44 years old [1]. While some of those risk factors are avoidable and modifiable (compared to characteristics like age, gender, and genetic factors), it's often difficult to implement changes that benefit patients in the long run. Once patients are ready to make lifestyle adjustments to reduce their risk or treat current chronic conditions—they need frequent monitoring to maintain accountability and motivation when trying to make long-lasting changes. This means even if patients are taking the right steps to reduce their chronic illness risk, continuous support by healthcare teams is still required through the use of both digital and in person resources and time to support patients along the arduous journey back to wellness. With an evident lack of access to many of these resources, reducing the global impact of chronic diseases using traditional healthcare models is not sustainable.

Chronic Diseases with Unique Challenges

It's no secret that chronic conditions and disease management come with a large economic burden. Chronic conditions require more spending and impart more financial strain than acute conditions, especially when patients have more than one

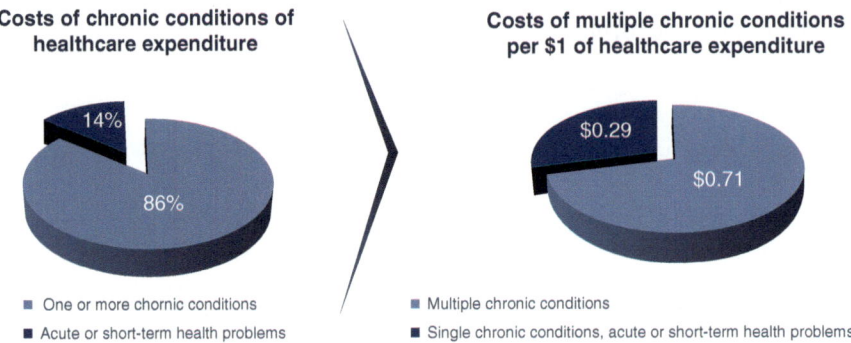

Fig. 10.2 Cost impact of chronic conditions on healthcare expenditure

chronic condition [8]. Figure 10.2 shows the tremendous cost impact chronic conditions have on the healthcare system. Eighty-six percent of all healthcare spending is spent on patients with one or more chronic conditions. This means only 14% of healthcare costs are made of acute or short-term health care problems [10]. The numbers are even more staggering for patients with multiple chronic conditions. For every US dollar spent on healthcare, $0.71 of that dollar is spent on patients with multiple chronic conditions [10].

People with multiple chronic conditions visit their physicians more frequently and account for 64% of all physician visits and 70% of all inpatient stays [10]. The financial strain of chronic disease management can be overwhelming to patients and healthcare systems. Patients with three or four chronic conditions visit their healthcare teams on average 12 times per year. If they have five or more chronic conditions, the visits increase to 20 per year [1]. In counties where access to chronic disease management is limited, patients often must spend a large portion of their income to cover costs. For example, in India, a patient managing diabetes may spend up to 25% of their household income to cover medical expenses [9]. This means that even if a person has only one chronic condition to manage, one-quarter of their entire household spending is going towards medical bills to cover it.

The economic burden for patients dealing with chronic illness varies worldwide, but what remains consistent is chronic diseases have the potential to greatly impact a household's (and by extension the entire healthcare system's) financial stability [7]. Not only do chronic conditions require frequent monitoring within healthcare systems and potentially require expensive prescriptions every month—but patients with multiple chronic conditions are admitted and readmitted to the hospital at a much higher rate [1]. Patients with five or more chronic conditions spend twice as much each year on healthcare compared to those with three or four conditions and spend *14 times* as much on health-related services than someone without any chronic conditions [1]. When looking at cardiovascular disease specifically, there is an enormous economic burden worldwide. Studies have found countries like India experience a predicted $2.4 trillion economic loss over less than two decades due to cardiovascular diseases. China is predicted to have an even larger loss of $8.8 trillion—and these reports occurred before the coronavirus outbreak in 2020 [10].

As emerging market economies develop, higher economic prosperity casts a shadow on community health and wellness. The number of people worldwide with chronic conditions continues to rise, as does the number of those living with multiple chronic conditions, further highlighting the need to implement innovative solutions to proper management [10]. Challenges to chronic condition management include both financial and logistical obstacles. Even if the economic toll of chronic disease management is removed—there is still a major gap in care management when it comes to juggling multiple comorbidities and the various therapies including medications and lifestyle changes required. A prime example of this is Germany, which has one of the most robust healthcare systems in the world that should lead to better chronic condition management. Unfortunately, Germany's increase in chronic conditions has mostly led to more hospitalizations and increased resource utilization [11]. As the average age of Germans increases (as it is globally) there must be a shift in improving how resources are utilized rather than simply providing them to be overused—increasing the economic and medical system burden.

There is also the challenge of multiple physicians providing treatment and monitoring (with some overlap no doubt occurring as a result). Not every health system provides integrated access to view prescription history, chronic disease progression, and treatment goals making it difficult for physicians to get an up-to-date picture to guide treatment decisions. Due to the potential physical, functional, and cognitive limitations caused by chronic conditions, many patients rely on caregivers for assistance throughout the day. Ensuring caregivers are included in the patient care loop is difficult due to the complexity of care, multiple providers prescribing care, and the ever-evolving status of patients (see Chap. 7 for more on hybrid models of caregiving).

These challenges showcase how complicated chronic conditions and disease management can be, but they also highlight how many steps within the treatment and care process can be improved upon by adopting a hybrid approach where both communication and data are optimized using digital solutions. Improving chronic care management creates a huge opportunity to improve the financial and medical burden for all parties involved. By improving how well the patient, caregiver, and physician communicate and improving the information shared amongst everyone— nearly every obstacle to safe and effective chronic disease management can be improved.

Digitalization and Innovative Health Technologies

The need to optimize time is crucial in improving patient care in the setting of chronic disease management. There continues to be incredible advancements in technology developing regarding communication, monitoring, and management for chronic disease which are slowly starting to matriculate into clinical practice. Such technology includes easier and non-invasive ways to detect diseases earlier and before they completely disrupt a patient's quality of life. Blood-based cancer screening is one example as well as blood-based progress tracking for patients with cancer.

Wearable technology is also becoming more prevalent and integrated into one's life. People are constantly accessing more information from their smartphones, fitness trackers, and sleep apps—and healthcare technology companies are using this access to collect more data outside of a clinic setting. With the fusion of wearable technologies and sensors, patients (and patient platforms) can access data analytics to generate biofeedback and improve treatment while physicians can track progress and implement interventions as necessary. This creates a partnership between the patient and physician providing care as well as a partnership between the physician and technology platform.

A hybrid approach to chronic disease management can provide a time-saving service for physicians while simultaneously increasing the focus and monitoring for patients who require long-term surveillance. Tracking medical information allows for passive data collection and interpretation by healthcare teams. This way a larger picture of a patient's health can be generated rather than a snapshot in a clinical setting which can contain multiple variables impacting results. There can also be an increase in assessing progress after medical interventions (as well as lifestyle interventions) have been implemented—both informing the healthcare team and potentially motivating the patient by visualizing the results of their efforts. Inversely, warning signs of deteriorating status can be identified earlier by using monitoring parameters within digital technology. As with most things, there are shortfalls in implementing digital solutions in a clinical setting. There can be a lack of human 'touch' and judgment when technology is left to interpret too much. This calls for a more standardized and specialized role of the physician when integrating digital tech and medical care.

The Continuously Advancing Role of Physicians

Physicians and other healthcare providers are faced with unique challenges when it comes to chronic condition management. Our traditional healthcare approach focuses on acute problems with acute treatments targeting a single disease or symptom at a time. However, with chronic diseases, especially multiple conditions, traditional methods need to shift into long-term treatment solutions while taking into consideration multiple comorbidities that can impact treatment choices and outcomes. Physicians have the burden of diagnosing chronic conditions that often are diagnosed late only when symptoms become excessively burdensome to patients. Physicians must also create acute treatment plans and initiate long-term treatment planning.

This multi-faceted approach is impossible to achieve in the typical siloed treatment approach by most traditional healthcare teams. Factors including patient understanding, financial constraints, medication adherence, and overall treatment adherence impact outcomes for patients with chronic conditions. Physicians must also consider other conditions and how the patient's multiple chronic diseases ebb and flow with each other depending on how well they are being managed. Time is limited for healthcare teams and continues to be constrained with an aging population and a lack of physicians to manage everyone. This sets up the risk for treatment gaps and failure to recognize a patient potentially starting to fall further behind in their chronic disease management. Communication within healthcare systems continues to be mediocre at best, despite efforts to create portals, hubs, and telecommunication avenues within the clinical setting. Not only do patients need to be able to communicate with the health care team, but their caregivers also need to be aware of changes in treatment or status—something often difficult to maintain [12].

With a lack of time and fluid communication, the risk for adverse reactions and events for patients with chronic diseases increases. A lack of time, data, and communication are all barriers to chronic condition management for physicians. These also happen to be areas where health technology and innovation can best support physicians. But it's not always as simple as applying a new device, adapting a new medical record, and implementing a new AI data analysis system.

Physicians have hesitations like any early adopter about how well technology can replace roles that were previously only completed by trained and experienced clinicians. With any new technology, there is always a learning curve, one that many physicians feel takes time away from the care of the very patients they are trying to heal. There also remains the Luddite concern of self-obsolescence due to technology. Physicians train for years and apply human judgment to their patient's ailments. Surrendering any critical thinking or data analysis regarding chronic disease management is a huge leap of faith for healthcare teams. These valid concerns and hesitations are what health tech companies must consider when developing novel hybrid healthcare solutions. The best tools are the ones that enhance the role of the physician rather than replacing it as outlined in Chap. 13 on Consumer Centricity. If a certain technology does not allow for human interpretation and follow through, this leaves room for error, lack of judgment as well as a lack of overall empathy towards the patient and their family.

When companies employ a hybrid technology approach that can work seamlessly alongside physicians, this is where the magic happens. The hybrid approach in Fig. 10.3 works best when technology supports physicians in task completion and data analysis which saves them time. Time to focus on their patients and their families, time to focus on management planning, and time to support the best outcomes for everyone involved. While digital healthcare solutions continue to enable personalized and detailed care for patients, a balance must be struck between machine and man when it comes to managing complex chronic conditions and diseases. A hybrid approach is required—one that seamlessly connects physical touch and attention with digital tools and innovations.

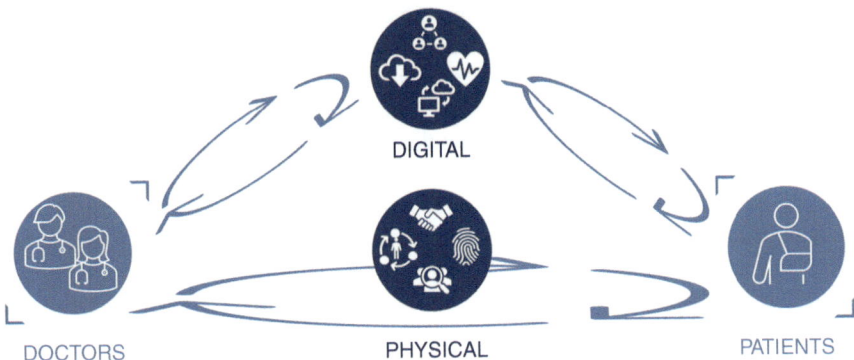

Fig. 10.3 Doctor–patient interaction in a hybrid way

The Promise of New Technology in Managing the Largest Chronic Diseases: Heart Health, Cancer, Diabetes

With new technology development, there is a renewed hope that chronic disease detection, treatment, and management can become an attainable goal for patients and healthcare systems. Advances in the world of cancer screening and treatment, cardiovascular status monitoring with wearable technology, and personalized diabetes management are all improving how chronic conditions are diagnosed, treated, and managed. Reliable remote monitoring has become even more important in the era of COVID-19. Remote patient monitoring programs can track symptoms, vital signs, and monitor for deterioration all digitally which is crucial when dealing with such a contagious disease [13].

Heart Health

Nearly 18 million people die from cardiovascular diseases worldwide, making it the most prevalent cause of death globally. Heart attacks and strokes make up the majority of these deaths, many of which are caused by preventable risk factors [3]. Smoking cigarettes, excess use of alcohol, poor diet, and limited exercise all contribute to a person's risk for developing heart disease and other chronic conditions that can lead to cardiovascular dysfunction [3]. A key aspect of successful cardiovascular disease management beyond treating modifiable risk factors, as with all chronic disease management, is prompt, accurate monitoring. Continuous monitoring of cardiac function as well as a patient's overall functional status can provide physicians with key metrics to assess response to treatment and predict outcomes when it comes to cardiovascular disease.

Pacemakers and other implantable devices have been around for a long time and even can transmit data remotely via a patient's smartphone. As far as wearable devices, the Holter monitor has been a standard in cardiovascular monitoring from an electrical standpoint, but the device is bulky and cumbersome to wear [14]. Due to its size and the requirement of at least two leads attaching to the chest, Holter monitors are not ideal long-term wearable device. There have been advances in wearable cardiovascular monitoring devices including devices as small as fitness bands, patches, headbands, and even necklaces to collect data [23].

Wearable technology and digital biomarkers are making their path quickly into the clinical field to support physicians: In a recent study, using biosensors and digital biomarkers assess Response to Cardiac Rehabilitation (CR), physicians found that when using wearable sensor technology, the differences in response of patients to cardiac rehabilitation can be characterized by means of commonly used heart rate parameters and digital biomarkers that are representative of cardiac response to exercise. These digital biomarkers, derived by innovative analysis techniques, allow for more in-depth insights into the cardiac response of cardiac patients during standardized activity [15]. These results give physicians the opportunity to more patient-tailored treatment strategies and potentially improve CR outcome.

But current wearable technology does not "only happen in the clinic". It has made its path into allowing physicians to "look into our everyday life" to monitor heart rate and rhythm, blood pressure, stress, respiratory rate, oxygen saturation, and more [23]. These devices use various types of technology to collect data including accelerometer-based approaches that interpret movement to predict parameters such as heart rate [23]. .The Zio patch by iRhythm is a continuous cardiac rhythm monitor in the form of a patch, which can be worn for up to 2 weeks and generates continuous data for the duration and has in many instances replaced the aforementioned Holter monitor as a new gold standard of cardiac care [16]. The downside is that the data cannot (yet) be interpreted in real time, but it substantially informs the patient/physician interaction [24].

The NUVANT Mobile Cardiac Telemetry monitor goes a step further and access patient data in real time and immediately inform the physician in case of abnormalities. The small wireless patch detects electrocardiography (ECG) activity and transmits it to a diagnostics laboratory for analysis [17]. It's one thing for the physician to view the information, but to give the patient both control and peace of mind can help improve overall compliance. It may also take away time burden from the physician as the patient gets enabled to monitor their own cardiac care.

In the case of the Apple Watch, patients are fully enabled and can react on the data the device provides. It can also help physicians treat heart disease. The Apple Heart Study assessed the smartwatch's ability to detect an irregular pulse to identify dangerous arrhythmias like atrial fibrillation [18]. Over 400,000 smartwatch wearers participated, and the results found the watch to have a positive predictive value 84% of the time. While the percentage of participants who had an irregular pulse notification was low, 76% of those who received an alert contacted their physician [28]. This shows the potential benefit of encouraging patients to contact their physicians and increasing engagement in patient driven care for cardiovascular conditions [28]. This feature of the watch has been cleared and approved by the federal Food and Drug Administration (FDA) therefore giving physicians the assurance of the quality of the data. Here, the benefit for patient and physician becomes most apparent: Essentially the data upgrades the protocol from a simple punctual examining to a continuous tracking and immediate detecting. It allows for self-assessment by the patient with clear evidence—it also allows the physician to essentially "go back in time" should the punctual data generated at the physician office not be conclusive, thus resulting in incredible improvement for patients.

Huma has even gone a step further and created a digital 'hospital at home' that uses real-time health data from smartphones to help patients and physicians to enable longer lives. The app does not only collect and analyzes data. It also shares it with physicians. In addition, it allows the patient and physician to interact via video calls. Therefore, the physician can provide the patient feedback on when data has been reviewed but also "jump on a video call" to discuss implications and decide on next steps—all by saving time and improving quality of care [26]. By using digital biomarkers, unbiased information about the patient status can be obtained to better predict outcomes and to create personalized treatment. And beyond that, the large volume of data collected can be used for further development of life saving and life improving applications for patients, especially in those with chronic conditions [19].

Beyond monitoring heart rate, also other technologies make their strive into the medical field to support physicians in their aim of taking care of their patients. They may be as simple as text messaging: Text messaging programs designed to support smoking cessation have been used for several years at this point. A systematic review found that patients who used a text messaging program were nearly twice as likely to quit smoking after 6 months compared to those not using the program [20]. Physical activity is also increased when text messaging programs are used to support patients. Step count and heart rate can both be monitored with wearable pedometers and accelerometers devices, and when patients use text messaging-based programs, there are significant increases in steps per day [29]. The 2015 TEXT ME study showed extreme promise in reducing several risk factors of chronic disease [29]. This study took place over 6 months and patients who used the text-based program had reductions in cholesterol, blood pressure, body mass index (BMI), reduced smoking rate, and increased physical activity [29]. Patients in the group were three times more likely to achieve control over multiple risk factors and participants found the program useful and engaging [29]. Not only are the specific results impressive. The ability to automatize the collection of longitudinal data opens new horizons for the physician: A better basis for decision making as data gets automated collected and curated but also: Potential indications for other comorbidities, focus on interpreting the data and discussing its implications with the patient and not on collecting it. It highlights one of the main levers to fight chronical diseases—the interaction between physician and patient. By using digital technologies, physician and patient maximize time together and can immediately react to changing conditions or challenges—even if it may only be a positive message and encouragement to keep trying to stop smoking.

With elderly patients, less "tech-savvy", physicians may experience more challenges to leverage data from an i-Watch or use texting apps to interact with. But here, too, physicians start to team up with new technologies: Ambient sensor systems are increasingly used to monitor seniors in their apartment not only for safety reasons but more recently to detect patterns indicating serious mental or physical problems. These sensors are unobtrusive and allow for privacy and independence. First findings indicate great potential of contactless pervasive computing systems for detection of early signs of serious health problems such as heart failure decompensation [21].

Apps, wearables, digital biomarkers and many more innovations are making their path into the "toolset" of the physician to treat heart disease. The biggest impact lies most likely in combing this arsenal of digital tools in a hybrid approach as they together provide a more much holistic picture of the state of a patient. By implementing wearing technology and interactive digital solutions, both the patient and physician gain valuable insight into maintain their chronic heart condition and avoiding slipping into an acute abyss.

Chronic Cancer Care

Cancer is one of the leading causes of death worldwide. Nearly ten million people died of cancer in 2020 with breast, lung, and colon cancer being the most diagnosed cancers [22]. Early detection can make the difference between curable cancer and one that causes chronic, life-threatening complications. By detecting and diagnosing cancer early with screening tools, more patients can be cured and avoid these complications, including an early death. The World Health Organization states that detecting cancer early should be a priority for all cancer programs, regardless of the cancer. By reducing delays and removing barriers to cancer-related care can reduce cancer mortality. This is done with early diagnosis as well as screening [13]. Increasing early diagnosis involves educating patients on signs and symptoms of cancers that should trigger an evaluation by a physician. It also entails providing timely access to diagnostic services and clinical evaluations [13]. Routine screening programs should be made available to at risk patients as another part of early detection. With digital and technological advances in cancer screening, many barriers including lack of resources or complex testing can be addressed [13].

By identifying cancer in its earliest stages and continuously monitoring it as show in Fig. 10.4, successful treatment and the potential for cure are much greater. Identifying pre-cancerous cells can be even more beneficial in truly preventing cancer from ever developing. Many health technology companies are working towards innovative ways to detect cancer before spread or even development. Not only is early detection the goal, but so is finding minimally invasive screening techniques.

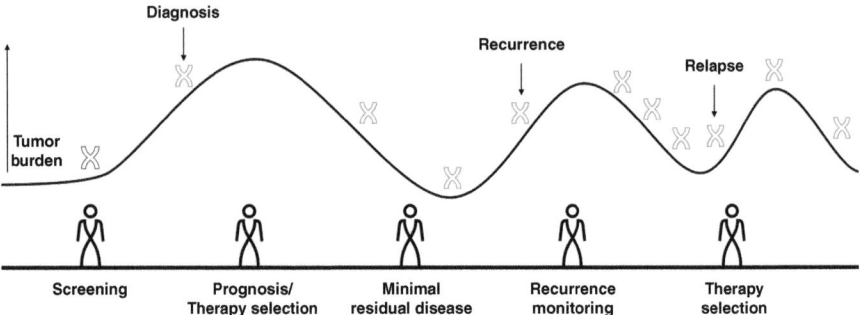

Fig. 10.4 Detecting cancer earlier at every stage, starting with screening [23]

Colorectal cancer is the third most common cancer worldwide [24]. Colorectal cancer is also one of the deadliest cancers and is the third most common cause of cancer related death in the United States [25]. Traditional screening methods, including digital rectal exams and colonoscopies are considered invasive and unpleasant. Colonoscopies carry the risk of complication for sedation, missing work for the procedure, not to mention the cumbersome full bowel cleansing required before the procedure [26]. There is also a risk of bowel tears and perforation during the test [16]. This leads to patients avoiding or delaying screening due to apprehension about the screening method itself. According to the American Cancer Society, only 56% of Americans aged 45 years and older reported being up to date with colorectal screening in 2018 [16]. Frequency intervals, which in the case of colonoscopy, can be up to 10 years make the physician's life harder: Less interaction with the patient, less data points and substantially decreased ability to detect illnesses early, e.g., miss the cancer developing from a pre-cancer state. Non-invasive blood tests can turn this around—from providing the physician information every 10 years with a colonoscopy, a simple blood test can provide information annually as part of the yearly health check-up. In addition, while a colonoscopy is only a visual exam, blood-based tests provide molecular information, enriching data sets for decision making at physician level.

Universal Diagnostics is one such company and is creating minimally invasive colon cancer screening tests to address this apprehension. Their Signal-C is a blood test that reaches accuracy for colorectal cancer detection at par with a colonoscopy but makes it much easier for physicians to convince patients to do it, as it is a non-invasive blood based test [27]. Therefore, physicians will spend less time convincing patients to "do it" and can use their time with the patient to focus on more essential topics.

By focusing on minimally invasive ways to screen for cancers, physicians can collect data on a much more frequent basis, providing more focused monitoring for at-risk patients. This data tracking also allows for a bigger picture analysis to make more informed treatment decisions. Results from blood tests like Universal

Diagnostics, Guardant Health, Grail, Burning Rock, and Freenome are simple to understand and highly accurate—providing a reliable tool for physicians to incorporate into their daily practice [19].

Proactive blood testing is also used in oncology to monitor patient progression and response to treatment. Rather than relying on colonoscopies as an invasive procedure in the case of colorectal cancer or imaging scans which require millions of cancer cells before being detectable—measuring minimal residual disease (MRD) allows physicians to monitor disease more closely.

MRD is commonly used to monitor blood cancer response including acute lymphoblastic leukemia as well as chronic leukemia and lymphoma. As the strongest prognostic indicator, MRD has become standard in oncology care to drive decision making including treatment and surveillance decisions [28]. Its testing frequently uses DNA sequencing including analyzing methylation profiles to measure disease. This same technique is being used to help determine risk as well. China's Burning Rock is exploring how DNA technology can help detect cancer early in the Pan-Cancer Early Detection Project [29]. Minimum residual disease tests substantially improve patient experience—often avoiding invasive procedures and improving data and information level for the physicians [26]. This is one of the main reasons why the Chinese lung commission endorsed a blood based tests to help predict risk for relapse for early stage non-small cell lung cancer patients [29]. It allows the physician to apply the data for a much more tailor made approach at scale, e.g. adjusting frequency, types of testing procedures depending on the status of the patient. As an example—minimal residual disease monitoring moves from "colonoscopy only" to "blood testing 2–3 times annually, year over year with a colonoscopy only when needed". The physician's role is enhanced in not only improving outcomes but also the patient experience. In addition, the physician can now spend more time with the patient which so substantially increases the patient experience as part of a hybrid healthcare approach.

Physicians are also supported in treatment decisions leveraging artificial intelligence techniques like deep learning and machine learning, more accurate interpretations of mammograms and magnetic resonance imaging (MRI) are possible. With AI technology, tumor and tissue characteristics can be more closely evaluated and characterized to assist with staging, segmentation, and even generating genomic data [30]. In order for the physician to effectively use all this information and tailor treatment plans for patients to improve the outcome versus creating a chronic cancer condition, it is important to create a holistic and always up-to-date view of the cancer patient's journey. The multidisciplinary care teams need to be supported by relevant technology, which enables them to focus on providing the best possible cancer care due to the oncology specific clinical decision support that brings together all relevant information for the patient, A.I., from the medical field, latest research, clinical trials and from the patients (including PROMs into the entire process).

Diabetes

Over 400 million people worldwide have diabetes with type 2 diabetes being the most prevalent compared to type 1 diabetes. Deaths related to diabetes have increased with a 5% increase in premature mortality related to diabetes from the year 2000 and 2016 [31]. Diabetes is a chronic disease and one that many people spend years attempting to manage. Consequences of unmanaged diabetes include vision and kidney problems, heart attacks, strokes, and lower limb amputations [29]. Uncontrolled diabetes can cause financial strain to patients related to medication costs, costs of managing complications, and loss of the ability to work due to disability [29].

Lifestyle modifications continue to be the best way to manage diabetes and prevent any related complications. Early diagnosis and screening can also improve blood sugar control and reduce the impact of complications related to uncontrolled diabetes. This includes blood sugar testing, retinopathy screening, kidney monitoring, and foot care [29]. Managing diabetes and the chronic complications caused by diabetes can be overwhelming for a physician and their team. Similar to cardiovascular disease, the amount of monitoring that must be done, often on a multiple times per day basis, can lead to manageable amounts of data to sift through.

There are several hybrid health companies focusing on diabetes management including remote monitoring and support for physicians and patients. Omada Health is one such company that provides a diabetes program to help patients seize control of their chronic disease and improve outcomes [32]. They provide members with access to a diabetes care team and coaches to address blood sugar control, medication management, physical activity, and much more. This is done via connected devices to monitor blood sugar and matching patients with certified diabetes specialists [30]. The app-based platform used is protected under health insurance portability and accountability act (HIPAA) compliant technology to share information securely [30].

Another approach is an initiative by medtech giant Medtronic called Diabeter, which is focused on improving remote diabetes management for type 1 diabetes which tends to affect children more often making them a unique patient population to manage remotely [33]. Remote blood sugar monitoring with or without an insulin pump is also incorporated. By enabling this remote monitoring, physicians can develop completely new approaches with their patient population: In this specific example, they can give children the opportunity to stay and play at home rather than spend time in physician practices. In fact, when patients use Diabeter, they have a decreased risk of hospitalization thanks to the increased support for both patients and caregivers at home. There could hardly be more encouraging news.

As with cardiovascular monitoring, providing patients access to their own information and data is a way to empower them to take control of their chronic disease. Far too often patients feel helpless and hopeless when it comes to chronic conditions that must be managed and prioritized for an indefinite period of time. Livongo (which was acquired by telemedicine pioneer Teladoc in 2020) provides diabetes as well as blood pressure remote management tools to patients and providers. By using their app, patients can track trends when it comes to their blood sugar, blood pressure, and weight [34]. Patients upload their information and instantly receive an automated tip or piece of encouragement. They can also send their information to their healthcare team if they choose [31]. Another benefit is that patients can potentially have access to free blood glucose monitoring supplies such as strips and monitors. This is possible due to insurance coverage or employer coverage [35]: To enroll in Livongo for Diabetes, a patient must have a diagnosis of type 1 or type 2 diabetes, and be eligible through his or her employer or health plan. For example, the Centers for Medicare and Medicare Services have recognized Livongo as an enrolled provider for Medicare Advantage members, making Livongo's diabetes management available to Medicare Advantage members receiving care through a Cambia Health Solution regional health plan [36].

South African insurance company Discovery offers its Diabetes Care Programme, together with registered General Practitioner to actively manage diabetes. The programme gives the patient and the GP access to various tools to monitor and manage the condition to track progress through personalized dashboards. The programme also unlocks cover for valuable healthcare services from healthcare providers like dietitians and biokineticists and access to diabetic retinopathy screening [37]. Many of these services are offered remotely. And studies continue to show the benefits of remote monitoring programs focused on supporting patients living with diabetes. Hemoglobin A1c (HBA1c) levels are improved, and treatment satisfaction is just as good for those using remote monitoring compared to if patients were attending a specialty diabetes center [38]. When patients use remote patient monitoring to manage their diabetes, patients are more engaged which leads to better blood sugar management [39].

The Future of Remote Health Monitoring

Remote monitoring and digital tools are currently being used to improve care for patients with chronic conditions. Health technology companies continue to revolutionize how patients and physicians use technology to connect, organize, and structure chronic disease care. Remote monitoring and remote chronic disease management combines patient-reported outcomes measures (PROMs) and biometric data to better inform everyone involved in the patient care setting. Health technology companies are taking monitoring a step further by combining PROMs with genomic advancements. These advancements contribute to the development of precision medicine for chronic disease and condition management. This also includes implementing a holistic approach to patient care. Just because something is based in technology, does not mean it omits the key factors of what makes humans, human; primarily empathy, emotion, and stress.

Calibrate is a health technology company focused on what they consider to be the 'four pillars of metabolic health'. This includes emotional health, diet, sleep quality, and exercise when it comes to weight management [40]. Their program is 100% virtual and consists of medication management, blood work and laboratory value management, and telehealth visits [35]. Intuition Robotics takes remote care a step further with their personalized care 'companion' ElliQ, which focuses on empathy, relationship building, and increasing patient engagement when it comes to health management [41]. ElliQ is targeted towards older adults who need assistance maintaining independence at home. Patient activity can be monitored, patients can communicate directly with their healthcare team through ElliQ and social companionship can be achieved with this innovative device [36]. Not only is patient engagement a focus but the device can also alert healthcare teams or caregivers if anomalies in behavior are detected. This can provide an additional layer of security if someone with a chronic condition lives alone as well as help them maintain independence without sacrificing safety [36].

Challenges to Technology Implementation

While technology devices and tools in healthcare help address common barriers to chronic condition management, new challenges to overcome arise. Sometimes, it may be as simple as lack of internet. Access to remote solutions may not always be available, especially in lower income counties and areas. As many of the digital technology and remote data sharing programs rely on internet access, either through home-based internet or cellular based access through smartphone carriers, access to digital healthcare solutions may in many cases be limited by the underlying internet access [42]. 4.66B people, 60% of the global population, have access to internet and as global economic development advances, so will internet access and healthcare.

These digital technologies generate an unprecedented amount of data, which needs to be understood, interpreted, and acted upon by both the patient and the clinical community. This responsibility largely stays with physicians—this is why the "teaming up" between physicians and technology is so essential. Those digital solutions that combine great value add and an outstanding user experience, will most likely thrive in the world of hybrid healthcare. Almost every physician is also a smart phone user in his/her private life and used to a seamless, easy to understand, and fast to use device—digital healthcare solutions should aim for that to enable teaming. For physicians, the evolving path of grabbing the innovative technologies, get used to them, and above all engage with them with a positive and open mindset are critical.

With the advent of a large volume of apps and platforms, the question of regulation, oversight and true clinical effectiveness comes into play—which will ultimately be linked to reimbursement. It should not be left to physicians and healthcare teams to determine which platforms and technology have been vetted and verified without spending time exploring every single option, but rather clear regulatory standards as in other fields of medical practice are needed.

While COVID-19 accelerated many of the regulatory processes for digital health solutions, there remains a gap in what is acceptable from both a legal and medical standpoint. Countries like the United Kingdom have implemented programs like the Accelerated Access Review which aims to prioritize technology innovations. This initiative pours money into programs to support technology advancements to try and implement tools as quickly as possible [43]. But the choice of what programs and what technology to use, ultimately falls to the physician and their clinical team. They must determine what programs they wish to utilize, what data to include, and how to best react to the data.

Integrated healthcare ecosystems such as Lilly Diabetes is a hybrid approach where patient data and physician intervention are more closely connected. Lilly hopes their Connected Diabetes Ecosystem will provide a platform to connect patients, caregivers, and physicians with the latest technological advances and medical management options available [44]. As is the case with most successful hybrid platform, there is strong consideration of human behavior. Patients and healthcare teams must both learn how to navigate the hyper connected environment and develop protocols to communicate effectively and interpret data safely.

Evolving the Physician's Role

The role of the physician and other healthcare providers continues to evolve with technology. Traditional methods of chronic disease management, although helpful, are proving to be unsustainable in an aging population requiring more resources and assistance. Technology provides solutions to compliment the physician role rather than replace it. There is already a surplus of patient needs, especially in the chronic condition patient population, so it can not be overstated that the role of health tech is not to replace but is to support. Health technology has the potential to save time and improve patient care, but, the physician will be needed even more. With massive amounts of data and organization needed, physicians will have an even closer look into the health of their patients—a look that was only a dream in the not too distant past.

By implementing digital health technology solutions, physicians must apply their data interpretation skills more rapidly, to include patients not on their clinic schedule for the day. Remote monitoring can close an information gap, but someone still has to take the time to interpret the data. And if the goal is to keep patients out of the clinic as often (and out of the hospital) as possible, more information will be coming to physicians and their staff regardless of the day or time. While AI algorithms and parameter settings can help manage large amounts of data, for digital healthcare to make a difference, integration is key. Studies continue to show if digital health solutions are created to support both the patient and the physician, outcomes improve across the board. An example is the use of digital glucose monitoring technology. Endocrinologists were enrolled in the trial to implement digital monitoring for their patients with long term diabetes and researchers found that care was more effective and more individualized with the digital technology [45]. Patient engagement and health outcomes were also improved. But the barriers of reimbursement and a lack of standardization continue to leave areas of improvement with this type of technology [40].

Addressing the obstacle of reimbursement, the joint project called Target:BP by the American Heart Association and the American Medical Association are providing tools to improve blood pressure control in Americans [46]. Target:BP focuses on accurate blood pressure measurement, rapid treatment plan intervention, and partnering with patients and physicians to control blood pressure. The self-measured blood pressure device allows patients to take control of their blood pressure monitoring and helps physicians better track and diagnose at-risk patients [41]. Creating platforms, ecosystems, and models that facilitate ways to organize this new level of connectivity often falls on the physician. This has become so vital that organizations like the American Medical Association (AMA) are creating networks to connect physicians and health tech companies [47]. The Integrated Health Model Initiative aims to improve health outcomes by partnering physicians with reliable health care data. This AMA initiative helps organize data from remote monitoring and other devices for physicians to access, exchange, and act upon [42].

In Germany, Dr. Jürgen Schäfer created thirty-one centers focused on rare disease management. By creating these centers, patients can be seen by a variety of specialists to help identify and diagnose difficult cases [48]. While these centers are providing a vital service for patients in the area, Dr. Schäfer admits that they have to limit the amount of inquiries they receive as they only have so many resources. His Center for Unrecognized and Rare Diseases could be a great example of how a multidisciplinary approach could benefit from integrating with digital health tools and tech.

Conclusion

When it comes to chronic disease management, digital technology solutions have the potential to unlock fantastic opportunities. But as with all advances, they are not the sole solution but rather a supportive tool for clinicians who must incorporate them into a hybrid approach. This means there will be growing pains and adjustments as clinical teams work to incorporate time saving and efficiency improving technology models into their daily practice. Digital tech in healthcare creates endless opportunities to support clinicians, not replace them. Robotic surgery devices in the operating room cannot (yet) provide complex surgical judgments but AI and other tech could still provide assistance to physicians inside the clinic. Technology, wearables, and AI can also provide much needed insight into the health of chronic patients. This insight can support physicians and their clinical decision making to create profound improvements and advances in the complicated world of chronic disease management.

This technology enriched hybrid approach may even 1 day help patients and physicians uncover underlying risk factors or even conditions before they have a chance to express themselves physically into symptoms, thus truly preventing disease and reducing the economic strain of chronic disease management. The future of chronic condition management includes incorporating hybrid health technologies and protocols so that clinicians are enable to spend more time with the patients, who need their guidance, empathy, and attention.

References

1. Buttorff C, Ruder T, Bauman M. Multiple chronic conditions in the united states. Rand Corporation; 2017. https://www.rand.org/content/dam/rand/pubs/tools/TL200/TL221/RAND_TL221.pdf. Accessed 10 Sept 2021
2. Centers for Disease Control and Prevention: about chronic diseases. 2021. https://www.cdc.gov/chronicdisease/about/index.htm. Accessed 10 Sept 2021.
3. World Health Organization: cardiovascular diseases. 2021. https://www.who.int/health-topics/cardiovascular-diseases#tab=tab_1. Accessed 10 Sept 2021.
4. World Health Organization: Cancer. 2021. https://www.who.int/health-topics/cancer#tab=tab_1. Accessed 10 Sept 2021.
5. Martin A, Hartman M, Lassman D, Catlin A. National health care spending in 2019: steady growth for the fourth consecutive year. Health Aff. 2020;40(1):14–24. https://doi.org/10.1377/hlthaff.2020.02022.
6. World Health Organization: Obesity and overweight. https://www.who.int/news-room/fact-sheets/detail/obesity-and-overweight. Accessed 10 Sept 2021.
7. Global alliance for chronic diseases. https://www.gacd.org/research/what-are-ncds/chronic-diseases-fact-sheet.
8. Agency for Healthcare Research and Quality: multiple chronic conditions chartbook. 2010. https://www.ahrq.gov/sites/default/files/wysiwyg/professionals/prevention-chronic-care/decision/mcc/mccchartbook.pdf. Accessed 10 Sept 2021.
9. Suhrcke, M, Nugent, R, Stuckler, D, Rocco, L. Chronic disease: an economic perspective. Oxford Health Alliance 2006. https://www.who.int/management/programme/ncd/Chronic-disease-an-economic-perspective.pdf. Accessed 10 Sept 2021.
10. Gheorghe A, Griffiths U, Murphy A, Legido-Quigley H, Lamptey P, Perel P. The economic burden of cardiovascular disease and hypertension in low- and middle-income countries: a systematic review. BMC Public Health. 2018;18:975. https://doi.org/10.1186/s12889-018-5806-x.
11. OECD: health at a glace 2017: OECD indicators 2017. https://www.oecd.org/germany/Health-at-a-Glance-2017-Key-Findings-GERMANY.pdf. Accessed 10 Sept 2021.
12. Brunner-La Rocca H, Fleischhacker L, Golubnitschaja O, Heemskerk F, Helms T, Hoedemakers T, et al. Challenges in personalized management of chronic diseases-heart failure as prominent example to advance the care process. EPMA J. 2016;7(1):2. https://doi.org/10.1186/s13167-016-0051-9.
13. Huma: Huma's remote patient monitoring solution. https://huma.com/covid-19/healthcare. 2021. Accessed 10 Sept 2021.
14. Sana F, Isselbacher E, Singh J, Heist K, Pathik B, Armoundas A. Wearable devices for ambulatory cardiac monitoring. J Am Coll Cardiol. 2020;75(13):1582–92. https://doi.org/10.1016/j.jacc.2020.01.046.
15. De Canniere, H. et al. Using biosensors and digital biomarkers to assess response to cardiac rehabilitation: observational study. 2020. https://www.jmir.org/2020/5/e17326/. Accessed 12 Sept 2021.

16. Zio by iRhythm: single-use cardiac monitoring. 2021. https://www.irhythm-tech.com/?utm_term=zio%20patch&utm_campaign=alwayson-branded&utm_source=google&utm_medium=cpc&utm_content=branded&hsa_acc=7527145821&hsa_cam=7130733808&hsa_grp=102556240540&hsa_ad=437862180880&hsa_src=g&hsa_tgt=kwd-513105067374&hsa_kw=zio%20patch&hsa_mt=e&hsa_net=adwords&hsa_ver=3&gclid=CjwKCAjwvuGJBhB1EiwACU1AiSSFHZMGKes-us6rnZ1_pbiIKOCuc546nP--uu_K_PvZoplAMz5ZgdxoCfnEQAvD_BwE. Accessed 10 Sept 2021.
17. Cardiac Monitoring.com: NUVANT mobile cardiac telemetry (MCT) monitor. 2021. http://cardiacmonitoring.com/mobile-cardiac-telemetry/companies/corventis/nuvant-mobile-cardiac-telemetry-mct-monitor/. Accessed 10 Sept 2021.
18. Perez M, Mahaffey K, Hedlin H, Rumsfeld J, Garcia A, Ferris T, et al. Large-scale assessment of a smartwatch to identify atrial fibrillation. NEJM. 2019;381:1909–17. https://doi.org/10.1056/NEJMoa1901183.
19. Huma: life sciences. 2021. https://huma.com/life-sciences/digital-biomarkers. Accessed 10 Sept 2021.
20. Santo K, Redfern J. Digital health innovations to improve cardiovascular disease care. Coronary Heart Disease. 2020;71. https://link.springer.com/article/10.1007/s11883-020-00889-x. Accessed 10 Sept 2021
21. Saner, H et al. Case report: ambient sensor signals as digital biomarkers for early signs of heart failure decompensation. 2021. https://www.frontiersin.org/articles/10.3389/fcvm.2021.617682/full. Accessed 12 Sept 2021.
22. World Health Organization: Cancer. https://www.who.int/news-room/fact-sheets/detail/cancer. 2021. Accessed 10 Sept 2021.
23. Exact sciences - detecting cancer earlier at every stage https://s22.q4cdn.com/877809405/files/doc_presentations/2021/Exact-Sciences_v3.pdf.
24. World Cancer Researcher Fund: colorectal cancer statistics. https://www.wcrf.org/dietandcancer/colorectal-cancer-statistics/. 2018. Accessed 10 Sept 2021.
25. Centers for Disease Control and Prevention: colorectal cancer statistics. 2021. https://www.cdc.gov/cancer/colorectal/statistics/. Accessed 10 Sept 2021.
26. American Cancer Society: colorectal cancer facts & figures 2020–2022. https://www.cancer.org/content/dam/cancer-org/research/cancer-facts-and-statistics/colorectal-cancer-facts-and-figures/colorectal-cancer-facts-and-figures-2020-2022.pdf. 2021. Accessed 10 Sept 2021.
27. Universal diagnostics: signal-C. 2021. https://www.universaldx.com/multicancer-platform#signalc. Accessed 10 Sept 2021.
28. Van Dongen JJM, van der Velden VHJ, Bruggemann M, Orfao A. Minimal residual disease diagnostics in acute lymphoblastic leukemia: need for sensitive, fast, and standardized technologies. Blood. 2015;125(26):3996–4009. https://doi.org/10.1182/blood-2015-03-580027.
29. Genomeweb: burning rock details plans for cancer monitoring assay, adds new data supporting early detection. 2021. https://www.genomeweb.com/business-news/burning-rock-details-plans-cancer-monitoring-assay-adds-new-data-supporting-early#.YT2N8p37Q2w. Accessed 12 Sept 2021.
30. Bi WL, Hosney A, Schabath M, Giger M, Birkbak N, Mehrtash A, et al. Artificial intelligence in cancer imaging: clinical challenges and applications. CA Cancer J Clin. 2019;69(2):127–57. https://doi.org/10.3322/caac.21552.
31. World Health Organization: Diabetes. 2021. https://www.who.int/news-room/fact-sheets/detail/diabetes. Accessed 10 Sept 2021.
32. Omada: Omada for diabetes. 2021. https://www.omadahealth.com/programs/diabetes. Accessed 10 Sept 2021.
33. Diabetes: who we are. 2021. https://diabeter.nl/en/about-diabeter/who-we-are/. Accessed 10 Sept 2021.
34. Livongo: take charge of your health. 2021. https://hello.livongo.com/GEN/TLD. Accessed 10 Sept 2021.
35. Livongo: diabetes made easier at no cost to you. 2021. https://hello.livongo.com/DBT?vwo=154_c. Accessed 10 Sept 2021.

36. CMS approves Livongo as enrolled provider for medicare advantage. https://www.mobihealth-news.com/content/cms-approves-livongo-enrolled-provider-medicare-advantage. Accessed 20 Sept 2021.
37. Discovery: diabetes care program. https://www.discovery.co.za/medical-aid/diabetes-cover. Accessed 20 Sept 2021.
38. Amante D, Harlan D, Lemon S, McManus D, Olaitan O, Pagoto S, Gerber B, et al. Evaluation of a diabetes remote monitoring program facilitated by connected glucose meters for patients with poorly controlled type 2 diabetes: randomized crossover trial. JMIR Diabetes. 2021;6(1):e25574. https://doi.org/10.2196/25574.
39. Su D, Michaud T, Estabrooks P, Schwab R, Eiland L, Hansen G, DeVany M, et al. Diabetes management through remote patient monitoring: the importance of patient activation and engagement with the technology. Telemed JE Health. 2019;25(10):952–9. https://doi.org/10.1089/tmj.2018.0205.
40. Calibrate: how it works. 2021. https://www.joincalibrate.com/how-it-works. Accessed 10 Sept 2021.
41. Intuition robotics: better care starts with empathy. 2021. https://www.intuitionrobotics.com/healthcare. Accessed 10 Sept 2021.
42. UNESCO: startling digital divies in distance learning emerge. 2020. https://en.unesco.org/news/startling-digital-divides-distance-learning-emerge. Accessed 10 Sept 2021.
43. Asthana S, Jones R, Sheaff R. Why does the NHS struggle to adopt eHealth innovations? A review of macro, meso and micro factors. BMC Health Services Researcher. 2019;984. https://bmchealthservres.biomedcentral.com/articles/10.1186/s12913-019-4790-x. Accessed 10 Sept 2021
44. Stat: the promise of technology to help solve chronic disease management challenges. 2021. https://www.statnews.com/sponsor/2018/03/07/technology-chronic-disease-management-lilly-diabetes/. Accessed 10 Sept 2021.
45. May S, Huber C, Roach M, Shafrin J, Aubry W, Lakdawalla D, et al. Adoption of digital health technologies in the practice of behavioral health: qualitative case study of glucose monitoring technology. J Med Internet Res. 2021;23(2):e18119. https://doi.org/10.2196/18119.
46. Target:BP: BP improvement program. 2021. https://targetbp.org/blood-pressure-improvement-program/. Accessed 10 Sept 2021.
47. American Medical Association: integrated health model initiative. 2021. https://innovation-match.ama-assn.org/groups/ihmi-community/pages/landing-page. Accessed 10 Sept 2021.
48. Research for rare: German networks on rare diseases. 2021. https://www.research4rare.de/en/centers-for-rare-diseases/. Accessed 10 Sept 2021.

Chapter 11
Industry Regulations and Approvals to Enable Hybrid Healthcare

Reenita Das and Deenah Zayed

Abstract The pandemic facilitated adoption of hybrid models across many different industries including healthcare. The difference in healthcare however was the need to provide a holistic and an integrated care experience across different settings (inpatient, outpatient, and home care departments) without losing any of the richness of the patient experience throughout the patient journey. This chapter discusses several debating points and challenges that stakeholders across the healthcare industry have been coming across in the past year and a half with the rise of hybrid healthcare. Many of those challenges do not have solid answers; however, the chapter sheds light on aspects that need to be zoomed into to enable us to build successful hybrid care models. Topics discussed revolve around workflows, staffing models, digital infrastructure, patient engagement and experience, and regulations & reimbursement:

- Workflows: what kind of workflows do we need for a successful hybrid care model and how do we integrate digital models into existing clinical workflows in a sustainable way?
- Personnel: how do we optimize staffing models, and ensure proper training to reduce resistance?
- Digital infrastructure: how do we build tools that are secure, interoperable, flexible, and user-friendly?
- Engagement and experience: what are some practical initiatives that healthcare providers can implement to enhance short-term patient involvement and long-term patient empowerment?
- Regulations & reimbursement: how do we ensure patients can afford hybrid health services? What regulatory changes are needed to continue to incentivize models that provide superior care at a lower total cost?

Keywords Integrated care · Resistance · Training · Data security · Data storage Interoperability · Experience · Engagement · Adherence · Regulations

R. Das · D. Zayed (✉)
Healthcare and Life Sciences, Frost & Sullivan, Dubai, United Arab Emirates
e-mail: rdas@frost.com

© The Author(s), under exclusive license to Springer Nature Switzerland AG 2022
M. Al-Razouki, S. Smith (eds.), *Hybrid Healthcare*, Health Informatics, https://doi.org/10.1007/978-3-031-04836-4_11

Introduction

The COVID19 pandemic has taught us a multitude of lessons in a few months that we would have otherwise learnt in three to 5 years. We first thought that telemedicine was easy, providers did it on a dime overnight and some even went from 2% telemedicine to 60% and everyone wondered why we never did this before. Then we started to realize that the difficulty behind it was putting together a holistic and an integrated care experience across inpatient and outpatient departments as well as those patients receiving care at home- all without losing any of the richness of the patient experience. That is when things got complicated and we realized how much more logistics, orchestration and a combined experience were required to make it effective [1].

This chapter will tackle several big questions and challenges that providers, payers, and innovators have been experiencing in the past year and a half and what still needs to be done to enable us to build successful hybrid care models [2].

These questions include

- Workflows: what kind of workflows do we need for a successful hybrid care model and how do we integrate digital models into existing clinical workflows in a sustainable way?
- Personnel: how do we optimize staffing models, and ensure proper training to reduce resistance?
- Digital infrastructure: how do we build tools that are secure, interoperable, flexible, and user-friendly?
- Engagement and experience: what are some practical initiatives that healthcare providers can implement to enhance short-term patient involvement and long-term patient empowerment?
- Regulations & Reimbursement: how do we ensure patients can afford hybrid health services? What regulatory changes are needed to continue to incentivize models that provide superior care at a lower total cost?

Workflows

It is crucial for organizations to establish comprehensive and interconnected patient workflows to support the combination of virtual and in-office appointments. Once telehealth services were implemented rapidly at the start of the pandemic, many providers faced challenges in keeping patient flow moving and making the process as simple as possible for patients, as they were learning to navigate between an in-person and virtual journey.

Patient scheduling is the first part of a patient's journey, but one of the most critical touch points. The first step required to enable patients to smoothly create, modify, or cancel appointments is to provide ways to educate them on how to use online scheduling tools effectively. This can be done through simple videos or brochures

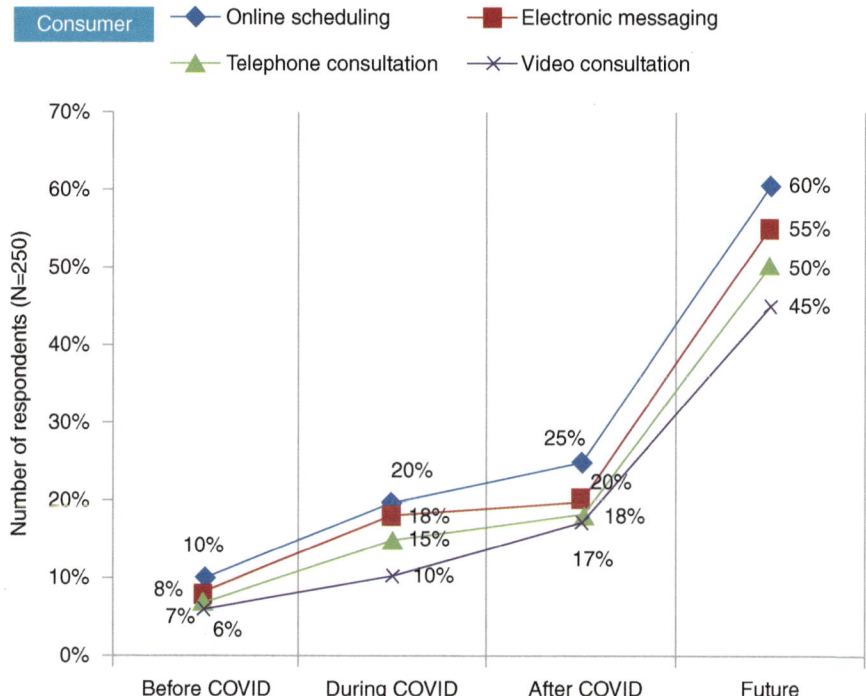

Fig. 11.1 Top digital health technologies, US, 2020–2025. Source: [3]

on providers' websites demonstrating the process. As shown in Fig. 11.1, based on Frost & Sullivan's analysis, online scheduling is the top digital health technology used by consumers and physicians before, during and after the pandemic and therefore providers should ensure that the process for scheduling an appointment is easy for patients, whether over the phone or through a computer or a smartphone. Another challenge that patients face is deciding which type of care needs could be met virtually and which ones need to be addressed in person. Thus, proper information collection when scheduling an appointment could make the process more efficient by directing patients to the proper channel of care.

Incomplete patient information is another sudden challenge that rose with the spike of telehealth services. Patient registration is needed to capture a wide range of data that is needed in both patient care and the billing process that follows. Patient registration during in-person visits is done by trained front desk staff and therefore all required data is captured. However, with virtual visits, due to the lack of digital tools, patients tend to provide incomplete forms and outdated payer information, leaving medical office staff scrambling for workarounds through manual processes and patient outreach. Based on best practices, capturing information should be done prior to a patient appointment, whether a patient is being seen virtually or in-person. To ensure a smooth registration process, online forms should be clear and easy to use and also have a shared interface across all platforms.

Providers who have already been using automated appointment reminders recognized the need to customize and provide proper directions for patients who are receiving care services via telehealth. Patient reminders no longer compromise the date, time, and physician's name only; the notifications should include a telehealth link or directions for the telehealth appointment as well. Reminders should also allow two-way communication to enable patients to confirm, reschedule, or cancel their appointments which in turn needs to be integrated to the scheduling system for automated workflows and easier access to patient replies.

Virtual waiting rooms are also confusing to patients when they wait too long. Unlike in-person visits, patients who wait for too long are not able to get reassurance that they are going to be seen and at the same time, they do not feel pressured to wait as they had not been through the inconvenience of making the journey to the doctor's office. Thus, when virtual waiting rooms are not managed properly, patients tend to drop out.

Other gaps in the workflow include proper communication between patients and providers. Quick and constant communication is key. Medical organizations who turned to a hybrid model struggle to keep patients informed about changes in their offices and ways to access care. Along with telehealth solutions, providers need means and tools to communicate which locations are seeing patients in-person and which ones have closed or are not accepting COVID cases. A great example as such is the Dubai Health Authority. They constantly communicate changes through their social media platforms and provide updates on all the public hospital offerings in Dubai from telehealth, home care services, and home delivery service. Similar to other industries, patients should be able to communicate with their medical providers and staff via text. Two-way patient communication is crucial during the transition into hybrid care so that patients are able to navigate through new processes in a simpler way and can have all their questions answered along the way [4].

Personnel

Having the right personnel on board and training them is essential for the safety and satisfaction of patients. It should be provided to all staff members who are expected to participate in the hybrid healthcare model. This includes personnel responsible and involved in in-person visits, virtual visits, virtual waiting room engagement (including the telehealth coordinator), care team members, and technical, billing, coding, and compliance staff [5, 6]. Although it completely depends on a health organization's needs, care team and staff members for a hybrid system often include the clinical roles and responsibilities shown in Fig. 11.2 [5, 6]. This challenge can be addressed by proper training on handling both clinical and social needs of patients regardless of where and how care is provided.

When looking at telehealth adoption, many believe the main challenge with providers is resistance to change especially amongst the less tech-savvy, older medical workforce. However, younger clinicians who are more open to accepting and

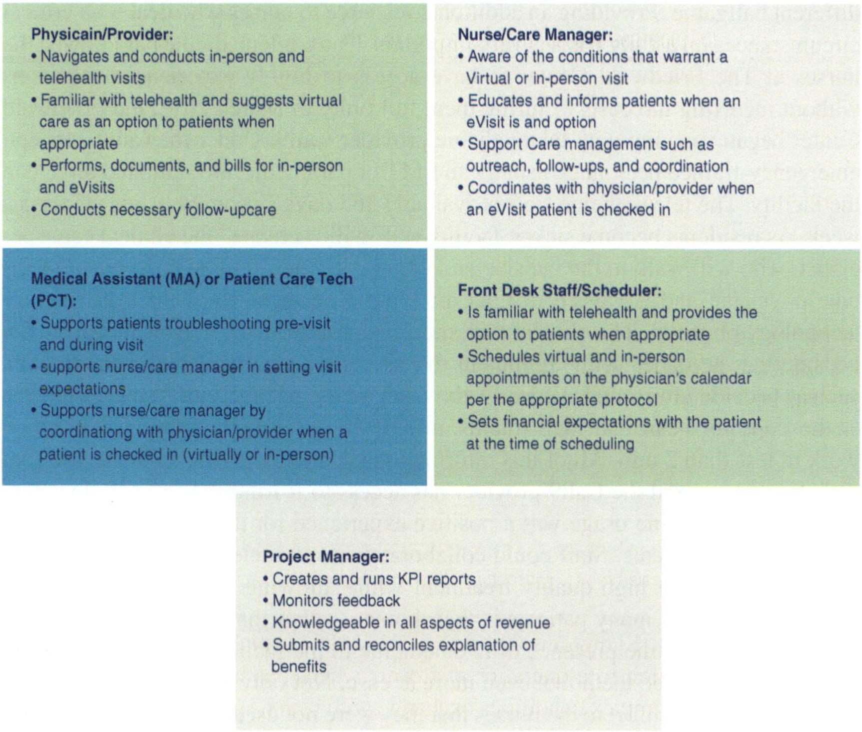

Physicain/Provider:
- Navigates and conducts in-person and telehealth visits
- Familiar with telehealth and suggests virtual care as an option to patients when appropriate
- Performs, documents, and bills for in-person and eVisits
- Conducts necessary follow-upcare

Nurse/Care Manager:
- Aware of the conditions that warrant a Virtual or in-person visit
- Educates and informs patients when an eVisit is and option
- Support Care management such as outreach, follow-ups, and coordination
- Coordinates with physician/provider when an eVisit patient is checked in

Medical Assistant (MA) or Patient Care Tech (PCT):
- Supports patients troubleshooting pre-visit and during visit
- supports nurse/care manager in setting visit expectations
- Supports nurse/care manager by coordinationg with physician/provider when a patient is checked in (virtually or in-person)

Front Desk Staff/Scheduler:
- Is familiar with telehealth and provides the option to patients when appropriate
- Schedules virtual and in-person appointments on the physician's calendar per the appropriate protocol
- Sets financial expectations with the patient at the time of scheduling

Project Manager:
- Creates and runs KPI reports
- Monitors feedback
- Knowledgeable in all aspects of revenue
- Submits and reconciles explanation of benefits

Fig. 11.2 Hybrid Care Staff & Care Team roles & responsibilities. Source: [5, 6]

adopting technology have faced the same challenge. For any kind of treatment, drug, medical device or even protocol, the medical community is heavily reliant on evidence-based practices. Similar to patients, the entire medical workforce was not keen on a hybrid health system previously as there was barely any proof of the effectiveness of telehealth services. When the pandemic came along however, and there was no other option, organizations started using telehealth services and they realized its effectiveness in terms of patient responsiveness as well as medication adherence which created an overall positive impact on their health outcomes. Now that health organizations had a taste of this success, acceptance has increased tremendously and more telehealth services and providers are coming up.

To examine this further, let us look at the example of how The Friedwald Center, a 180-bed skilled nursing facility in New York City, optimizes operational resources with telemedicine. Across the US, there are more than 15,500 skilled nursing facilities providing rehabilitation-based care and assisting with Activities of Daily Living (ADLs) to over 1.35 million patients according to Commonwealth Medicine [7].

The Friedwald Center wanted to use telemedicine to grant its patients faster access to high-quality clinicians who are familiar with acute care. A nursing home doctor or medical director is typically a family practitioner who is well-versed in nursing home rules. That's a far cry from emergency medicine and a completely different ballgame. Providing an additional resource to nurses who deal with critical circumstances on a daily basis is very important. Thus, telemedicine has allowed the nurses at The Friedwald Center to have access to highly experienced clinicians without incurring the costs of hiring them full time. In March 2018, the Friedwald Center began working with telemedicine provider Call9. Under the Call9 concept, emergency-trained personnel, usually an EMT or paramedic, are stationed on-site in the facility. The telemedicine staff is available 365 days a year, 24 h a day, 7 days a week. As residents become sicker, facility staff will "activate" the clinical care specialist, who will walk to the bedside and connect to their remote emergency medicine physician and advanced practice provider care team via Call9's proprietary technology platform. The clinical care specialist also brings a diagnostic cart to the bedside that is loaded with equipment that is not usually available in the facility, such as bedside ultrasound, 12-lead EKGs, telemetry, pacing, vital signs, electronic stethoscope for heart and lung sounds, urinalysis, and on-site point-of-care blood work in less than 2 min. All of this information is entered into the clinical care specialist's system, and the Call9 provider has access to it from their remote location. Overall, telemedicine usage was a positive experience for the center and a significant benefit to patients. Staff could collaborate with the telemedicine team to provide residents with high-quality treatment while allowing them to remain in the facility—which for many patients is their home—rather than travelling to the hospital. Furthermore, the presence of telemedicine in the facility has boosted nurses' confidence and made them feel even more at ease. Not only did it educate and provide a degree of comfort to the nurses that they were not used to, but it also provides that extra level of support [8]. Although Call9 cared for tens of thousands of people and reduced unnecessary hospital transfers by approximately 80%, it was not able to receive proper reimbursement due to restrictions in telemedicine payment back in 2019. The pandemic however caused Medicare and the Federal Government to realize the life-saving value of solutions like Call9, and to approve reimbursement for services provided remotely. Thus, Curve Health was founded in March of 2020, amidst the Covid-19 pandemic and expanded on the Call9 platform. Curve Health not only enables telemedicine, but establishes a true virtual hospital-level care experience for patients and providers in nursing facilities [9].

Digital Infrastructure

Technology plays a critical part in the growth of the hybrid healthcare market. Sensors, communication technology, Big Data, and artificial intelligence have come a long way in terms of infrastructure and equipment. Whether the usage of technology is linked to improving the accessibility of care, or overall reduction of healthcare costs, lack of proper data connectivity, interoperability, security, and lack of ICT infrastructure is proving to be a major impediment in the general adoption of new-age technologies for successful hybrid healthcare deployment.

Given the complexity and amount of interconnected systems, cyber security is becoming increasingly important. Patient adoption of telemedicine is hampered by concerns regarding confidentiality, data security, and storage, as the lack of rigorous data protection legislation and data sharing regulations may lead to commercial or malevolent use of patient data. Early on in the pandemic, it became evident that several services, such as Zoom, were not up to HIPAA security standards. Patients require their clinicians to use encrypted, password-protected platforms, despite Zoom's security improvements. Despite the existing HIPAA flexibility, providers should maintain strict standards in protecting patient privacy and security to maintain patient trust. It is vital to implement a system to detect and prevent breaches when sending electronic Protected Health Information (ePHI). All potential dangers to the integrity of ePHI, particularly virtual environment modifications or end user hazards, must be considered. If a provider or third-party contractor works from home and is connected to a hospital network, it is vital that they are properly safeguarded against cyber-attacks. VPNs are one of the most prevalent, secure solutions for accessing remotely to an enterprise network, according to HEALTH IT SECURITY. However, despite repeated warnings and accessible updates, corporations have been failing to address core vulnerabilities detected in some of the most popular VPNs. Thus, to provide extra protection against cyber-attacks, providers could consider using two-factor authentication. They should also have a clear plan in place to handle security and privacy issues, as well as ways to preserve patient security and soothe potential fear [5, 6]. It is also important to note that patients, like clinicians, require data-privacy education and training when accessing their Wi-Fi network for a telehealth session. They should make sure that the bare minimum clinicians who are needed to treat their disease have access to their information [10].

Increased access to quality care and the development of a successful hybrid health ecosystem requires ubiquitous, adequate, and affordable broadband to facilitate telehealth and health information exchange. This, on the other hand, is a universal challenge that everyone is working to address. As such, in rural areas of the United States, the Federal Communications Commission started enrolling qualified households in its Emergency Broadband Benefit ("EBB") program. Eligible households can receive a $50 monthly discount on their internet plans (or a $75 monthly discount if they live on tribal territories). The EBB also includes funding for a one-time discount of up to $100 for qualifying households on a tablet, computer, or other specified equipment. The EBB initiative also provides a long-term opportunity to prioritize the extension of broadband connectivity in the United States, particularly in rural areas where infrastructure is weak [11].

In addition to security and data connectivity, interoperability is another technology related hurdle for implementing a successful hybrid health care system. Interoperability is the ability to transmit data between applications such as electronic health record (EHR) systems and other health IT applications like clinical decision support (CDS), computerized physician order entry (CPOE) systems, and other healthcare-related systems. With data management and AI-powered analysis, tech companies have attempted to improve data sharing, but providers and payers continue to struggle with securely and effectively sharing medical data. Interoperability can be achieved in several ways. The most effective approach is to use Application programing interface (APIs). APIs can be established to allow access to everything from basic data collections to entire program operations. Other methods of data exchange rely on the interchange of data files that are formatted in a standard way. The US Department of Health and Human Services has issued new standards and promoted the Fast Healthcare Interoperability Resources (FHIR) standard in healthcare. FHIR is a data exchange framework developed by the High Level 7 organization that, while currently limited in its capacity to handle unstructured data, provides a platform on which to build more robust data exchanges. Finally, several EHR application and data analysis providers are beginning to embrace interoperability as a core part of their legacy IT products. EMR vendors are leaving no stone unturned to demonstrate superior data interoperability features in accordance with the needs of payers, providers, and government agencies, whether through integration with multiple healthcare information exchange (HIE) platforms or the development of third-party applications through open API architecture.

The healthcare interoperability growth is driven mainly by regulatory constraints that tend to favor IT pathways that allow for smooth patient data exchange, transfer, and download across the treatment continuum as shown in Table 11.1. For many health IT applications, interoperability has become a significant consideration as major healthcare stakeholders around the world recognize the need to invest in digital infrastructure capabilities that enable cross-continuum patient information interchange and scale-up evidence-based care [3].

Engagement and Experience

Patient-centered engagement methods have become more crucial to hospitals and medical practices as a result of the emergence of healthcare consumerism (discussed in more detail in a later chapter). Any channel of care, regardless of its scale, staffing structure, or patient demographics, should be designed to engage patients in their own care, empower them to modify lifestyle behaviors, and give them more control over their condition. It is common to assume that a virtual visit will lack a sense of human connection and cause patient satisfaction concerns, as patients and clinicians communicate through a video screen, and visits are shorter than traditional in-person appointments. Therefore, it is the need of the hour to implement effective engagement tools and strategies with all current and future patient characteristics in mind.

Assessing individual needs and tailoring information to each patient are key goals of not just providers, but also payers, pharmaceutical companies, and medtech companies. Figure 11.3 shows how patient engagement can help deliver measurable business outcomes for all healthcare stakeholders. For the sake of this section however, we will only look at some digital solutions that healthcare providers can use to increase patient engagement in a hybrid system ([13].

Table 11.1 Healthcare interoperability market: drivers of interoperability, global, 2019–2024

Regions	Major Drivers of Healthcare Interoperability	Revenue contribution in 2019	Revenue contribution in 2024	CAGR (2019–2024)
North America	• Regulatory mandates and incentives for patient-centric care and quality reporting • Improved patient awareness about the need to access medical records pre, during, and post care • Prevalence of cloud-based digital health platforms that drive population, health management and chronic condition management at a regional level • Adoption of visionary healthcare interventions (e.g. precision medicine) that thrive on multidisciplinary patient data	$2854.8 Million	$5112.8 Million	12.4%
Europe	• Regulatory requirements, coupled with centralized governance and incentive framework (primarily UK and Scandinavian countries) for cross-country healthcare interoperability • Positive consumer opinion about General Data Protection Regulation (GDPR) aiding provisions for standard healthcare interoperability guidelines	$623.8 Million	$1264.7 Million	15.2%
Asia-Pacific	• Public funding to build national healthcare interoperability infrastructure (India, Japan, Singapore, China) • Ad-hoc investment in localized healthcare interoperability solutions by large hospitals, major players, and top ICT companies	$397.3 Million	$988.2 Million	20.0%
Latin America	• Public policies that drive adoption of cloud-based healthcare solutions for the purpose of connecting regional electronic medical records (EMRs) that allow multiple payers and providers to collaborate with each other	$83.3 Million	$151.7 Million	12.7%

Note: Base year is 2019. Rest of World (RoW) contributes $208.4 million in 2019 and will contribute $447.7 million in 2024 at a CAGR of 16.5%
Source: [3]

Patient engagement in hybrid systems has become more attainable due to digital technologies. Digital health tools that enable and strengthen patient engagement include online patient portals, mobile health applications, wearable devices, remote monitoring devices, telehealth services, electronic health records (EHRs), and other integrated tools, as well as medication adherence/reminder solutions.

So how can providers harness technology to improve patient engagement in a hybrid system?

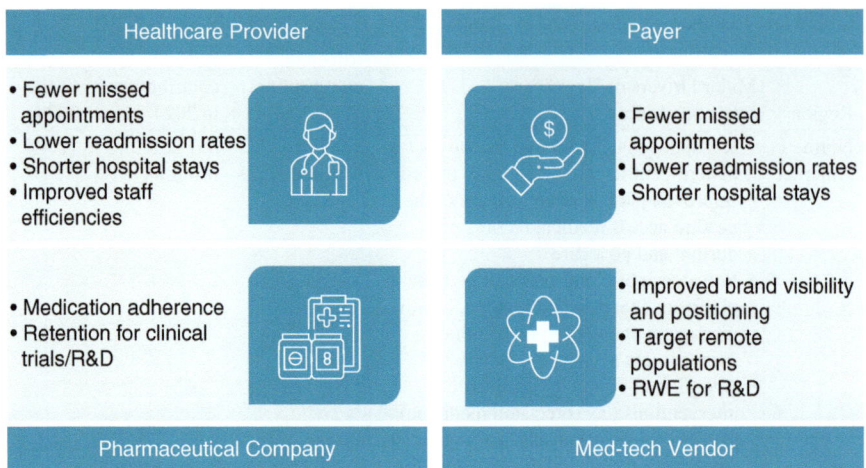

Fig. 11.3 Outcomes of patient engagement on various stakeholders. Source: [12]

Providing digital tools for accessing and managing care: Consumers expect to interact and transact through the internet. They're used to seamless, intelligent, and technologically enabled experiences like receiving suggestions based on past purchases or securely transferring payments via a smartphone app. That is the norm to which all healthcare providers must adhere. During COVID-19, many providers used apps to help triage and streamline care, allowing patients to use digital solutions to choose the right channel, book an appointment, check symptoms, initiate online visits, access their health history, manage prescriptions, get preventive care reminders, monitor their health, and estimate health care expenses.

Delivering care anywhere, anytime: We live in an instant-gratification, on-demand environment. Although not all healthcare can be provided on those terms, new entrants to the industry are focusing on how to match consumer demand for convenience. Extending and tailoring in-home monitoring to an individual's needs is one example. Providers can use wearables and new generations of in-home equipment to capture and set baselines for a single person, then monitor for data that are unusual for that person. Identifying and examining signs that are specific to a person, such as small changes in blood oxygen levels, would set new standards for engagement, early intervention, and improved outcomes. Therefore, forward-thinking companies are exploring new hybrid care models that combine telehealth, in-home care, Rx fulfillment, and traditional care delivery to provide consumers with what they need, when they need it, regardless of channel.

Simplifying billing for patients: Following severe losses from deferred elective and wellness procedures, healthcare providers are retooling their business offices to improve cash flow. Healthcare businesses can use contemporary revenue cycle management (RCM) to help patients better understand their financial obligations, read bills, make payments, take advantage of tailored payment plans, and receive other communications—all through a convenient, online experience. This also has a potential to be part of a more automated, end-to-end RCM procedure that enhances the financial health of the provider [14].

Regulations and Reimbursement

When discussing regulations related to hybrid healthcare, virtual care is the main concern. Every country has its own set of regulations for virtual care. For the sake of simplicity however, let us examine the regulatory landscape in the United States specifically. Even then, it is important to note that Telehealth policy trends vary from state-to-state, with no two states alike in how telehealth is defined, reimbursed or regulated. Before looking at where the country stands now, let us take a quick review of telehealth regulations:

- Bipartisan Budget Act 2018: A federal law that makes telemedicine treatment and coverage more widely available. It primarily concerns Medicare, and it outlines telemedicine care for kidney and stroke care in particular.
- Home Health Payment Innovation Act of 2019 (pending): The bill would grant Medicare enrollees' access to in-home healthcare services while also paving the way for new ways to use these services. It makes a number of modifications to how home health services are reimbursed and covered under Medicare and Medicare Advantage.
- Creating Opportunities Now for Necessary and Effective Care Technologies for Health Act of 2019 (pending): The act would allow the secretary of health and human services to waive any telehealth restrictions (geographic, originating site, modality limitation, provider type, and service requirements) given it would reduce spending without reducing quality of care or improve quality of care without increasing spending, or if it would apply to telehealth services furnished in originating sites. The secretary would be expected to develop a process for stakeholders to submit comments on the waivers and to post specific information about the waivers on the Centers for Medicare & Medicaid Services (CMS) website every 2 years.
- Interstate Medical Licensure Compact: Qualified physicians can now acquire licenses to deliver treatments in multiple jurisdictions according to the compact. The agreement will cover 29 states, the District of Columbia, and the US territory of Guam as of 2020. Patients in underserved or rural locations will benefit most from the growth in the number of eligible care providers because telehealth services will provide them with access to specialist care.
- Opioid legislative efforts: Several bills presented in Congress to combat the burgeoning opioid epidemic would expand access to telehealth services for Medicare drug abuse treatment.

On January 31, 2020, once the federal government declared COVID-19 a countrywide public health emergency, CMS added 135 services to Medicare telehealth, including emergency department visits, initial inpatient, nursing facility visits, and discharge day management services. The 2021 Physician Fee Schedule was then updated to indicate that 20 min of interactive communication time can include time spent examining and analyzing RPM data and care management via both in-person and connected channels. Both developments support a hybrid care model, with many hospitals attempting to take advantage of the reimbursement changes.

Despite the enormous value propositions a hybrid model could give, determining whether the costs will be borne by consumers or providers/payers is a significant challenge. Employers, insurers, and providers, rather than customers, are expected to pay for the majority of the technology, according to much consumer-led research. Telemedicine reimbursement and coverage that is similar to in-person services is a major cost for the industry and payment parity between telemedicine and in-person health care is not guaranteed. Even in the 28 states where payment parity rules have been enacted, there is no system in place to implement them. This might possibly negate the goal of telemedicine, which is to lower health-care costs and increase access to services, as well as deter clinicians from giving telehealth because similar remuneration is not assured [15].

The applicability of having a hybrid health care system has been inhibited for years due to state and federal funding constraints, which has been cited as a major hurdle for telemedicine initiatives. However, there has been tremendous progress in recent years. Previously, Medicare billing criteria required that the telehealth visit take place in a Health Professional Shortage Area (HPSA) and at an approved originating site, such as a doctor's office, hospital, or skilled nursing facility. This completely negated any benefit of telehealth as a home option, virtual care visit, or reimbursement that was limited to specific HCPCS and CPT codes. CMS temporarily increased Medicare reimbursement for applicable services in response to the COVID-19 outbreak, allowing all Americans to access telemedicine. This increase now allows Medicare to pay for virtual visits regardless of location, even at a patient's home, and allows a larger range of providers to offer these virtual visits. Furthermore, congress provided $200 million in funding to healthcare providers to create and implement virtual care services, thus strengthening the future of telehealth [5, 6].

Some regulatory reforms established during COVID-19 that made telehealth more accessible have been made permanent. In the final rule for the 2021 physician fee schedule, CMS, for example, made telehealth coverage permanent for a number of current procedural terminology (CPT) codes. When the public health emergency ends, however, some telehealth restrictions may revert to pre-COVID-19 levels. In addition, a waiver for public health emergencies permitted Medicare beneficiaries outside of rural areas to receive telehealth services from their homes rather than from a provider's office. It is yet to be seen what will happen to these measures after the public health emergency is over [12].

Figure 11.4 shows a country-by-country comparison of telehealth uptake, reimbursement relaxation, and stakeholder buy-in on telehealth continuity after COVID

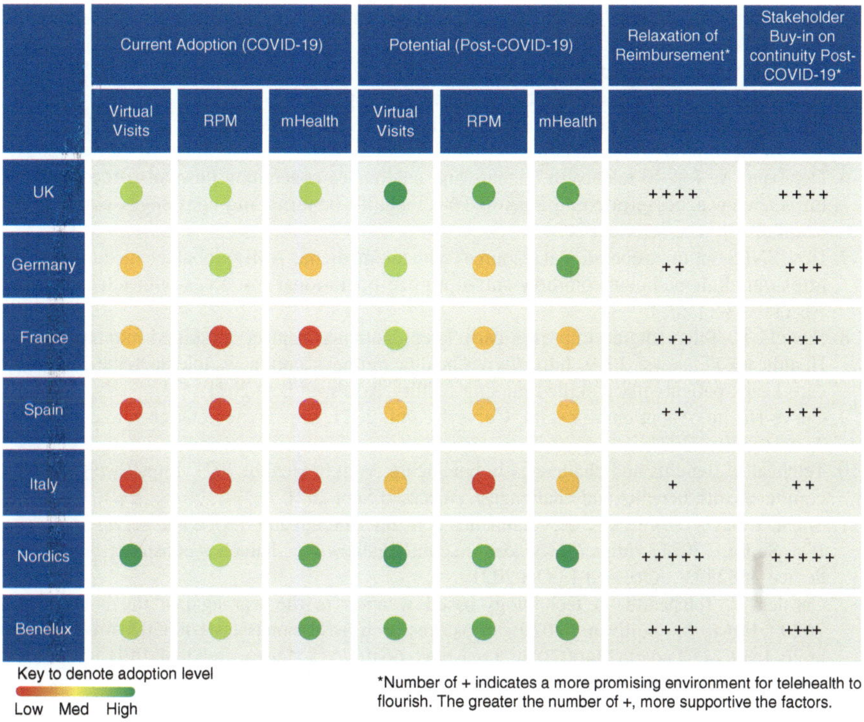

	Current Adoption (COVID-19)			Potential (Post-COVID-19)			Relaxation of Reimbursement*	Stakeholder Buy-in on continuity Post-COVID-19*
	Virtual Visits	RPM	mHealth	Virtual Visits	RPM	mHealth		
UK	Med	Med	Med	High	High	High	+ + + +	+ + + +
Germany	Med	Med	Med	Med	Med	High	+ +	+ + +
France	Med	Low	Low	Med	Med	Med	+ + +	+ + +
Spain	Low	Low	Low	Med	Med	Med	+ +	+ + +
Italy	Low	Low	Low	Med	Low	Med	+	+ +
Nordics	High	Med	High	High	High	High	+ + + + +	+ + + + +
Benelux	Med	Med	High	High	High	High	+ + + +	+ + + +

Key to denote adoption level

Low   Med   High

*Number of + indicates a more promising environment for telehealth to flourish. The greater the number of +, more supportive the factors.

Fig. 11.4 Telehealth market: country comparison, Europe, 2020–2025. Source: [16]

across Europe. While the Nordics excelled out in terms of telehealth adoption during COVID-19, thanks to strong reimbursement and regulatory requirements that are likely to last post-pandemic, the UK is expected to dominate in virtual consultation adoption and Germany in mHealth adoption post-COVID-19.

In conclusion, connection, integration, and collaboration are the guiding principles to developing a successful hybrid care system, and patient engagement and outcomes should exist at the core. The points tackled in this chapter do not have simple solutions. Each organization has its own strategy and priorities. But solutions exist and innovation is occurring.

References

1. Holland M. Hybrid care is healthcare's future. SearchCIO. 2021. https://searchcio.techtarget.com/feature/Hybrid-care-is-healthcares-future. Accessed Sept 2021.
2. Antall P. Telehealth and the future of hybrid care. Oliver Wyman. 2020. https://health.oliver-wyman.com/2020/10/the-future-of-hybrid-care.html. Accessed Sept 2021.
3. Pathak R. United States healthcare consumerism growth opportunities. Frost & Sullivan. 2021. https://research.frost.com/assets/1/f0a502e4-4463-11e8-b626-1aa9f74f20ad/59dfdd38-

e065-11eb-a584-623587aee387/research?eui=9f91d4e6-40ff-11ea-9aa1-3e00d11ca22elogi
nas=falsesessionId=null.

4. Catron J. What is a hybrid patient care model and how to implement it. Relatient. 2020. https://
    www.relatient.com/hybrid-patient-care/. Accessed Sept 2021.
5. Delabano A. Best practices for building a telehealth team now. Accessfm. 2020. https://www.
    accessefm.com/blog/best-practices-for-building-a-telehealth-team-now. Accessed Sept 2021.
6. Delabano A. Top 10 telehealth benefits and challenges concerning hospitals. Access. 2020.
    https://www.accessefm.com/blog/top-10-telehealth-benefits-and-challenges-concerning-
    hospitals-0. Accessed Sept 2021.
7. How SNFS optimize operational resources with telemedicine. AMD global telemedicine. 2021.
    https://amdtelemedicine.com/how-snfs-optimize-operational-resources-with-telemedicine/.
    Accessed Sept 2021.
8. Siwicki B. Telemedicine improves care, keeps patients in place at skilled nursing facility.
    Healthcare IT News. 2019. https://www.healthcareitnews.com/news/telemedicine-improves-
    care-keeps-patients-place-skilled-nursing-facility. Accessed Sept 2021.
9. Curve Health. About curve health. Curve Health. 2021. https://www.curvehealth.com/about.
    Accessed Sept 2021.
10. Telehealth: Benefits and challenges in healthcare. Welkin Health. 2021. https://welkinhealth.
    com/telehealth-benefits-and-challenges/. Accessed Sept 2021.
11. Spencer-Davis C., Clerk L. FCC launches consumer broadband device and service program.
    JD Supra. 2021. https://www.jdsupra.com/legalnews/fcc-launches-consumer-broadband-
    device-3682893/. Accessed 13 Oct 2021.
12. Camlek V. Telehealth—a technology-based weapon in the war against the coronavirus,
    2020. Frost & Sullivan. 2020. https://research.frost.com/assets/1/f0a502e4-4463-11e8-
    b626-1aa9f74f20ad/cfa23460-885c-11ea-b0f1-66af07635d4c/research?eui=9f91d4e6-40ff-1
    1ea-9aa1-3e00d11ca22eloginas=falsesessionId=null. Accessed Sept 2021.
13. Kijne J. Tips to ensure telehealth patient engagement. HRS. 2020. https://www.healthrecov-
    erysolutions.com/blog/ensuring-telehealth-patient-engagement. Accessed Sept 2021.
14. Brock J. Using tech to improve patient engagement in the new normal. Becker's Hospital Review.
    2020.   https://www.beckershospitalreview.com/using-tech-to-improve-patient-engagement-
    in-the-new-normal.html. Accessed Sept 2021.
15. Challenges in the telehealth industry: UIC Health Informatics. UIC Online Health Informatics.
    2020.   https://healthinformatics.uic.edu/blog/challenges-facing-the-telehealth-industry/.
    Accessed Sept 2021.
16. Innovative business models powering the telehealth market in Europe. Frost & Sullivan. 2021.
    https://research.frost.com/assets/1/f0a502e4-4463-11e8-b626-1aa9f74f20ad/4ff3a7f8-6f
    2e-11eb-90ac-261f142dfec6/research?eui=9f91d4e6-40ff-11ea-9aa1-3e00d11ca22eaugSearc
    hTerm=telehealthpagename=homessokey=loginas=falsesessionId=. Accessed Sept 2021.

Part III
The Future of Hybrid Healthcare

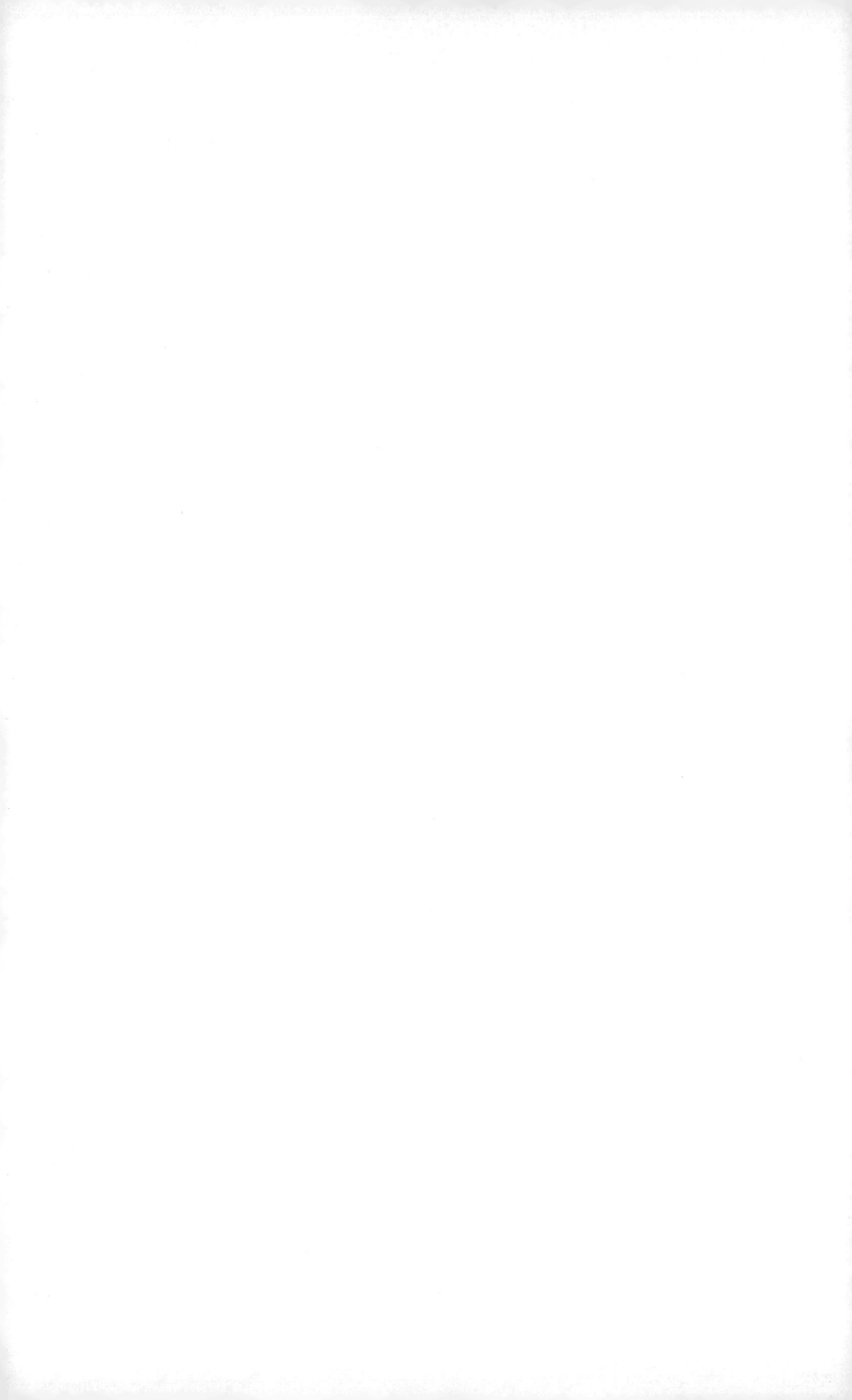

Chapter 12
Hybrid Genomics

Tariq K. Al-Shimmari

Abstract Genetic medicine has been long promised as the holy grail of precision, personalized medicine that has the capacity to treat most of humanity's bodily afflictions. The cost-reduction of direct-to-consumer (DTC) genotyping and sequencing technologies has led to greater consumer involvement with aspects of their health at extremely high resolution. Not only is personal genetic information accessible and available in a user-friendly manner, but it is pushing healthcare practitioners to hone their skills to deliver high-quality care. The impetus for pharmacogenomics developments is due, in large part, to how popularized DTC genotyping has become. DTC genotyping coupled with much publicized gene therapy tools such as CRISPR/Cas has spurred developments at unprecedented speed in the biopharmaceutical industry. Typical bottlenecks to these technologies are fast becoming a non-issue and humanity is on the way to fully realizing true precision, personalized medicine, and perhaps even one day erase our need for any form of healthcare, even the hybrid in nature.

Keywords Genomics · Gene editing · Gene therapy · Gene insertion · Crispr Genotyping · Direct to consumer (DTC) · Pharmacogenomics · Silencing

Introduction: The Human Instruction Manual

The Delphic maxim, *"Know thyself,"* is just one of 147 maxims ingrained in stone at the Temple of Apollo in Delphi yet has remained in our collective conscience for millennia. Some of the other aphorisms are hardly relevant to our futuristic, cognizant global society. *"Admire oracles"* or *"Master wedding-feasts"* have been cast to humanity's trash bin long ago. They did not communicate essential truths relevant to the species long-term. Indeed, *"Know thyself"* borders on a vapid platitude,

T. K. Al-Shimmari (✉)
Kuwait City, Kuwait

© The Author(s), under exclusive license to Springer Nature
Switzerland AG 2022
M. Al-Razouki, S. Smith (eds.), *Hybrid Healthcare*, Health Informatics,
https://doi.org/10.1007/978-3-031-04836-4_12

163

but reminds us of an essential learning: to keep our eyes (and mind) open so that we can tame our chaotic universe.

This is profoundly true in human health, where our control over wellbeing dwindles as our awareness of biology falters. We can't all be expert pathologists or surgeons and employ corrective measures when things go awry with our health. That doesn't mean non-experts are powerless—quite the contrary in today's world.

Health, like rocket science or advanced physics, can be probed by the billions of people on this Earth with their smartphones and wearable devices. Humans can gain an understanding of their biology at a level their ancestors could not fathom. This is real power, and we are undergoing a significant shift in this understanding with our knowledge of the human genome—the panoply of genes that comprise *us*. To *"Know thyself"* is becoming easier as technological and scientific advancements enable all of us to take charge of our own health and care.

Overview

It was only in 2003 that the Human Genome Project was declared "complete" (even though around 6% of has yet to be sequenced) after 15 years of work and three billion dollars. Until then, scientists and clinicians did not have a satisfactory picture of genes that make up our species. The reason for such an investment is clear: *the fundamentals of cellular processes are governed by DNA, so it follows that disease states are also governed, in large part, by DNA.* By leveraging newfound knowledge of human genetics, we can make strides in medicine only dreamed of by our forebearers, such as:

- Detecting predisposition to disease
- Improving treatment protocols for disease and delivering customized medicine
- Potentially curing disease

There is a whole host of applications to having such knowledge, especially outside the realm of human health. However, stewardship of genomic information comes with a large responsibility. The scope of this chapter is not to discuss the philosophical ramifications of genetic medicine, in the present or the future, but to inform you that genetic medicine is *here* and many of the concepts for future applications of it are inevitable. This chapter will emphasize how the traditional patient-physician relationship is changing drastically as patients are empowered with the ultimate data: their personal instruction manual.

The genetic medicine and information industry have a key responsibility to communicate what patient/customer genetic information means. Possessing genetic variants that predispose you to Alzheimer's disease (such as *APOE-ε4*) does not condemn you to this disease with 100% certainty. Alzheimer's disease is a coalescing of environmental/lifestyle factors in addition to genetics. Meanwhile, there exist single-gene diseases that can, in fact, condemn someone to a certain disease such as hemophilia, a disorder in which sufferers lack proper clotting factors to stop bleeding and heal wounds. Communication is important because millions now have access to cheaper genetic tests offered by companies like 23andMe. Thanks to these direct-to-consumer (DTC) genetic tests, genetic information has become democratized and is now a simple tap of the finger away for many. Yet, these DTC genetic tests are not useful for diagnostic or clinical applications. Either the science behind results is not in agreement, or the DTC technology itself is not completely accurate.

Despite these shortcomings, DTC genetic tests are still being utilized by consumers to inform them of their respective lifestyles. Many genetics and genomics apps on the market today are marketed as "wellness" apps that avoid making clinical assertions of the user's health and instead provide lifestyle suggestions [1]. Despite a lack of FDA approval and strict clinical relevance, wellness apps encourage users to take responsibility for the minutiae of their health. This not only serves the consumer, but the various stakeholders that have access to this valuable data. A nascent push to integrate genetic information with environmental data is underway which seeks to attain a greater scope of the human machine.

The mobile health (mHealth) industry produces wearables that track multiple health and non-health metrics (i.e. heartbeat and GPS location), enabling us to see both sides of nature versus nurture in relation to disease etiology. Coupled with powerful data analytics and machine learning algorithms, health data is invaluable and provides a more comprehensive picture of human health not only for the intended end user, but for healthcare professionals and researchers [2]. DTC services and genetics/genomics apps simplify data collection for researchers especially and allow better screening for candidates involved in clinical research. Predicting if a patient will react poorly to a specific drug is also an enormous asset that can streamline the time it takes for new treatments to arrive at market. Humanity's treatment protocols are becoming exceedingly diversified to not only utilize chemical pharmaceuticals, but to speak the language of human biology a little more clearly.

Gene therapy research, which was first initiated in 1989 presents a unique opportunity to alter the one-size-fits-all model of medicine [3]. The resolution of our biological understanding is far improved, so it follows that our treatment options also improve. Although gene therapy underwent a tumultuous and slow-going past, it is experiencing a renaissance due to widely publicized technology like CRISPR/ Cas that quicken the developmental pace. The ~5000 single-gene disorders in the human species are the low-hanging fruit we can collect in the coming years [4]. Multi-gene disorders, like Alzheimer's, Parkinson's, cancer, arthritis, type 1 and 2 diabetes, are vastly more complex and more time is expected for gene therapy to have clinical relevance with these conditions [5]. Gene therapy is only now making it to the clinic, and by extension in many patient's field of view. DTC services and genetics/genomics apps have enabled awareness of gene therapy, and in the coming year will play an essential role in hybrid healthcare.

In the coming years, will we "Know thyself" and leverage newfound knowledge ethically with eyes open? Or will we take the path that we have with our corn, tomatoes, and wheat and modify our most basic units?

Direct-to-Consumer Genotyping and Whole-Genome Sequencing

Direct-to-Consumer Genotyping

There is much debate over the disclosure of a patient's genetic information and the potential psychological harms it incurs [6]. Yet, people generally strive for a sense of control, even if illusory—having this sense of control over health can especially influence wellbeing [7]. A recent meta-analysis explored psychological outcomes of genetic test result disclosure and found patients generally desire information on their genome sequencing results even in the context of cancer, Alzheimer's, and Huntington's disease diagnoses [8–10]. Further, patients do not experience increased anxiety and depression from results disclosure. Interestingly, a trend towards *decreased* anxiety was noted in patients after they learned of their sequencing results. It is deceptively counterintuitive yet no small wonder that people prefer to feel a sense of control over their condition and treatment than to be subject to uncertainty.

Realizing the consumer's interest in their own genetic information, various companies have entered the genetic testing industry starting around 2007. Increased commercial investment in personalized genetic testing has now provided individuals with low-cost genetic data for the first time in human history. Direct-to-consumer (DTC) genotyping meant users did not have to visit a healthcare professional and spend exorbitant amounts of money to gain insight into their genetics, they simply had to spit in a tube and send it off to services like 23andMe and AncestryDNA. Saliva contains the user's DNA, which is then analyzed for single nucleotide polymorphisms (SNPs, pronounced "snips"). SNP genotyping is touted as a low-cost alternative to fully sequencing one's whole genome and involves taking "snapshots" of places in DNA that vary among human beings. Those variations can translate to functional differences in our biology. SNPs can affect how humans develop diseases and can provide insight into how an individual will respond to medications, vaccines, and even pathogens. Certain SNPs, for example, are associated with higher incidence of type 2 diabetes and high blood pressure [11].

DTC genotyping can be a robust way of informing users of health predispositions. 23andMe, for example, can notify users of genetic variants that are linked to increased or decreased risk for age-related macular degeneration, celiac disease, late-onset Alzheimer's disease, and more. DTC genotyping services stress their services are not for diagnostic purposes, and that lifestyle, environment, and family history play a significant role in disease pathogenesis. For diagnostics, users must obtain clinical confirmation through rigorous testing, as DTC genotyping is more prone to false-positive results; DTC genotyping also rarely test for all genetic variants related to a disease [12].

Despite DTC genotyping's clinical shortcomings, it has become a popular way to inform "wellness" practices. DNAfit, a DTC genotyping service, only reports to their customers of SNPs relevant to diet and exercise such as carbohydrate sensitivity and not SNPs that may be pathogenic. In this manner, laypeople are increasingly mindful of the abstract idea of genes and make subjective alterations to their lifestyles because of them. In everyday life, we are accustomed to categorizing physical features of one another, or ourselves, which are influenced by genetics. *"You have the eyes and nose of your father!"* Yet disease etiology concerning genetics is difficult to fathom—it is rarely visible. DTC services help in conceptualizing genes in the context of disease and are thus an invaluable asset to human understanding of health, which enables consumers to take ownership of their wellbeing. While DTC genotyping offers limited resolution compared to whole-genome sequencing (WGS), it offers cheap genetic information regarding an individual's propensity for diseases and traits. The logical next step in the consumer market, however, is to ask for more information that DTC genotyping cannot offer.

Whole-Genome Sequencing

DTC genotyping is limited in detail, as only a few locations in well-known genes are analyzed for SNPs. Whereas WGS provides information on the entire genetic data of an individual. Compared to the "snapshots" of DNA from DTC genotyping, WGS offers "high-definition video" of DNA that is ultimately more useful for conveying information to the end user.

The cost of sequencing the entire genome made more exceptional resolution of disease susceptibility nigh impossible in the past. The National Human Genome Research Institute (NHGRI) has tracked the cost of sequencing a human's genome since 2001, where the price per genome was upwards of $100,000,000. Now, roughly 19 years later, at the time of this writing, the cost per WGS is less than $1000, depending on the services used and is almost on par with the cost of DTC genotyping [13]. In the coming years this is important because customers will demand higher resolution and accuracy of their genetic makeup as the monetary divide between DTC genotyping and WGS sequencing narrows.

Companies like Veritas Genetics have streamlined WGS, making it progressively more cost-effective. In 2019, Veritas Genetics offered $200 WGS tests via clinics, which includes access to their user interface and video genetic counseling services. Customers gain access to all services touted by SNP genotyping, but also obtain more clinically relevant information about their health such as a more complete risk analysis for Alzheimer's. However, the drawback with WGS services is they require physician consultation to obtain.

WGS delivers much more practical information that can be used in the clinic, as it collects data on ~3bn base pairs as opposed to several million SNPs. The so-called "diagnostic odyssey" that patients with rare genetic diseases experience in trying to determine the cause of their disorder can be the most considerable impetus for WGS. This issue becomes exceptionally relevant in countries with poor access to expert physicians and high healthcare costs. In Mexico, WGS has been used as a first-tier test to elucidate rare pathologies [14].

Recently, the Rady Children's Institute for Genomic Medicine in San Diego utilized rapid WGS (rWGS) to reduce the mortality rate in infants with varied pathologies. rWGS enabled quicker detection of disease etiology, translating to reduced management costs (~$800k-2m saved) and reduced infant mortality [15]. The power of genetic medicine, and especially WGS, is limited by the availability of genetic counselors and the ability of healthcare professionals to understand, communicate, and make measured inferences about genetic data [16].

As sequencing technologies become cheaper, and the customer experience delivered by genetic medicine companies becomes more seamless and integrated with everyday life, there will be an inflection point. At this point, consumers will be heavily involved in understanding their health and can make more informed decisions for their treatment.

The All of Us Program

The private industry has been the arbiter of genetic medicine to the public and is reflected by the commercial successes of SNP genotyping. Still, the US government has initiated the ambitious All of Us research program that aims to improve precision medicine broadly. The program is unique in that it will integrate mobile and web apps, interactive voice response, and wearable sensors with genomics data and environmental/lifestyle data of one million participants (20% of which have signed up). The need for the program stems from a simple ethos: individual differences among the population must be accounted for to deliver better, more personalized care.

The roots of the All of Us program is in the Precision Medicine Initiative (PMI) working group under the Obama administration. The PMI working group identified the current need for concerted precision medicine developments, pointing to the fact that there are four billion prescriptions per year in the United States. Yet, there are varying responses to such drugs [17]. Furthermore, around 50% of hospitalizations due to adverse drug responses have no preventable cause, pointing to genetic differences in drug metabolism. The cost of adverse drug reactions is around $30bn per year globally [18]. Patients and the healthcare industry itself cannot afford to be imprecise any longer.

In 2019, the first 20% of participants had signed on to be a part of the All of Us program. The projected participation of one million citizens in the United States is a strategic number to reflect population demographics in the country accurately. The goal of the All of Us program will integrate vast data on human health to improve precision medicine with the direct involvement of the participants. The one million participant cohort will have complete access to their health record in the program and are encouraged to communicate their condition to healthcare professionals. The accessibility and transparency aspect of the program points to the shifting patient-physician policy, ushering in principles of hybrid healthcare where patients assume a more active role in the treatment and are treated as reputable sources of data for their care.

Pharmacogenomics

Pharmacogenomics (PGx) is a relatively nascent field examining how the human genome influences drug responses in patients. PGx measures two main principles influencing drug action: firstly, is pharmacokinetics or how an individual processes a drug, and second is pharmacodynamics or how a drug affects an individual's physiology. These two indices describe how drugs are handled by human physiology, but they can vary depending on genetics. A key enzyme for drug handling, for example, may possess a disadvantageous structure for certain drugs and thus an individual with such variation is sensitive to those drugs. This simplified example illustrates a fact: drug response is highly variable among the general population due to genetic variability [19].

Common nonsteroidal anti-inflammatory drugs (NSAIDs, specifically COX-2 inhibitors) have response rates of around 80%, while typical chemotherapy cancer drugs have a meager response rate of approximately 25% [20]. Indeed, many pharmaceuticals only possess physiological response rates of 50–75% in the general population. The varied response rates by physiology are also reflected in patient perception—only around 50% of patients believe their medication is helping their condition [21]. Taken together, drug response is a serious issue that affects treatment efficacy and patient wellbeing.

Response rate is not only an issue for patients who are receiving improper dosages of drugs, leading to adverse responses but also hospitals and clinics that lose resources and time on patient care. Since adverse drug responses are the sixth leading cause of death in the United States, it is paramount interest of the consumer and healthcare practitioner to break from the standard roles in the patient-healthcare professional relationship [22].

There are a variety of PGx services marketed to consumers directly, though most are offered through healthcare professionals and institutions. The single direct-to-consumer PGx assay is inclusive in products from 23andMe, which remains the only FDA approved DTC PGx test. However, information from 23andMe PGx is minimal and DTC PGx tests have been criticized for their accuracy, quality, and the high chance for misinterpretation of results, thus sabotaging patient engagement [23]. Therefore, the industry has been comprised of "direct-to-physician" PGx tests that are used by healthcare professionals to augment their patient care. The demand for DTC PGx tests has been high, though, and instead of limiting consumers' access totally so they cannot conceptualize their biology, some experts suggest keeping physicians as the gatekeepers of PGx test *approvals* [24]. Physicians must have an active role in PGx testing lest patient information is misinterpreted by patients on their own.

PGx tests are typically patient requested, as clinicians are apprehensive about employing PGx for a variety of reasons. Clinicians mainly cite a lack of knowledge of PGx and concern over long-term responsibility for their prescriptions informed by PGx [25]. Physician training and policy must be in place for PGx usage, as the benefits for the patient are vast. Recently, PGx aided physicians in the UK and Sweden personalize doses of warfarin (an anticoagulant) for their patients. The trial showed fewer incidences of excessive anticoagulation and kept patients in the optimal therapeutic range for the drug [26]. These trials conducted in the UK and Sweden show that physician guided PGx must be made available to patients or they may seek imprecise alternatives.

A Third Party Loophole?

Third party services that compete with typical physician guided PGx services are available with patient DTC genotype data. Indeed, clinically relevant data can be garnered from PGx tests offered by physicians, but consumers are not picky with their data and how applicable it may be to them—as long as they can glean *something*. As such, DTC genotyping customers are combing through their "raw" data, which is easily obtainable from vendors, to draw conclusions about their personal PGx. The raw data is uploaded to third party services such as Promethease or Codegen, which link genetic data to databases on genetic variants. Many of these services relate relevant studies behind specific genetic variants that strengthen the reliability of data, and help customers learn about how nuances of their biology compare to others. For example, examining a tiny variation in the coding of the FTO gene (the "fat gene) *may* inform customers of their potential for obesity.

In many cases, users will resort to online forums to discuss their results with other users or even trained professionals who provide informal guidance or discussion. Such discussion is happening despite the disclaimers from third party services that their service is not intended for any medical application or other. Despite the somewhat paradoxical relationship between consumers and third party PGx services, they may present a powerful tool in the genetic medicine arsenal 1 day and complement recent advances in true precision medicine: gene therapy.

Gene Therapy

"Gene therapy" is an umbrella term describing the use of genes to prevent, treat, or correct human disease and offers the potential for long-lasting curative strategies. As science advances and ethical issues are resolved, gene therapy promises more precision-based and personalized medicine. Gene therapy advancements discussed here concern somatic gene therapy (SGT) and *not* germline gene therapy (GGT). SGT targets cells in the body that *do not* carry genetic information to the next generation, while GGT targets cells that *do* (i.e. sperm and egg). GGT is banned in many countries and thus has not been pursued— the dubious ethical tensions surrounding GGT have crippled its advancement. SGT presents a clearer path.

The techniques used in gene therapy are broadly composed of three main branches—gene insertion, gene silencing, and gene editing—each of which involve encouraging patient cells to function non-pathogenetically, typically by providing functional genes to cells or stopping the use of pathogenic genes (Fig. 12.1.). Each practice has its merits, and some technologies are more developed or hold more

Fig. 12.1. Gene therapy broadly classified based on three techniques. All techniques utilize varying delivery procedures and experimental design, but the end goal is the same: to make lasting changes to the way a cell or organism functions. (**a**) Gene insertion involves providing cells of a patient with a functional or non-pathogenic copy of the gene of interest. (**b**) Silencing involves quelling a pathogenic process in the cell from occurring, either at the aberrant gene, RNA, or protein that confers a disorder. (**c**) Gene editing basically translates to the removal or changing of an aberrant gene. Note that the figure only shows gene replacement

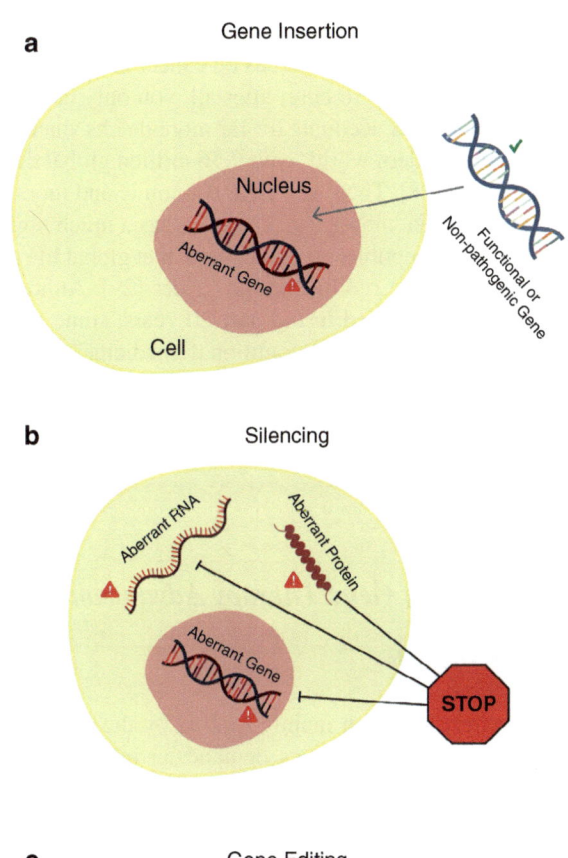

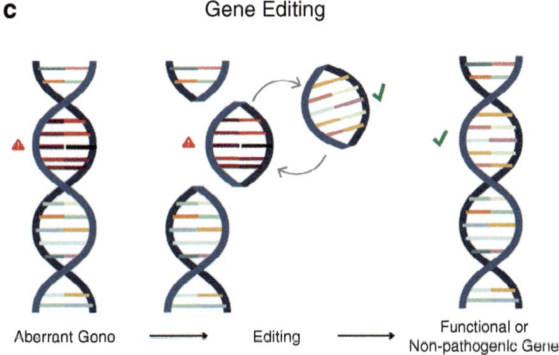

Illustration by Alexandra Budarina

promise than others. Many hurdles remain to be overcome before gene therapy reaches the masses, but clinical trials in the past two decades have seen success.

As of 2017, there have been around 2597 gene therapy clinical trials in 38 countries, most of which target cancer (65%). In contrast, monogenic diseases, and infectious diseases account for less (11.1% and 7% respectively) [27]. This large number of clinical trials has led to the approval of 17 gene and cell therapy products approved by the FDA. The focus on cancer may seem paradoxical since monogenic diseases are "easier" to cure; after all, you only need to target a single gene to see results. Yet, cancer accounts for far more deaths since it is the number two cause of death in the modern world, with 9.56 million global deaths in 2017 after cardiovascular disease [28]. There is a clear economic and moral reason for this.

Cancer, unlike monogenic diseases, has a much higher prevalence, and virtually everyone is susceptible, especially now that global life expectancy is higher as aging is the number one risk factor for cancer [29]. Although treatment for cancer has considerably improved in the past 20 years, some types of cancer have a smaller chance of responding to traditional medicine such as pancreatic cancer [30]. Reduced treatment efficacy spurs patients to find alternative therapies of their own—around 67% of cancer patients seek complementary and alternative medicine practices (CAMs) [31]. Thus, the need for gene therapy is clear. Yet, it is not without its limitations.

Limitations of Gene Therapy Advancements

Delivery Methods

Gene therapy has been mainly limited by the delivery vectors (tools) available to scientists. Gene therapeutics demand an intelligent way of inserting therapeutic DNA into patients. This can be done in vivo or ex vivo (Fig. 12.2). Each vector has its benefits and limitations. Adeno-associated viral (AAV) vectors, for example, are small viruses that do not cause an immune response in patients. Yet, the amount of DNA they can contain is limited due to their size. Actual adenoviruses (AVs) can hold much more DNA, but their immunogenicity can be of concern.

In 1999, during a gene therapy clinical trial studying a urea cycle disorder, a volunteer named Jesse Gelsinger died after being injected with 34 trillion AV virus particles meant to target his liver. Only around 1% of the therapeutic DNA to be delivered by the virus particles made it to the liver, and the rest of the DNA made it throughout the body. Shortly after the initiation of gene therapy, Jesse died from multiple organ failure [32]. This case highlights the dangerous consequences of gene therapy gone awry. Scientists are still working on the best delivery methods that can be used safely by all.

Off-target or Unintended Effects

Another limitation of gene therapy advancement is predicting off-target or unintended effects. Many types of gene therapy involve using retroviruses to integrate therapeutic DNA into a patient's cells. Controlling *where* this therapeutic DNA integrates into the host's DNA is an issue, especially in the recent past. Furthermore, the

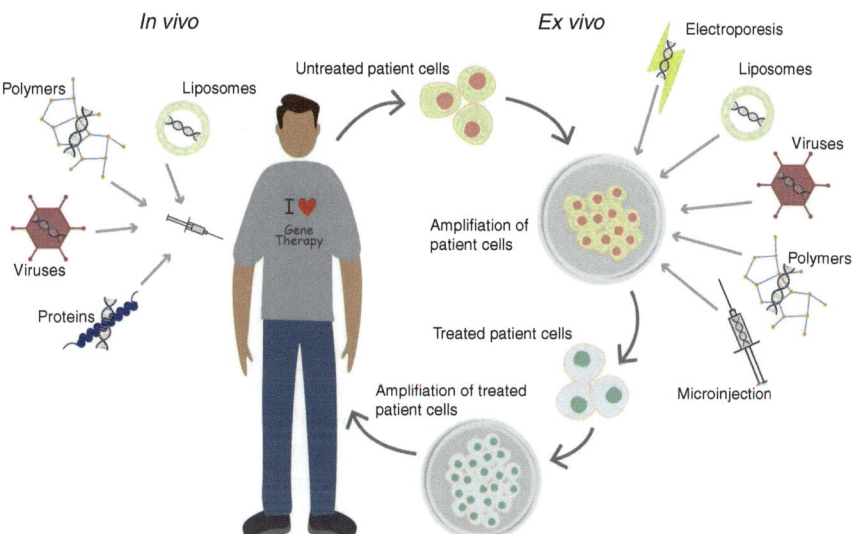

Fig. 12.2 In vivo or ex vivo gene therapy methods. In vivo delivery has inherently more risk and involves injecting therapeutic DNA directly into the patient. Ex vivo techniques involve removal of a patient's own cells followed by treatment. Ex vivo is generally safer and enables the experimenter to filter any gene therapeutics gone wrong. Both types of delivery utilize similar vectors depicted

consequences of off-target effects can sometimes manifest later, outside the clinical observation period. A clinical trial involving 16 infants with X-linked severe combined immunodeficiency proved successful, with 13 of the infants essentially cured of their monogenic condition [33]. Three years later, three of the infants developed leukemia, and the cause was attributed to *where* the retrovirus put the therapeutic DNA in the patients—it activated cancer. Most of the infants did not develop cancer, but this case illustrates that despite rigorous control over an experiment, there can still be unintended consequences.

Weissmann Barrier

The Weissmann barrier refers to the distinction between somatic cells (that compose us) and germline cells, which carry our genetic information to the next generations. Gene therapies must be expertly designed to target only somatic cells and not cross the Weissmann barrier to make alterations to germline cells. If the Weissman barrier is crossed, even accidentally, severe ethical qualms would persist around the field and further restrictions could hamper development processes. If gene therapy were to make it to the clinic in a more accessible way than is described here, it will certainly not cross this barrier [34].

Multigene Disorders

As previously stated, many diseases that afflict the population involve multiple genes and a variety of factors such as environment and lifestyle. Gene therapy must first cross the threshold to the clinic, which will be marked by the treatment of monogenic diseases and well-characterized cancers. Only then can gains in multigene disorders be made. Companies are far less likely to fund and focus on gene therapy for multigene disorders due to complexity.

Development Time

A limitation that has only recently been considered a lesser issue is that of development time and cost of some proteins (called nucleases) to target and cut sites in DNA. Proteins that bind to specific locations in patient DNA are arduous to create and very time-consuming. However, a nascent technology called CRISPR/Cas is widely publicized as a solution. CRISPR/Cas still involves the use of protein to cut DNA at specific sites but relies on RNA to home in on those sites as opposed to engineered proteins. Manufacturing RNA to target DNA sites is much easier than creating proteins to do the same. This RNA-DNA interaction (as opposed to protein-DNA interaction) is why CRISPR/Cas has received much media attention. It revolutionizes the speed of development and even the efficacy of gene therapeutics, which will translate to the clinic.

Types of Gene Therapy and Associated Successes

Gene Insertion

Broadly, gene insertions are defined as providing functional copies of a pathogenic or non-functional gene to ameliorate a condition (Fig. 12.1.a), and this can be further characterized in vivo or ex vivo. Ex vivo is much more common to all types of gene therapy clinical trials since it allows experts to control potential harms to the patient. Instead of administering gene insertion therapy to a patient and worrying excessively about the off-target or unintended consequence for the entire human system, it is much more controllable to deliver the treatment outside the patient's organism in a specific set of the patient's cells; this method enables more control and is generally safer for the patient.

The best case of gene insertion therapy was published in 2009 when two patients suffering from X-linked adrenoleukodystrophy (ALD) were treated with a retrovirus. ALD is an inability to handle a certain type of fatty acid (long-chain) because of a protein deficiency, which leads to a buildup of fatty acids in the brain. These fatty acids can damage the white matter in the brain quite quickly, leading to a vegetative state. ALD was corrected in patients by inserting a functional copy of a gene that helps them process the fatty acids [35].

More recently, a novel biopharmaceutical by Spark Therapeutics Inc. called Luxturna® had received FDA approval after phase III clinical trials. Luxturna® uses an AAV to deliver functional copies of a gene involved in light sensing to the retina. Luxturna® is meant for people with Leber congenital amaurosis, which causes loss of vision from birth; it is a one-time treatment that helps patients improve their quality of life. Many patients included in the clinical trials have grown in their ability to navigate a dim room. The pricing of this therapy is steep however, with a treatment cost per eye at around $425,000. Indeed, for gene therapy to make sense for the consumer there must be lower cost as only around 30 people have been treated with Luxturna®. Yescarta®, another type of gene therapy for cancer treatment, has been used on at least 7500 patients with non-Hodgkin lymphoma; the treatment is comparatively ~$200,000 [36].

Silencing

Genes and their products (RNA, which translate to protein) can be silenced which is favorable when a patient produces a pathogenic protein with aberrant function (Fig. 12.1.b). Silencing is done typically for monogenic diseases but also well-characterized cancers. Cancers develop multiple mutations in critical genes, which leads to an aberrantly functioning cell. Silencing or eliminating those mutated genes can make traditional chemotherapy more efficacious, as it inhibits the ability of cancer cells to survive [37].

Recently, the FDA hastened the approval of a biopharmaceutical named nusinersin (brand name Spinraza®) for spinal muscular atrophy (SMA) [38]. SMA is a genetic disease that results in progressive muscle wasting, which severely affects development and functioning. The cause is multifaceted but culminates in a nonfunctional protein required for motor neuron survival and maintenance. Nusinersin helps guide the proper production of a functional protein so motor neurons can develop and maintain connections to muscles. So far, nusinersin is available now in nearly 42 countries but is extremely expensive. This is one of the more recent advancements in the gene silencing therapy domains, but there are a multitude of clinical trials in the pipeline set to tackle a variety of disorders [27].

Gene Editing

Gene editing, unlike insertion or silencing, may present a better long-term strategy to treat or cure disease for the patient. Gene editing, in the most straightforward explanation, is to apply corrective measures to pathogenic DNA in a patient. Gene editing can involve the removal of a pathogenic gene or replacement of a nonfunctional gene with a functional one (Fig. 12.1.c).

Traditional gene-editing technologies have been limited, as previously stated, by the cost, time, and difficulty of producing nucleases. These systems, however, are far from old-fashioned. The first gene editing clinical trial ever conducted involved a type of nuclease called "Zinc-finger nucleases," or ZFNs for short. This trial excised the *CCR5* gene in HIV+ patients' immune cells, which codes for a co-receptor used by HIV to gain entry to cells. In this way, the patients retained a population of immune cells that cannot be infected with HIV, which may grant them the ability to stay off antiretroviral drugs [39].

Newer gene-editing tools like CRISPR/Cas have been well-publicized, and rightly so. As mentioned previously, CRISPR/Cas enables work in the lab to proceed at a much faster pace, which translates to quicker availability of this technology in the clinic. Instead of designing nucleases to attach to a certain area in a gene (a protein-DNA interaction), CRISPR/Cas works by designing short, complementary RNA sequences to bind to DNA of interest (RNA-DNA interaction). Producing RNA that binds to DNA is much simpler than the former.

The first-ever phase I clinical trial involving CRISPR/Cas gene editing recently published results; the trial involved editing the immune cells of three cancer patients, with CRISPR/Cas technology, to recognize refractory cancer tissue and attack it [40]. Of the three patients, only one demonstrated tumor regression. This is far from a failure, though, as all three patients' immune cells attacked their specific cancer cells for an extended time (9 months). The fact that cancer in two patients did not regress indicates our knowledge of cancer's power is lacking, or that the gene-editing technology still needs work. Either way, these are promising initial results and signal that the much-awaited CRISPR/Cas revolution is upon us.

A Word on Accessibility

Given how costly and recent these treatments and trials are relative to the publication of this text, it is easy to surmise that the gene therapy field still has much ground to cover to make it to the clinic, much less in the hands of patients. Once these therapies develop further, it should be cheap for *anyone* to attain gene therapy and correct their afflictions. Perhaps when this occurs, patients will have several options to treat their maladies and thus be compelled to perform their due diligence to take matters in their hands. Regulation around these technologies is restrictive, but for good measure as they possess immense power to alter our biology. In contrast, pharmaceuticals are designed to be processed by the human body and pass through in a certain time frame; not so with gene therapies, which tout lasting therapeutic potential.In the same way Moore's Law predicts advancement of integrated circuits and, by extension, the lower prices of such circuits, it follows that gene therapeutics also follow this trend; CRISPR/Cas, for example, has already demonstrated to be much cheaper than other gene editing techniques and offers more control over lab-based gene editing procedures.

The Near Future of Genetic Medicine

Recently, Dr. He Jiankui, a scientist in Shenzhen, China, sparked a vitriolic international response when he conducted unsanctioned gene editing experiments using CRISPR/Cas technology during an IVF procedure. The resultant twin girls born to the unwitting mother were allegedly born healthy [41]. Dr. Jiankui used CRISPR/Cas to remove the *CCR5* gene in the embryos, which was intended to give the babies some resistance to HIV infection. The use of this was called into question, especially since the mother was HIV negative and there was no pressing genetic dangers in the embryos. Did the CRISPR/Cas editing have any off-target effects? If so, what are the long-term consequences for the children? The myriad of functions the *CCR5* gene has is still being elucidated. For example, removing *CCR5* in mice was recently found to enhance memory and learning [42]; how will this translate in these two girls? Dr. Jiankui crossed a stigmatized threshold: permanently changing the germline of humanity. It must be stressed that even in the most carefully planned clinical trials, vetted by brilliant minds, and overseen by tight regulation, we are at the mercy of biology—we simply do not know enough.

Despite this unfortunate event, genetic medicine is advancing at a fever pitch, especially with CRISPR/Cas. Typically, CRISPR/Cas involves severance of both DNA strands to edit a segment of DNA, which severely limits the success rate of editing genes. CRISPR/Cas relies on the cell to make the appropriate repair it incurred to deliver the desired outcome, which is the technology's Achilles' heel. The chance of success can be increased with several modifiers, but recently the lab of Dr. David Liu demonstrated a new method to accurately edit DNA without double-stranded breaks: *prime editing* [43].

Prime editing involves the replacement of DNA sequences with single-strand breaks as opposed to double. DNA strands stay together, so the chance of faulty CRISPR/Cas is reduced. Prime editing is still being developed and has yet to see therapeutic application but is anticipated to be widely used due to laboratory success compared to traditional CRISPR/Cas.

Another recent advancement involves delivery vectors which, as previously stated, severely limit the efficacy of gene therapeutics because delivery of a DNA payload to the nucleus of a cell can be difficult.

As such, researchers have recently devised clever polymers to contain a therapeutic payload and deliver it to the cell nucleus [44]. The synthetic polymer encapsulates therapeutic DNA and delivers it to pathogenic cells by hijacking a type of protein signal that instructs the cell to transport the polymer to the nucleus. This type of technology could eliminate the need for viral vectors as it has an exceptionally low chance of eliciting an immune response. The previously mentioned biopharmaceuticals such as Yescarta® may cause a slight fever, difficulty breathing, chills etc. All these symptoms are a result of immune response.

Outside of the laboratory, initiatives across the world are gaining traction to increase awareness and practice of pharmacogenomics among healthcare practitioners. Pharmacists, and increasingly physicians and nurses, are required to complete PGx education modules for graduation [45]. The electronic tools that aid healthcare practitioners in understanding PGx is sorely lacking however, and there is a call to consolidate PGx data to streamline its employment [46]. One of the largest impedances to PGx employment is a lack of data on cost-effectiveness per patient. Yet, PGx screening of 10,000 patients in the Pharmacogenomic Resource for Enhanced Decisions in Care and Treatment (PREDICT) program helped identify risk-associated medications in 42% of the cohort, undoubtedly saving potential cost of future adverse reaction events [47]. It is predicted PGx will be covered by insurance providers of the coming years.

Closing Remarks

Genetic medicine is multifaceted and complex, and this fact makes it difficult for laymen to understand what kind of precision therapies are available to them. DTC genotyping services, the true tinder behind the new demand for genetic medicine, have evolved to provide the general population with an understanding of their biology. DTC genotyping has bridged a gap between healthcare practitioners and patients: that of technical understanding. PGx technology is a natural result of widely available information that aims to further personalize care. Point-of-care PGx has the potential to further involve patients, especially with accessible databases that are being developed by research entities, like the All of Us program.

On the horizon is a major change in the way we view our afflictions. Could gene therapies permanently alter our relationship with the numerous genetic and multidimensional diseases that cause much of human suffering? Will gene therapy simply erase our need for any form of healthcare including hybrid healthcare? Promising tools are at our disposal, such as CRISPR/Cas, that may be the harbinger of this new age in humanity. And lastly, will patients take part in their own gene therapy in much the same way they access their genotyping data through DTC services? Time will tell.

References

1. Talwar D, Yeh Y, Chen W, Chen L. Characteristics and quality of genetics and genomics mobile apps: a systematic review. Eur J Hum Genet. 2019;27(6):833–40.
2. Raghupathi W, Raghupathi V. Big data analytics in healthcare: promise and potential. Health Inf Sci Syst. 2014;2(1):3.
3. Rosenberg S, Aebersold P, Cornetta K, Kasid A, Morgan R, Moen R, et al. Gene transfer into humans — immunotherapy of patients with advanced melanoma, using tumor-infiltrating lymphocytes modified by retroviral gene transduction. N Engl J Med. 1990;323(9):570–8.
4. Foss D, Hochstrasser M, Wilson R. Clinical applications of CRISPR-based genome editing and diagnostics. Transfusion. 2019;59(4):1389–99.

5. Todd J. Interpretation of results from genetic studies of multifactorial diseases. Lancet. 1999;354:S15–6.
6. Gallo A, Angst D, Knafl K. Disclosure of genetic information within families. AJN Am J Nurs. 2009;109(4):65–9.
7. Rodin J. Aging and health: effects of the sense of control. Science. 1986;233(4770):1271–6.
8. Robinson J, Wynn J, Biesecker B, Biesecker L, Bernhardt B, Brothers K, et al. Psychological outcomes related to exome and genome sequencing result disclosure: a meta-analysis of seven Clinical Sequencing Exploratory Research (CSER) Consortium studies. Genet Med. 2019;21(12):2781–90.
9. Heshka J, Palleschi C, Howley H, Wilson B, Wells P. A systematic review of perceived risks, psychological and behavioral impacts of genetic testing. Genet Med. 2008;10(1):19–32.
10. Crozier S, Robertson N, Dale M. The psychological impact of predictive genetic testing for huntington's disease: a systematic review of the literature. J Genet Couns. 2014;24(1):29–39.
11. Sakamoto Y, Inoue H, Keshavarz P, Miyawaki K, Yamaguchi Y, Moritani M, et al. SNPs in the KCNJ11-ABCC8 gene locus are associated with type 2 diabetes and blood pressure levels in the Japanese population. J Hum Genet. 2007;52(10):781–93.
12. Tandy-Connor S, Guiltinan J, Krempely K, LaDuca H, Reineke P, Gutierrez S, et al. False-positive results released by direct-to-consumer genetic tests highlight the importance of clinical confirmation testing for appropriate patient care. Genet Med. 2018;20(12):1515–21.
13. Wetterstrand K. The cost of sequencing a human genome [Internet]. Genome.gov. 2020 [cited 25 February 2020]. https://www.genome.gov/about-genomics/fact-sheets/Sequencing-Human-Genome-cost
14. Scocchia A, Wigby K, Masser-Frye D, Del Campo M, Galarreta C, Thorpe E, et al. Clinical whole genome sequencing as a first-tier test at a resource-limited dysmorphology clinic in Mexico. NPJ Genom Med. 2019;4(1):5.
15. Farnaes L, Hildreth A, Sweeney N, Clark M, Chowdhury S, Nahas S, et al. Rapid whole-genome sequencing decreases infant morbidity and cost of hospitalization. NPJ Genom Med. 2018;3(1):10.
16. Hamilton J, Abdiwahab E, Edwards H, Fang M, Jdayani A, Breslau E. Primary care providers' cancer genetic testing-related knowledge, attitudes, and communication behaviors: a systematic review and research agenda. J Gen Intern Med. 2016;32(3):315–24.
17. Sovey C. United States tops 4 billion annual prescriptions: is our health improving? - HealthyConsumer.com [Internet]. 2020 [cited 1 March 2020]. http://www.healthyconsumer.com/911/united-states-tops-4-billion-annual-prescriptions-is-our-health-improving/.
18. Classen D. Adverse drug events in hospitalized patients. Excess length of stay, extra costs, and attributable mortality. JAMA. 1997;277(4):301–6.
19. Wilkinson G. Drug metabolism and variability among patients in drug response. N Engl J Med. 2005;352(21):2211–21.
20. Spear B, Heath-Chiozzi M, Huff J. Clinical application of pharmacogenetics. Trends Mol Med. 2001;7(5):201–4.
21. Brown M, Wastila L, Baras C, Lasagna L. Patient perceptions of drug risks and benefits. 3rd ed. University of New Hampshire; 1990.
22. Becquemont L. Pharmacogenomics of adverse drug reactions: practical applications and perspectives. Pharmacogenomics. 2009;10(6):961–9.
23. Carere D, VanderWeele T, Vassy J, van der Wouden C, Roberts J, Kraft P, et al. Prescription medication changes following direct-to-consumer personal genomic testing: findings from the impact of personal genomics (PGen) Study. Genet Med. 2016;19(5):537–45.
24. Filipski K, Murphy J, Helzlsouer K. Updating the landscape of direct-to-consumer pharmacogenomic testing. Pharmacogenom Pers Med. 2017;10:229–32.
25. Unertl K, Field J, Price L, Peterson J. Clinician perspectives on using pharmacogenomics in clinical practice. Pers Med. 2015;12(4):339–47.
26. Pirmohamed M, Burnside G, Eriksson N, Jorgensen A, Toh C, Nicholson T, et al. A randomized trial of genotype-guided dosing of warfarin. N Engl J Med. 2013;369(24):2294–303.

27. Ginn S, Amaya A, Alexander I, Edelstein M, Abedi M. Gene therapy clinical trials worldwide to 2017: an update. J Gene Med. 2018;20(5):e3015.
28. Roser M, Ritchie H. Cancer [Internet]. Our world in data. 2020 [cited 29 February 2020]. https://ourworldindata.org/cancer.
29. Hyde C. Age: the biggest cancer risk factor [Internet]. Cancer Research UK - Science blog. 2018 [cited 1 March 2020]. https://scienceblog.cancerresearchuk.org/2018/06/20/age-the-biggest-cancer-risk-factor/.
30. Arruebo M, Vilaboa N, Sáez-Gutierrez B, Lambea J, Tres A, Valladares M, et al. Assessment of the evolution of cancer treatment therapies. Cancer. 2011;3(3):3279–330.
31. Mao J, Palmer C, Healy K, Desai K, Amsterdam J. Complementary and alternative medicine use among cancer survivors: a population-based study. J Cancer Surviv. 2010;5(1):8–17.
32. Marshall E. Clinical trials: gene therapy death prompts review of adenovirus vector. Science. 1999;286(5448):2244–5.
33. Strauss B, Costanzi-Strauss E. Combating oncogene activation associated with retrovirus-mediated gene therapy of X-linked severe combined immunodeficiency. Braz J Med Biol Res. 2007;40(5):601–13.
34. Sabour D, Schöler H. Reprogramming and the mammalian germline: the Weismann barrier revisited. Curr Opin Cell Biol. 2012;24(6):716–23.
35. Cartier-Lacave N, Ali R, Ylä-Herttuala S, Kato K, Baetschi B, Lovell-Badge R, et al. Debate on Germline gene editing. Hum Gene Ther Methods. 2016;27(4):135–42.
36. Mullin E. Tracking the cost of gene therapy [Internet]. MIT Technology Review. 2017 [cited 6 May 2020]. https://www.technologyreview.com/2017/10/24/148183/tracking-the-cost-of-gene-therapy/.
37. Ren Y, Zhang Y. An update on RNA interference-mediated gene silencing in cancer therapy. Expert Opin Biol Ther. 2014;14(11):1581–92.
38. Wurster C, Ludolph A. Nusinersen for spinal muscular atrophy. Ther Adv Neurol Disord. 2018;11:175628561875445.
39. Tebas P, Stein D, Tang W, Frank I, Wang S, Lee G, et al. Gene editing ofCCR5in autologous CD4 T cells of persons infected with HIV. N Engl J Med. 2014;370(10):901–10.
40. Stadtmauer E, Fraietta J, Davis M, Cohen A, Weber K, Lancaster E, et al. CRISPR-engineered T cells in patients with refractory cancer. Science. 2020;367:eaba7365.
41. Cyranoski D, Ledford H. Genome-edited baby claim provokes international outcry [Internet]. Nature.com. 2018 [cited 19 February 2020]. https://www.nature.com/articles/d41586-018-07545-0.
42. Zhou M, Greenhill S, Huang S, Silva T, Sano Y, Wu S, et al. CCR5 is a suppressor for cortical plasticity and hippocampal learning and memory. elife. 2016;5:e20985.
43. Anzalone A, Randolph P, Davis J, Sousa A, Koblan L, Levy J, et al. Search-and-replace genome editing without double-strand breaks or donor DNA. Nature. 2019;576(7785):149–57.
44. Zelmer C, Zweifel L, Kapinos L, Craciun I, Güven Z, Palivan C, et al. Organelle-specific targeting of polymersomes into the cell nucleus. Proc Natl Acad Sci. 2020;117(6):2770–8.
45. Nutter S, Gálvez-Peralta M. Pharmacogenomics: from classroom to practice. Mol Genet Genom Med. 2018;6(3):307–13.
46. Hockings J, Pasternak A, Erwin A, Mason N, Eng C, Hicks J. Pharmacogenomics: an evolving clinical tool for precision medicine. Cleve Clin J Med. 2020;87(2):91–9.
47. Van Driest S, Shi Y, Bowton E, Schildcrout J, Peterson J, Pulley J, et al. Clinically actionable genotypes among 10,000 patients with preemptive pharmacogenomic testing. Clin Pharmacol Ther. 2013;95(4):423–31.

Chapter 13
Consumer Centricity in a Hybrid Age

Michael Schelper

Abstract The healthcare industry is at a tipping point and at the verge of fundamental disruption. Whether the next era will be shaped from within, by industry-
external players, or a combination thereof, remains the question. An undeniable fact
is the shift towards consumer-centric healthcare and the aim for proactive and preventative health management, enhanced with precision medicine. The way patients
and consumers interact with the healthcare system has to change, expectations are
rising, and a more seamless integration of healthcare services into the individual's
life is desired. Technological advancements serve as an enabler for healthcare professionals to deliver more timely, personalized, and better care. Yet, the pace of
adoption of such advancements is slow in healthcare. It needs to be understood that
technology, artificial intelligence and machines will not replace the jobs of medical
professionals. They rather take on tasks a machine is superior to perform. That
being said, healthcare practitioners need to embrace new technologies to obtain the
superhuman power required to advance into the next era of healthcare provision. In
this new era, human interaction is more required than ever. The needs of consumers
have to be understood, new services have to be defined upon those, and the doctor-
patient relationship needs to become a true partnership. These steps will serve as the
foundation to achieve the consumer-centric shift the healthcare industry is in defi-
nite need of.

Keywords Consumerism · Disruptive innovation · e-Patient · e-Consumer
Internet of Thing (IoT)

M. Schelper (✉)
Anvano, Dubai, United Arab Emirates
e-mail: michael.schelper@anvano.com

M. Al-Razouki, S. Smith (eds.), *Hybrid Healthcare*, Health Informatics,
https://doi.org/10.1007/978-3-031-04836-4_13

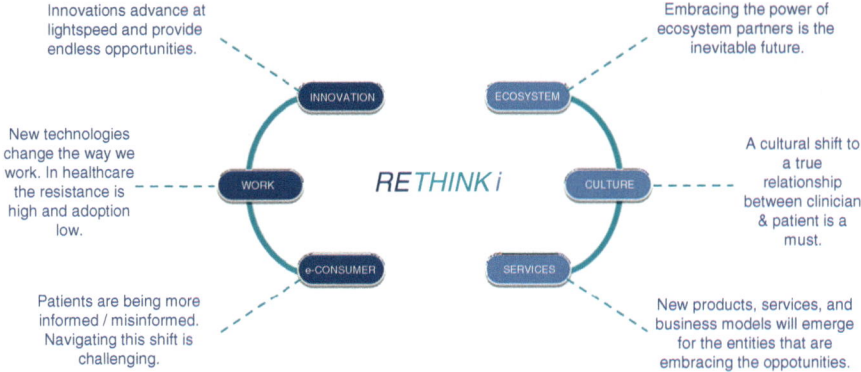

Fig. 13.1 The six drivers towards a consumer centric approach in a hybrid healthcare world

Tides of Change

The rate of innovations coming to the market is ever increasing. Technologies integrated into our daily lives are advancing at lightspeed. Living a healthy lifestyle has become the new norm. Though when interacting with the healthcare system, we rarely see the same level of innovations making it into daily use, it rather feels that one is sent back into the past. Why are some industries able to cope with the advancements and others are not? What is driving or in some cases hindering adoption? How can we overcome this tipping point and prepare for a consumer or patient centric healthcare provision in a hybrid healthcare world? As outlined in Fig. 13.1, we need to **RETHINK!** how to best provide care, whom we serve, what paths are most aligned with the ever-increasing expectations of all of us, whether you are on the provider or consumer side.

The Hybrid Dilemma we are facing is that the older and younger generations have to be served simultaneously, though they do require different interactions and services. At the same time, we are in a transitional period from the analog to the digital age in healthcare. Ask yourself how many of the services your institution is providing are still analog and how many are truly digital? If you are a consumer/patient, which interactions truly made a difference for you and increased your interest to experience these services from the same institution in the future?

Innovations Are Changing Our Expectations

Despite all the technologies surrounding us, when it comes to our health we strive to seek advice and reassurance from a medical professional rather than from a computer. Why are we not yet comfortable to '*trust*' a machine with something that is so intimate to us? We are seeking and trusting advice every single day from such machines, just think about how many times today you 'googled' something or used digital means for payments?

Clayton Christensen[1] was a pioneer in how to manage disruptive innovation, which has extremely high relevance to what we are experiencing in healthcare. There are three dimensions a service has to cater to, or three jobs-to-be-done, a consumer would hire a product or service to do—the functional, social and emotional job. When we translate this to the healthcare field the functional job a sick patient 'hires' the healthcare system to do is to identify the root cause, i.e. diagnose what is going on with the patient's health, and then obtain the right guidance to treat the medical condition. Clearly in many cases Artificial Intelligence could take over this job for the majority of cases and refer to a clinical practitioner when in doubt. However, the second dimension, the emotional job, is that we desire the empathy from and value a relationship with a medical practitioner when our health is concerned. Third, the social job is that you want to be seen by society as getting the best perceived advice, which in this case is from a medical practitioner to enable you to live a healthy and active life.

It is imperative to understand that we all strive for personalized experiences in our daily lives and this is no different when interacting with the healthcare system. It starts with how we can interact and book an appointment, over the registration, the interaction with the practitioners, the examinations and all the way to the communication and support post any episode.

During the COVID-19 pandemic we experienced how technology enabled many businesses and its employees to continue to effectively function utilizing a virtual environment. Technology is deeply and seamlessly integrated into each of our lives. Think about a time when your smartphone battery was empty and no possibility to recharge it in sight. The anxiety that quickly builds up is making it clear how heavily we rely on this 'black mirror' in our pocket, which gives us access anytime and anywhere to most of the services we need or want. This right-here-and- right-now-expectation is becoming more of a reality when interacting with the healthcare system and a positive impact of the pandemic was the accelerated adoption of such technologies in healthcare catering towards the consumer. How many times were you frustrated to find a PCR testing facility, where you don't have to commute for a long time, wait to get the test done, and then wait again to obtain the results, as you needed them to travel, go back to the office, or enter a public facility. This has quickly become our new normal due to the pandemic we are experiencing. We have swiftly seen digital technologies being adapted to streamline this experience, enabling us to digitally receive and carry the results, enabled with contact tracing to keep us and the communities at a lower risk. Telemedicine apps have also quickly become more accepted, also from a regulatory standpoint, and they enable us to more seamlessly obtain the advice we need when we are not feeling well. These services are increasing in adoption as technology serves as the enabler to the interaction with the medical practitioner, whom we naturally trust more; a human being

---

[1] https://www.christenseninstitute.org/jobs-to-be-done/

Fig. 13.2 Defining trends
of consumer centric
innovation in healthcare

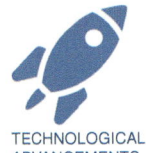

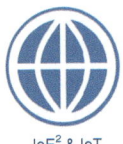

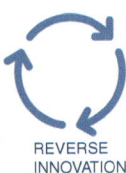

TECHNOLOGICAL   IoE² & IoT   REVERSE
ADVANCEMENTS   INNOVATION

who caters to our emotional desire of human interaction. Though, if we can't reach the source of our trust, we would rather take the next best alternative, than not to get any advice. With the Internet of Eyes and Ears being omnipresent (Fig. 13.2) like 3D depth analysis smartphone cameras or the digital assistants that are automating our homes, we do have access to such services with technology at our fingertips and around the environment we live in that enables us to receive high quality feedback instantaneously.

Early adopters experimented with innovative technologies in healthcare in non-life-threatening situations, such as the HIPAA conform Amazon Alexa Skill Kit[2] which companies and providers are increasingly using, like Boston Children's Hospital with their ERAS[3] skill to connect parents of children after they got discharged with the care team to update them on the recovery process and follow-up appointments, or Livongo's Blood Sugar Lookup[4] that helps diabetic patients to keep track of the blood sugar checks and receive personalized guidance. Adopting innovations from other industries such as blockchain, as elaborated in Chap. 3, to create a system that has a holistic overview of one's health, or the Internet of Things (IoT) with sensors embedded in clothes monitoring our well-being and implants in the not too distant future that will directly act in the case of a rising medical condition, will most likely be very normal to us soon. The world has become accessible from our fingertips, though innovations sometimes are not adopted or take too long for a widespread adoption due to a stigmatism in our society. If one of your loved ones were to experience a medical condition and you are offered by your healthcare provider two treatment options with the same level of outcomes (1) from a world renown medical institution and (2) from an entity in Cambodia or Senegal, at 1/100th of the cost, which one would you choose if you can afford both? Now ask yourself the question 'Why did you choose the more expensive treatment from the world renown organization'? It has exactly the same quality outcomes as the other option. This is the perception we have to overcome. Expensive does not mean that it is a better option. The outcomes that can be attained is what matters.

A multitude of advancements is making it into our lives every single day. Though the speed of adoption in healthcare is slow, albeit accelerated through the COVID-19 pandemic. Why is that? Naturally, new innovations will have some problems in the infant stages and mature over time. Which in turn means we cannot experiment with

---

[2] https://developer.amazon.com/blogs/alexa/post/ff33dbc7-6cf5-4db8-b203-99144a251a21/introducing-new-alexa-healthcare-skills

[3] https://accelerator.childrenshospital.org/portfolio/voice-in-healthcare/

[4] https://www.amazon.com/Livongo-Health-Blood-Sugar-Lookup/dp/B07QHF76RN

such technologies if a patient's life is at risk. The race to find a SARS-CoV-2 vaccine has showcased that technology can enable advances in a timeframe never seen before. Given the severe impact on a patient's life, the approval hurdles are rightfully in place, particularly given the impact a mistake could have on the world's population. However, there are many ways in non-life-critical situations where the trial-and-error path might be a possibility. We are thankfully seeing an increasing pace of reverse or trickle-up innovations, where great solutions and services, developed under resource constraints by medical practitioners or patients from developing economies, get adopted faster and more broadly. The foundation here is an open mind and humility. Great solutions, services or treatments don't need to be expensive or only come from the most renowned researchers, institutions, or companies. Already in 2009 Botswana-based company Deaftronics[5] pioneered the first solar-power rechargeable hearing aid which lowered the needed audiologists visits dramatically, particularly important, as these healthcare professionals are a scarce resource in Botswana. Due to a severely lower price-point they quickly expanded beyond the country's borders and one can only speculate whether this development sparked Sivantos'[6] work on an inductively charged hearing aid or whether it had an impact on the wireless rechargeable headphones each of us is using on a daily basis.

To tackle the rising problem of counterfeit medication mPedigree[7] from Ghana, launched in 2008, initially provided pharmaceutical producers with software to attach labels to their medications so that patients can simply validate the authenticity of the drug via a simple text message. They expanded not only globally but also into other verticals such as farming supplies, fabrics and cosmetics. There are many more examples which out of need and under resource constraints developed amazing solutions that had a profound impact on the worldwide healthcare environment.

With all these advancements, naturally health facilities will undergo a shift to cater to changes in expectations and demands of patients. The sensors, implants, nanobots, pills that dispense medication when needed, are helping or will help each of us to become more proactive in managing our health. Would this mean that health facilities in the future are only needed for specialized care and other more routine services will integrate into the lives of the patients and consumers in a hyper-personalized and seamless way? What has the COVID-19 pandemic taught us about the use-cases of technology in healthcare, how it can support healthcare professionals in delivering the needed care, and, more importantly, about the value, convenience, and insights that can be created with it?

---

[5] https://deaftronics.com/
[6] https://www.sivantos.com/
[7] https://mpedigree.com/

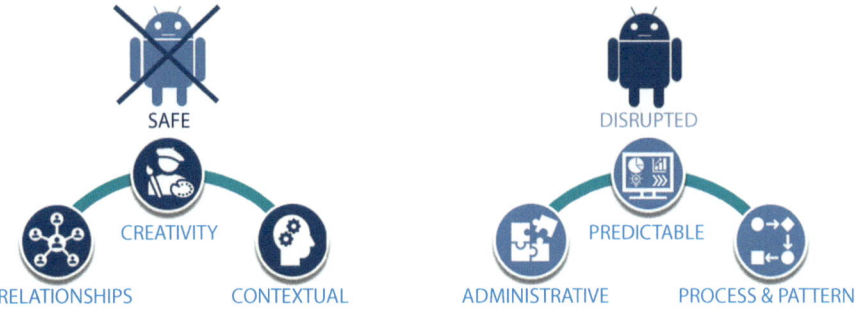

Fig. 13.3 Overview of tasks responsibilities of humans and machines

Reinventing Our Work

What was your dream-job when you were a little kid? Did this goal change while the years passed by? For most of us it did change. Maybe you have a job now that did not even exist in this form a decade ago. The fourth industrial revolution[8] is our new daily reality and is no different in the way it disrupts our lives like previous ones. People are scared about being replaced by machines and losing their jobs. Though this is not really true. Everything in our society over the last centuries is a result of human intellect, compassion, our ability to dream, build, think, solve problems and continuously advance ourselves. This does not necessarily change, but rather will continue at a faster pace due to technologies enabling us to do so. The important point to embrace is that technology is an enabler and does not replace our jobs in entirety, as shown in Fig. 13.3. This will impact more than half of the people in the worldwide economy. However, certain tasks will and should be performed by highly capable machines, in order to free up the time of the medical practitioner to focus on what is important, the patient. Robots are already disinfecting surgical rooms, supporting the doctors in performing procedures and much more. During the COVID-19 Pandemic we have witnessed an increased utilization of these automatic helpers for food delivery to infected patients and virtual consultations such as BeamPro,[9] Teladoc Health,[10] and others. Combining the functional capabilities of technologies with the core competencies of medical professionals to use the scarce time as best as possible is key. Imagine a surgeon with a VR headgear navigating a nanobot through the patient's body performing the surgery aided by artificial intelligence to get the right information at the right time.

We are facing a severe shortage of physicians and clinical staff, precious time is consumed by administrative tasks, which in turn results in burnouts of the medical practitioners and dissatisfaction of the patients when interacting with the healthcare

---

[8] https://www.weforum.org/focus/fourth-industrial-revolution

[9] https://suitabletech.com/products/beam-pro

[10] https://www.teladochealth.com/

system. We need to 'employ' technology for tasks that are repetitive, predictable, pattern oriented or administrative, so that the right focus can be put on the relationship between the patient and the medical professional. This is important to tackle the increasing lack of trust between doctors and patients, as well as to improve the care provision during the short time typically allocated for the consultation. The average citizen interacts five to six times a year[11] with the healthcare system for approximately 20 min. This leaves another 364 days and 23 h each year, where each of us is living our life, taking decisions impacting our well-being, making choices for our lifestyle, and ultimately generating a lot of data that can yield important insights. These digital breadcrumbs will enable not only us to live a healthier life, but also the medical practitioners to make more informed decisions and serve us better. Though, for this, these data points need to be consolidated in a meaningful manner to develop digital biomarkers and generate the insights that yield a positive impact. A task impossible to be performed by humans, so let machines do the data crunching and pattern recognition to provide your healthcare professional with a more holistic view on your health. The foundation would be that each consumer, each patient, needs to take an active role in managing one's life, also in the digital sphere, which seems to be an obstacle. It is the responsibility of each and every one of us to continuously advance ourselves, in every aspect of our life.

Don't Ignore the e-Patient or e-Consumer

Consumers, particularly patients, are more informed than ever and, in many instances, more misinformed than ever. The rise of the e-patient or e-consumer though can't be ignored. What does the 'e' stand for? Is it electronic, equipped, enabled, empowered, engaged or the expert patient? Most likely it is a combination of all of these due to the characteristics of the e-consumer or e-Patient as shown in Fig. 13.4.

It is natural to us to utilize a multitude of data sources that are at our fingertips in order to educate ourselves. We don't use a scientific encyclopedia or contact a doctor in our trusted circle when we experience some sort of medical condition, but we rather use what we have immediate access to, such as search engines, read through articles, discussion boards, wearables information, or medical advice pages on the internet. The phenomena that then occurs is very similar to the medical school syndrome,[12] where the medical students perceive themselves of having the symptoms of the disease they are studying. For the e-Patient seeking advice from Doctor Google can have adverse effects, increased anxiety, and in drastic cases fatally wrong decisions. Certainly, the readily available tools are improving in efficiency to provide initial

---

[11] https://ec.europa.eu/eurostat/statistics-explained/index.php/Healthcare_activities_statistics_-_consultations

[12] https://en.wikipedia.org/wiki/Medical_students%27_disease

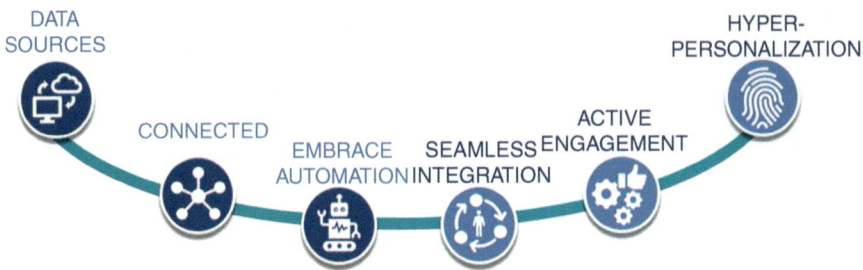

Fig. 13.4 Key characteristics of e-Patients/e-Consumers

guidance such as the Symptoms Checker at WebMD,[13] which applies more medical contextual information to a query, or platforms where patients that are undergoing lengthy and often complex conditions exchange with peers, such as PatientsLikeMe[14] or CureTogether,[15] whereas the latter was acquired by Genomic-Testing company 23andMe. However, in most instances the right next step is to obtain professional guidance from a medical practitioner. The e-Patient is, as you and I, living in this hyper-connected world, where most of the services that we consume and appreciate are seamlessly integrated into our lives. Why would our expectations be any different when seeking medical advice? This is where the dilemma starts, as a vast majority of services are still provided the same way they have been for decades. In a business environment, it is completely natural to send voice notes or WhatsApp messages to clients and business partners. Working from home has become the norm due to the COVID-19 pandemic and many companies already communicated the adoption on a permanent basis as flexible work arrangements are valued more by employees than for example a higher paycheck. We happily maintain our digital avatars on various platforms in order to have a more personalized experience. The e-Patient wants to take an active role in hers/his health management, but is being handcuffed from the start, trying to make sense of behavioral, social, healthcare, wellness, and wearables data-points without the right guidance. Why are we facing resistance and where do we go from here? How can we close the loop and enable the e-Patient to be more proactive in managing hers/his health?

Unleashing the Power of Ecosystems

Transforming the current healthcare delivery to cater to increased expectations is not only scary and difficult for many institutions to perform, but it also does consume substantial financial resources, which in turn can't be invested where they are

---

[13] https://symptoms.webmd.com/default.htm#/info

[14] https://www.patientslikeme.com

[15] https://curetogether.com/

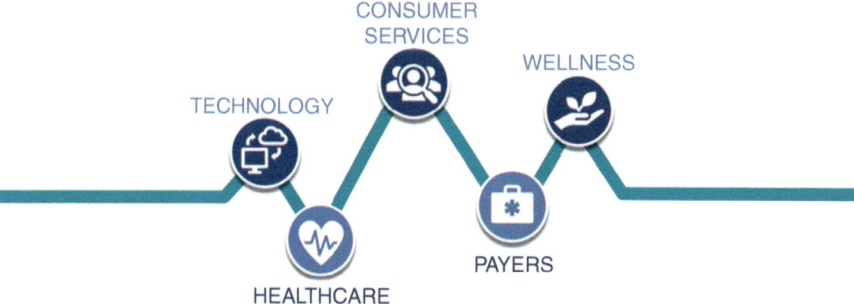

Fig. 13.5   The players of an integrated proactive health management ecosystem

needed today. Does this mean a gridlock situation for the majority of healthcare systems? It most certainly does not.

The entities that are very interested in enabling their members to live as much a healthy life as possible are the insurance companies (Fig. 13.5). Naturally, a healthy member will have less need to interact with the healthcare system for expensive medical conditions and in turn will generate lower claims to be paid. Many of the insurance companies, besides their own activities to provide their members with mainly virtual guidance for improving their health, are heavily working together with partner organizations from startups, to established companies, public and private healthcare providers and all the way up to the regulators, in order to provide different means of interacting with consumers and patients, as well as supporting healthcare providers on specific use cases. Bupa, for example, has partnered with Teladoc Health[16] to provide 'Global Virtual Care',[17] a service where consumers can connect via a smartphone telehealth app with doctors to obtain advice. The same goes for Aetna, AXA, Cigna, and others. Besides the more seamless integration into the lives of the consumers, who receive the appropriate guidance, it also positively impacts healthcare providers that have void capacity amongst their physicians in some locations and can, via this approach, maximize the impact of their medical staff members. Cleveland Clinic, a world-renowned healthcare provider in the United States, expects over half of all outpatient visits to be conducted online within the next 5 years.[18] Till this becomes reality, to tackle the current problem of 'no-shows', which has drastic operational costs and losses of revenue for health facilities, Mobility-on-Demand services Lyft as well as Hitch Health partnered with healthcare providers in the United States to provide non-emergency medical transport[19] and realized during the 1-year study a reduction by 27% of patients that

---

[16] https://teladochealth.com/en/

[17] https://www.bupaglobal.com/en/broker/news/global-virtual-care

[18] https://www.fastcompany.com/90450883/cigna-will-now-let-you-go-to-the-doctor-on-your-phone

[19] https://www.healthcaredive.com/news/lyft-hitch-health-nemt-pilot-reduced-no-shows-by-27/528401/

previously missed appointments and generated an almost 300% ROI. Further integration directly into the clinical workflow has been realized by partnerships of Lyft with electronic medical record vendor Allscripts and Uber with Cerner Corporation's electronic health record system.[20] Besides the operational efficiencies, these partnerships also have a more holistic impact on the healthcare environment, as the time to treatment is being shortened, which in turn improves the clinical outcomes, lowers the costs of treatment in many instances, and also enables more patients to be effectively consulted by a medical professional.

Doctors are recommending more services to patients that can positively impact the recovery, help in educating a patient, or provide personalized guidance post an intervention. Services like Medicus.ai,[21] which is an A.I. platform that converts your blood test results and medical reports into personalized and understandable explanations. They also directly integrate with an increasing number of laboratory providers around the world, help to demystify health information and transform it into actionable tasks for the regular consumer. The transferability of such technologies has been showcased by Medicus.ai with their support of aviation companies such as Etihad Airways[22] for COVID-10 triaging, as well as businesses and governments with rapid antigen testing, so that we all might get quicker back to a less restricted normality. For diabetic patients, MySugr[23] helps to lower the daily challenges of managing the condition by connecting to smart glucometers and guiding the patient throughout the daily routines.

Whichever partnerships are being created, the ultimate goal is to get you, a provider, payer, startup, (bio-)tech company closer to the consumer to provide better care by complementing your products, services, and skills with partners that can fill a void and improve the holistic patient experience, ultimately striving towards a proactive health & life management. Some entities are still skeptical or scared about the economic impact, as partnering could in many instances mean to give up a piece of one's potential business. Whereas, the overall opportunity will become hundred-fold, if done properly. When we have accomplished this in the future and ultimately enable the practitioners with all the technologies, wearables, implants, services to proactively and remotely manage a person's health, making sure her or him to never really feel sick, would this bring a behavioral shift of not caring anymore about taking good care of one's health? The risk is there. Also the foundation to guide, educate, and enable the patients' needs to be put in place today by performing one of the most difficult tasks: We need to change the culture of how we interact with each other in healthcare, incorporating the patients' needs into our daily routines.

---

[20] https://www.modernhealthcare.com/patients/lyft-uber-expand-reach-healthcare

[21] https://medicus.ai/

[22] https://www.etihad.com/en-ae/news/etihad-airways-partners-with-medicus-ai-to-launch-covid-19-risk-assessment-tool-across-digital-platforms

[23] https://mysugr.com/en

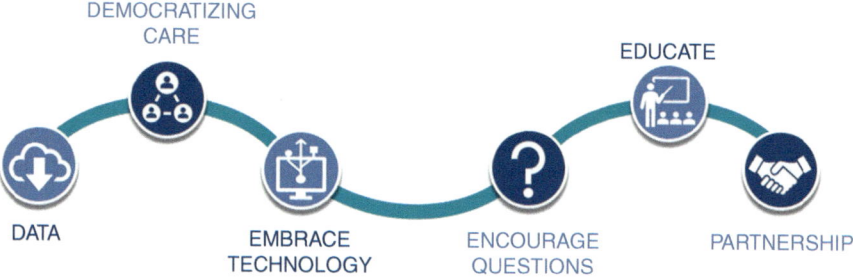

DEMOCRATIZING
CARE

EDUCATE

DATA

EMBRACE
TECHNOLOGY

ENCOURAGE
QUESTIONS

PARTNERSHIP

Fig. 13.6 Drivers for a cultural shift towards consumer centric healthcare provision

Culture Eats Strategy for Breakfast

With the e-consumer or the e-patient, data is not only available to the medical professional, which leads to a perceived democratization of care as we know it. Though,
the intervention from a physician is in most cases more required than ever, in order
to put the patient on the right path, to interpret the found data-pieces the right way,
and to relate them to the condition the patient is experiencing. However, healthcare
professionals do not have the possibility of using and analyzing all the digital breadcrumbs each of their patients is creating every day while living their lives. Neither
can clinical staff members perform this task, despite the fact that important insights
can be yielded from such data points. This is where technology needs to be embraced
and deeply embedded in the daily routines as an enabler to support the clinicians in
their work, as data is becoming easier to collect and easier to analyze with the right
tools. Doctors practicing in an old-school way will most definitely get replaced, but
not by machines. They will get replaced by doctors recognizing the value of technology and who dare to use the services available to support their work, to free up
time for patients, to reduce or even eliminate physician burnouts, and to then provide an increased level of care. In a nutshell, become the Superhero Doctor we need,
who values a true partnership with consumers/patients, as showcased in Fig. 13.6. A
biotech company, called Universal DX,[24] is set out to revolutionize the early detection of cancer, a global pandemic killing ten million people annually.[25] They have a
bold vision of making cancer a curable disease by detecting it early via a simple
blood draw. They may even be able to detect the pre-cancer stage, hence preventing
cancer altogether. The test is seamlessly integrated into the patient's annual check-
up and with the result the physician will decide if further medical procedures should
be taken, so that a proactive plan can be defined together with the patient to cure the
identified disease or to stay healthy. I doubt anyone would feel comfortable or well-
equipped without the guidance of a specialist in that field to define the next steps, if

[24] https://www.universaldx.com/

[25] https://www.who.int/news-room/fact-sheets/detail/cancer

we were to just be presented with the findings of the A.I. for something as life-impacting as cancer.

Data privacy is certainly of utmost importance. Misuse of personal health information has to be avoided and the right governance structures need to be put in place. However, we are currently facing too drastic limitations on free dataflow, which is hindering the obtaining of essential information that can save lives. Two of the most personal and most precious areas of our life are our health and our finances. Ask yourself the question 'Why are you comfortable to use credit cards around the world, access your bank account via apps or online banking despite the risk of fraud and cyber-crime'? Now think about 'Why do you have your health information either locked away or separated in various silos?', which prohibits a holistic view of your health status, when needed. Let's take it to an even more extreme level, if you were facing a severe medical emergency, where having all relevant information about your health available to the paramedics could save your life and the lack thereof would result in death, what would you choose? Thus, it becomes a required mindset shift for the patient, the healthcare industry, and regulatory bodies alike, to ensure the right maintenance and distribution of health-related information is performed, supported by a solid governance structure and world-class cyber-security, very similar to what has been accomplished in the financial industry. With this, doctors can become the Superheroes that help patients the best way possible and the foundation for the desired shift towards proactive or even preventative healthcare will be in place. Imagine such a scenario with the COVID-19 pandemic and what difference it could have made in the response efforts. Could a pandemic have been entirely avoided?

Patients need to be encouraged by doctors to ask questions, as they consulted or will consult Doctor Google anyway. They need to share what they have learned from their research, their thoughts and worries that arose from it, so that with the expertise, intuition and empathy from a healthcare professional the right path towards a swift recovery will be taken. Enabling patients to feel comfortable and safe to ask such questions and share their thoughts is also a very important step towards (1) educating the e-patient on how to search for relevant information effectively and (2) to build the foundation for an active engagement that positively impacts the episode of care. Learning went from classrooms to virtual classrooms and then to mobile devices. Which means that information is on the fingertips of the patient at any point in time. However, navigating without guidance through the vast amount of available services and sources is often resulting in resignation. This is one reason why medically vetted advice is very crucial to help and educate the patients, by using the right ecosystem partners and services that complement the care provided. In the mental health field, we see an increased utilization of services such as the chatbot WoeBot[26] or digital therapist platforms like Bloom.[27] The former is doing the same triaging a medical professional would do in the form of a chatbot

---

[26] https://woebot.io/

[27] https://www.enjoybloom.com/

and is very popular amongst the younger generations like high school and university students. The latter rebuilt the therapy experience in a digital way with personalized on-demand video sessions based upon cognitive behavioral therapy to make it more affordable and accessible. Thus, enabling the user to get educated on specific topics she/he is experiencing and directly work on a betterment is key, albeit being seamlessly integrated into the life of the consumer. Guiding the user in the time of need or worry towards the right path, which could mean as a next step to schedule an appointment with a healthcare professional. Particularly, with the enforced lockdowns and home confinement, Bloom experienced a surge in demand, as people needed guidance, but didn't have the possibility and/or financial means to consult a medical professional. Patients want to take an active part in positively impacting their health, they want to be properly prepared for the next doctor's appointment, as they are living with the condition and thoughts every single hour of the day. The common goal is to recover from a medical condition as best and fast as possible. With the right guidance, patients can become a very valuable asset in their health recovery journey.

The current relationship between the doctor and the patient has to be lifted up to a true partnership. Think about the worst customer relationship experience you faced with a regular consumer service or company in the last year. Most likely this experience aggravated you, you might have regretted having bought the product or availed the service, and the likelihood of becoming a return customer was very low. Now think about a great and maybe surprisingly positive experience you had in the last 12 months. What were the actions that made the difference?

Most likely you were able to get in touch with the service provider in a seamless way when you needed to address the pains you had. You got a response either immediately or in due time that acknowledged the problem, valued you as a customer, and either provided directly a resolution or a path to solving the problem with defined next steps, which are the gains you desire as outlined in Fig. 13.7. You felt that someone cared about you and that you were not left alone. In such a comfortable state we are calmer and more open to suggestions. All these together relieve the pain, create the value and ultimately are addressing the jobs-to-be-done framework from section "Innovations are Changing our Expectations" functional, social, and emotional jobs a customer is hiring a service or product for. This is no different in healthcare. A right step to be taken is that communication with the patient needs to change. This means proper online and offline communication, available when needed, to get this often very short piece of advice that enables the e-patient to continue hers/his active participation in their health management. During offline interactions, adding technologies integrated into the clinical workflow that also solve the pains and create the gains for the clinical practitioners, is another part of the equation. Services such as Nuance Dragon Medical Virtual Assistant[28] or Amazon's Transcribe Medical[29] services capture the doctor-patient interaction and directly

---

[28] https://www.nuance.com/healthcare/ambient-clinical-intelligence/virtual-assistants.html

[29] https://aws.amazon.com/transcribe/medical/

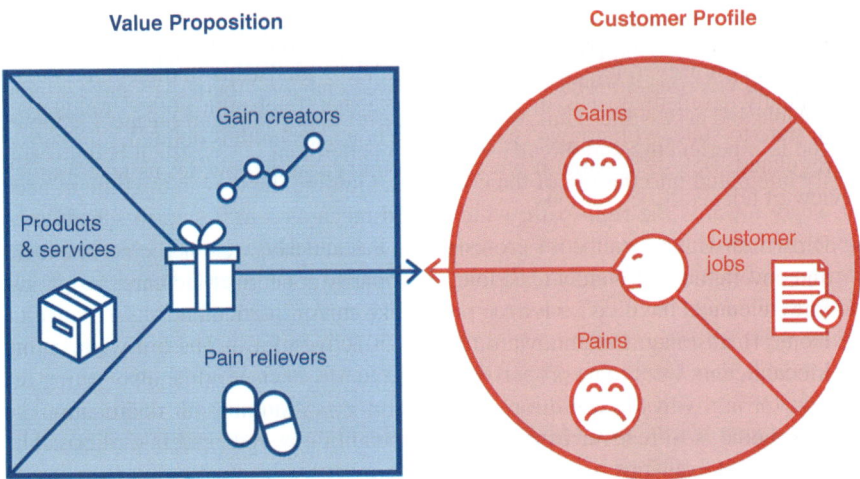

Fig. 13.7 Value proposition canvas (https://www.b2binternational.com/research/methods/faq/what-is-the-value-proposition-canvas/)

integrate into the clinical workflow via electronic health records (EHRs), provide the right information, at the right time and aid the examination by the doctor. In the near future, more artificial intelligent services, as outlined in Chap. 2 will amplify this trend and also enable healthcare providers to learn more from their patients, offline and online. However, if the trust basis is not established, nothing much will happen. We constantly need to learn from the patient / consumer the same way they and machines learn from medical professionals. A practitioner is constantly receiving advice from various sources in the healthcare system, but when are insights and advice obtained from the patients / consumers, besides a 'satisfaction survey' that might be sent out? How many healthcare providers have patients in their advisory boards? These cultural and mindset changes can yield many new services, lower costs, and improve the highly desired outcomes. Sadly, in many areas the pioneers that want to drive this change and make healthcare futureproof, are facing roadblocks and mindsets that can't be easily changed.

The Rise of New Services and Delivery Models

It needs to be understood what the consumer and the patient really want, the jobs-to-be-done. At the same time, an environment has to be established that enables clinical practitioners to cater to those demands, alleviate the challenges they are facing in the daily routines, and let technology, as an enabler, take over tasks where possible. Thus, supporting the healthcare professionals in their workflow and letting them unleash hidden potentials. This can't be done in isolation and an effective ecosystem of partners, that provides complementing value adding services to complete the patient experience, is imperative for success. Only then it is possible to craft new services, experiment, pivot, and pioneer them for a more holistic approach to the ideal proactive patient experience.

I mentioned earlier that cancer is a global and very personal tragedy. Why is that the case? On the one side, there is not yet the one single cause for cancer, or specific types thereof, identified. It is believed that a combination of different factors, such as environmental, lifestyle, genetic or specific characteristics of the individual can produce cancer.[30] In addition to that, no single doctor can be a specialist in diagnosing or treating every type of cancer as best as possible. The complexity of the disease is supporting this struggle, though there is an unbelievable high amount of scientific, clinical, and research information available that could potentially support an oncologist in these tasks. Technology is imperative in this field to bring all available information about a cancer patient together, apply A.I. to the information given by the multidisciplinary care team and then crawl relevant data points from research reports, medical journals, clinical studies and more to provide potential diagnoses with an estimate of how reliable the hypothesis for each is back to the clinicians. This enables a more personalized therapy plan thereafter and reduces the potential for medical errors in medication and treatment. Leveraging technology to do what it does best and to support medical professionals in what they do best, can only be a winning proposition we need to follow. Particularly in the case of a life-threatening disease, I believe we all would like to get the attention from a doctor we trust, the empathy we desperately need in such a situation, and the dedication that might increase our chances to win the fight against cancer and other diseases.

In less critical situations, consumers want to obtain advice, they want to be guided, utilize services such as artificial intelligence wherever they can to achieve an experience more seamlessly integrated into their lives, as shown in Fig. 13.8. It is understood that the doctor of their trust can't be available 24x7. Though this would rarely be needed anyway. Technology can gladly bridge the gap and virtual interactions can imitate the desired personal exchange so that the time is not wasted by the patient to drive to a health facility, if it is not really needed. Ideally, a 360-degree life concierge that takes us on the hand in this hyper-connected world, guides us through our health & life and eliminates the uncertainty, takes off the burden that is sitting on our shoulders and enables us to proactively manage our health in a seamlessly integrated manner. Just imagine an appointment will be scheduled for you automatically in the location where you have a break between two meetings so that your soon to be overdue vaccinations can be refreshed, or if that is not suitable a drone will be dispatched to administer the shot at your office. Until this becomes possible, it needs to be ensured that the services provided are mobile enabled, as the chance of adoption will otherwise be extremely low or they will entirely fail and waste precious resources along the way. This way, a more seamless integration into the life of the patient can be achieved and needs to be

---

[30] https://stanfordhealthcare.org/medical-conditions/cancer/cancer/cancer-causes.html

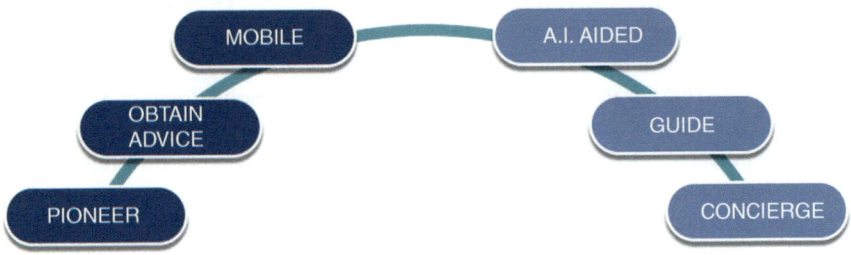

Fig. 13.8 Consumer needs to craft new services

complemented with hyper-personalized services, as we are used to and expect customized guidance catered to our specific situation.

Where best to get inspired for new services then by going where the potential
future users are. Sadly, a common pitfall is that services are designed without the
clinicians or patients in the loop. We need to take advantage of these great assets and
include them from the idea to solve a specific pain, throughout the ideation and
design, product / services development, all the way to the launch and also establish
a continuous feedback loop for further enhancements. Very similarly to any startup
or product, the target customers need to get identified right from the beginning so
that the most value creating services can be defined. With this in mind, it is clear that
a one-size-fits-all approach is not possible. The old and young generations require
different services, interactions, and experiences.

Why did for example Amazon acquire PillPack,[31] despite their dominant position
in online retail? It would have been a fairly simple task for them to build an online
retail pharmacy. The simple answer for the acquisition is that their desired target
customers were there! Changing established behaviors and relationships is a very
challenging task. Thus, understanding the key drivers of your target customers'
behavior and the value they want to obtain from a potential service is key.

Figure 13.9 outlines the key components for consumer centric services.
Consumers need empathy, time, and attention. Though, with the physician burnout
epidemic how can this be provided where over 50% of physicians worldwide are
showing some sign of burnout? How can the negative health impact be eliminated,
how can more time get freed up, how can patient care provision get improved?
Technology needs to be leveraged to support the work of clinicians, to take the burden away from the physicians to craft a true partnership that is accessible at all
times, that is hyper-personalized to the patient, it has to augment what the patient is
doing and it needs to be a holistic experience to enable everyone to live a healthier
life. Think about the impact A.I. can have for providing world-class care in rural
areas, where a care provider is complemented with it to enable less skilled professionals to provide a higher level of care and connect seamlessly to the specialists,

---

[31] https://www.cnbc.com/2019/05/10/why-amazon-bought-pillpack-for-753-million-and-what-happens-next.html

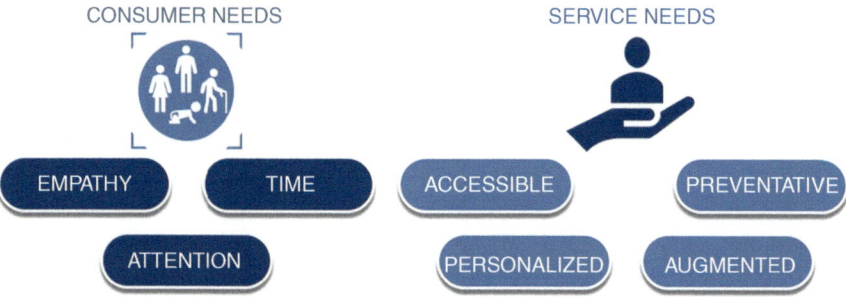

Fig. 13.9 Key components to consumer centric services

when required. With this the highly relevant insights can be obtained, transformed into actionable tasks to influence behavior, of both the patient as well as the physician.

In 5 years' time, none of us will just book an appointment with a doctor. We need to select whether the booking will be in person, via video consultation, a messaging service, or maybe in virtual reality. The initial triaging will get conducted by artificial intelligent services to guide the patient in the most effective way through the healthcare system. This will save time that then can be dedicated to more complex cases, where the expertise of a medical professional is highly required. The empowered consumer will fully rely on sensors of wearables, implants, health apps, A.I. and online resources for simple medical advice and guidance.

The good news is that the future lies in all our hands to be shaped and to make it our reality. Let's lift up the doctor-patient relationship to a true partnership to enable the entire healthcare ecosystem to thrive and each of us to live a healthier life.

Chapter 14
Quantum Computing and Digital Twins

Chengyi Lin and Paul Critchley

Abstract The quantum world has an indeterministic nature, which, with extreme difficulty, can be harnessed by quantum computers to provide unimaginable computing power. Once quantum computers can be built that are powerful enough, a new era of information technology and computational modelling in the medical space will begin.

With the development of quantum computing among new digital technologies, data analytics and computational models will not be limited to one disease or therapeutic area. In other industries, the combination of data collection, cloud hosting, and machine-learning-aided data analysis have already made it possible to generate "digital twins" for physical objects such as ocean vessels.

In this chapter we discuss the bases of quantum computing and the application of digital twins across industries. The evolution in these areas could have a profound impact on how we understand health and deliver healthcare in the future.

Keywords Quantum · Computer · Probability · Indeterministic · Deterministic Qubits · Bits · Digital twins · Mirror world · Data · IoT · Cloud computing · Digital health · EHR

C. Lin (✉)
INSEAD, Fontainebleau, France
e-mail: chengyi.lin@insead.edu

P. Critchley
Institute of Physics, London, UK
e-mail: paul.critchley@vodafone.com

© The Author(s), under exclusive license to Springer Nature
Switzerland AG 2022
M. Al-Razouki, S. Smith (eds.), *Hybrid Healthcare*, Health Informatics,
https://doi.org/10.1007/978-3-031-04836-4_14

Quantum Computing

Intro to Quantum Physics: No Scary Maths (Well Almost)

"If you think you understand quantum mechanics, you don't understand quantum mechanics." R. Feynman—The Character of Physical Law—(Anon 2014) (a father of quantum physics).

Quantum processes are the fundamental building blocks of everything around us. However, we rarely experience any of the effects of quantum physics. The everyday world, from a physical point of view, is deterministic, that is to say, event A causes event B. For example, Newton's classical laws of motion are deterministic and can be modelled to a high degree of accuracy, but this is not the case in the quantum world. Instead of deterministic behaviour, the quantum world is indeterministic and therefore only probabilistic behaviour can be modelled: event A may cause event B by some associated probability. An example of indeterministic behaviour is the Heisenberg Uncertainty Principle (described in detail below).

Many of the events in the quantum world are to some extent random, so it is somewhat illogical that on a macro scale we live in a physically deterministic universe. In reality, it is the sum of the quantum probabilities that leads to our deterministic universe. However, there remain infinitesimally small probabilities that a quantum effect could occur on a macro scale, albeit it would take more than the duration of the known universe to be observable. This is one of the many strange outcomes of the quantum world.

The classical view is that the world is made up of atoms, which are made up of electrons, neutrons and electrons that are typically thought of as particles. However, in the quantum world, these particles are also waves and are more accurately treated mathematically as probability distributions.

Figure 14.1a shows a classical dot cross diagram of hydrogen (a favourite of chemists) with an electron orbiting the proton. The reality of the quantum world is shown in Fig. 14.1b. Figure 14.1b shows some of the same features as the dot cross diagram, but the electron (the ring) is in fact a probability distribution denoted by

Fig. 14.1 (a) Classical view of a hydrogen atom shown using a dot cross diagram; (b) the reality of the quantum world showing a hydrogen atom, wherein the intensity of shading indicates the probability that the electron or proton is at any given location

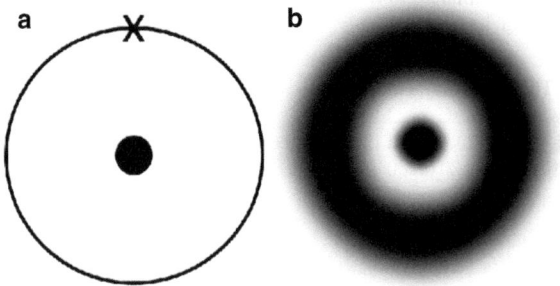

the intensity of the shading of the ring. The electron is not in any one place but exists as a probability cloud around the proton, and the proton itself occupies a probability cloud in the centre of the atom. Of course, a hydrogen atom is the simplest atom that exists. The energy levels and hence probability distributions of the electrons and nuclei become increasingly complex for atoms with a greater number of electrons, protons and neutrons (and in higher energy states).

Schrödinger's Cat

Schrödinger's cat is a thought experiment that illustrates a paradox of quantum superposition. The question is, if the cat is put into an opaque box with a mechanism that has a 50% chance of causing the cat's death, is the cat dead or alive? Obviously, the answer cannot be known without observing the cat: there is a 50% chance the cat is dead and a 50% chance it is alive. In physics this is known as a superposition of states. Mathematically speaking, the cat is both dead and alive simultaneously, that is until the observer opens the box to observe it. Once it is opened, the superposition of the two states collapses and the outcome of the cat's fate is known.

The purpose of this thought experiment is to demonstrate how physicists handle quantum physics mathematically to gain useful information. In fact, this is how a quantum computer works mathematically, as described in more detail later in this chapter.

The (Lesser Known) Heisenberg Uncertainty Principle

The renowned quantum physicist Werner Heisenberg demonstrated that there are some quantities which are not possible to know simultaneously. As indicated below, for any given particle, the proven equation where h and π are constants and Δx and Δp are the uncertainty in position and momentum of the particle respectively demonstrates that it is not possible to know the exact position and the momentum of the particle, because the greater the certainty in the position of a particle (i.e. the lower Δx), the greater the uncertainty in momentum. Other equally related quantities are time Δt and energy ΔE. It is not possible to know precisely both the time at which an event happened and the energy of the event simultaneously (further explanation of this principle is beyond the scope of this book).

$$\Delta x \, \Delta p \geq \frac{h}{4\pi}$$

Quantum Physics in Everyday Use

Despite its apparent strangeness, some aspects of quantum physics have already been harnessed for everyday use. For example, lasers are based on aspects of quantum mechanics where atoms have discrete energy levels. For this reason, lasers only ever emit one colour at a time of a very specific wavelength. Examples of their everyday use include CDs, DVDs, Blu-ray and Ultra-HD players. Many of these use a strained silicon laser, which itself relies on properties of quantum physics. The transistors used in every computer are made of semiconductor material that functions on the principles of quantum physics.

Light-emitting diodes (LEDs) rely on discrete atomic energy levels to produce light of a specific frequency from semiconductor material. You may recall that white LEDs took far longer to achieve than blue and red LEDs. This is a direct consequence of the atomic energy levels in LEDs being very well defined. White LEDs require a mixture of LEDs operating across the spectrum, or alternatively, fluorescent coatings to down convert the frequency of blue photons in order to produce white light.

Organic light-emitting diodes (OLEDs) also rely on the discrete nature of atomic transitions to produce the red, green and blue components for screen technology so that the entire rainbow of colours can be reproduced, as well as quantum energy transfer processes between the organic and inorganic parts of the OLEDs.

Fibre optics such as those used in medicine and telecommunications also rely on quantum effects. These effects rely on light waves being guided, rather than reflected, along the length of a fibre optic cable.

Magnetic resonance imagery relies on the concept of quantum spin. In this quantum phenomenon, every atom and fundamental particle exhibits a quantum spin that generates a small magnetic field. In MRI, a powerful magnet is applied to the atoms of the body, which can align the protons due to the small magnetic field they generate. There are further quantum effects such as spin splitting, where atoms cannot occupy the exact same energy state (again, this goes beyond the scope of the book). Once the protons are aligned by the applied magnetic field, a radio frequency is used to probe the energy states of the atoms.

Intro to Quantum Computing

Schrödinger's Cat: Bits to Qubits

In traditional computing, the fundamentals of the computer are binary, that is, information is contained in bits, where each bit can have one of two values, either a 0 or a 1 (Fig. 14.2a). You may be familiar with computer bytes and one byte consists of 8 bits—for example, 01001001 is equal to the decimal number 73. Each bit (0 or 1) is multiplied by 2 to the power of its order from right to left starting from 0. Of course, 0 multiplied by anything is still 0, so taking just the 1s (from right to left) the value is $(1 \times 2^0) + (1 \times 2^3) + (1 \times 2^6) = 73$.

Fig. 14.2 Diagrammatic expression of (**a**) a classical computer bit which has discrete binary states; (**b**) a quantum bit (qubit) which has some mixing of the binary states

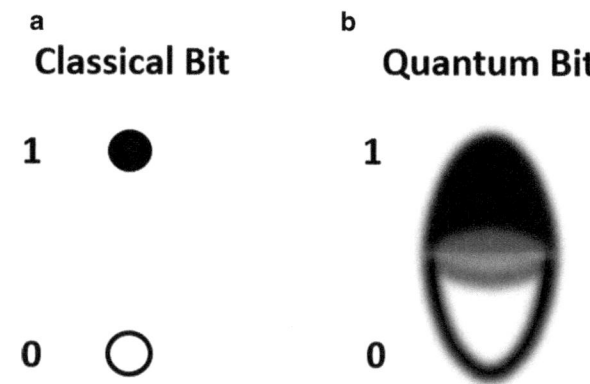

We generally come across bytes in the context of the storage capacity of a computer or mobile phone. For example, smartphones are sold with 64GB, 128GB, or 256GB (GB stands for gigabyte, a GB being 1×10^9 bytes). A smartphone with 64×10^9 bytes of storage is 5.12×10^{12} bits of storage.

The purpose of this is to demonstrate that a single bit (which can be a 0 or a 1) is not particularly useful on its own, but combining bits in large numbers can be very useful. In traditional computing, the lowest number of bits grouped together is 8, as in the byte mentioned above. Nearly every computer on the planet relies on there being 8 bits in a byte.

Beyond storage capacity, computer processors operate in a very similar way. At its most fundamental, a processor is a large collection of switches (known as transistors) which may be on (1) or off (0) each time they perform a calculation. The speed of a computer depends on several factors, but the clock speed is how many processes the millions of transistors can perform per second. For example, a central processing unit (CPU) with a clock speed of 2.9 GHz executes 2.9 billion cycles per second.

Unlike everyday experiences, when a switch is either on (1) or off (0), in the quantum world switches can be both on and off simultaneously. Like the Schrödinger's cat illustration above, if we take the cat to be a single bit, when we observe the cat it is either alive (1) or dead (0). However, when it is in the opaque box (before observation) mathematically the cat is both alive (1) and dead (0), a superposition of states that allows the cat (or bit) to occupy both simultaneously.

In the quantum computing world, this bit is called a quantum bit, or qubit (Fig. 14.2b). Again, the same principles of bits apply: we can collect 8 cats in boxes and form a byte with 8 qubits—or qubyte. However, to be a true qubyte, each of the qubits must be entangled (another strange property of quantum physics), meaning that the state of each box (qubit) in the entangled qubyte can feel the states of the remaining boxes (qubits), such that the boxes (qubits) cannot be described in any meaningful sense independently of one another.

It is largely the issue of entanglement and the closely-related effect of quantum coherence that makes quantum computers so hard to construct.

Classical Computers and Their Limitations

In classical computers, the central processing unit (CPU) consists of millions of transistors which are binary—they can only have a value of 1 or 0. For example, the Intel i7 chipset is thought to consist of approximately three billion transistors.[1]

One of the earliest-ever computers, Colossus, was developed in 1943 during World War 2 (and featured in the film Imitation Game), has approximately 1500 vacuum tubes[2] (the equivalent of today's transistors).

The best way to think about how a classical computer solves a problem is by imagining a 4-digit combination lock. To crack the combination (without prior knowledge of the solution) you have to try every possible combination of numbers. A logical approach is to start at the lowest possible combination (0000) and work iteratively through every possible combination 0001, 0002, 0003... (without using clever programming, hacking or other shortcuts). The computer solves the problem by trying every possible value in turn, one after the other. So if the combination is 3268, the computer will have tried 3269 combinations. This is fundamentally how a classical computer operates.

Today's fast computing is possible because of the sheer power of the computers around us—there can be three billion transistors on a single chip. The above combination would be relatively trivial for today's powerful computers to break. However, instead of a 4-digit combination, imagine a one million alphanumeric combination lock—that would take far longer to solve. And even harder cryptographic locks exist, on which internet banking relies, that would take a classical computer centuries to break (without using hacks or shortcuts). For example, it would take a classical computer 300 trillion years to break an asymmetric Rivest–Shamir–Adleman(RSA)-2048 bit encryption key[3]—far too long for it to be possible in any meaningful way. Take modelling a caffeine molecule. In this case, the amount of information needed to represent the caffeine molecule in binary would require 10^{48} atoms, which is roughly the number of atoms on the entire Earth (10^{49}).[4]

From this, the benefits of quantum computers over classical computers start to become apparent. We can see that there are limitations to classical computers, even if most of us do not experience them in everyday life.

Quantum Computers and Their Benefits

The advantage of quantum computers is rooted in the quantum superposition of states and the quantum entanglement mentioned earlier.

---

[1] https://www.tomshardware.com/reviews/intel-core-i7-8086k-cpu-8086-anniversary,5658-2.html

[2] https://newscentre.vodafone.co.uk/features/five-facts-colossus/

[3] https://www.quintessencelabs.com/blog/breaking-rsa-encryption-update-state-art/

[4] https://www.technologyreview.com/2019/10/23/102523/google-ceo-quantum-supremacy-interview-with-sundar-pichai/#:~:text=Caffeine%2C%20with%2024%20atoms%2C%20can,has%20about%201,010%20bits

Going back to Schrödinger's cat, instead of having billions of transistors each operating independently and discreetly (i.e. forming a result of 1 or 0), quantum computers have the ability to occupy all states simultaneously. Just as the cat is both dead and alive simultaneously in a superposition of states, our qubits are in a superposition of states of 1 and 0. Taking a qubyte (our eight entangled qubits), this means that a quantum computer is able to exist in every possible permutation of the byte simultaneously.

Analogously, when we look at the cat in the box, or our qubits, the superposition of states collapses to a known value that is the solution to our value.

Solving the Numerical Padlock: The True Power

Furthermore, if we had enough qubits, our quantum computer would be able to occupy every possible numerical combination simultaneously. So although it may not take long for current computers with three billion transistors to solve our four-digit combination lock, with enough qubits our quantum computer would be able to solve this problem instantaneously. Thus the quantum computer arrives at 3268 instantaneously—without having to wait for it to try every preceding combination. Here we begin to see the true benefit of quantum computers.

When applied to the RSA-2048 bit encryption key, which may take a powerful classical computer 300 trillion years to solve, a quantum computer with enough qubits would be able to solve this instantaneously.

Revisiting our example of a caffeine molecule which would require 10^{48} atoms to represent in binary, it is possible to represent caffeine with just 160 qubits.[5]

Quantum Supremacy: A New Era

The ability of a real life quantum computer to instantly solve a problem that the most powerful classical computer would take years to solve is known as 'quantum supremacy', a term coined by John Preskill in 2012 to indicate the true beginning of the quantum computing era.

Quantum supremacy is currently the goal of many companies and quantum computing researchers, and is a highly sought-after prize. In 2019, Google produced a Nature Paper[6] that claimed their quantum computer, which has 53 qubits, had solved a problem in seconds that would take a classical computer 10,000 years to solve. Shortly afterwards, IBM demonstrated that in fact a classical computer could solve the same problem in in 2.5 days.[7]

---

[5] https://venturebeat.com/2019/07/14/ibm-research-explains-how-quantum-computing-works-and-could-be-the-the-supercomputer-of-the-future/

[6] https://www.nature.com/articles/s41586-019-1666-5

[7] https://www.ibm.com/blogs/research/2019/10/on-quantum-supremacy/

As of early 2021, we are still not in the quantum supremacy era, and by some estimates it is still years away. It is thought that a quantum computer with less than 60 qubits can be simulated by a classical computer fairly easily.[8]

What Are the Advantages of Quantum Computers: And How Do They Help Healthcare?

We have already seen some of the general advantages around computing times and cryptography. However, these few examples show that quantum computers may not benefit the average computer user. We do not need a quantum computer to load Microsoft Word, PowerPoint or Excel—existing computers are good enough.

However, we can see the benefits of faster computing and envisage where these advantages can best be realised. The example of cryptography is important because it is key to the functioning of society. The new field of quantum cryptography already exists, where governments, banks, and also healthcare providers use it to protect the valuable information they hold and the transactions they perform.

Advantages of Quantum Computers in Hybrid Healthcare

In a future era of hybrid healthcare, quantum computers would offer radical benefits.

A new drug typically takes 10–15 years from discovery to launch, and the costs can exceed $2 billion, with a success rate of less than 10%.[9] Drug design on a computer takes a huge amount of processing power, and researchers are limited by the power of the super computers they use. Quantum computers will see the birth of supersonic drug design, especially with respect to the BioCloud (covered in Chap. 4) where quantum computers can generate results from various permutations almost instantly. Once quantum computers are mainstream, we can expect to see a huge rise in companies like BenevolentAI and a shift away from traditional drug design practices in the lab.

It will be possible to run clinical trials entirely in-silico, that is to say simulating the drug trial process in its entirety. This would have huge repercussions on the speed and cost at which clinical trials are run. Rather than taking months, a quantum computer could potentially generate output results in hours, and the drug would never have to be produced before trials begin, merely modelled. Furthermore, no patients for studies would be needed, making medical trials completely safe.

Sequencing and analyzing DNA will become a relatively trivial task as the power of quantum computers outperform classical computers by several orders of magnitude; giving the medical profession incredible insights into possible treatment

---

[8] https://www.newscientist.com/article/2246940-honeywell-claims-it-has-built-the-most-powerful-quantum-computer-ever/

[9] https://www.bcg.com/publications/2019/quantum-computing-transform-biopharma-research-development

pathways, as well as the development of highly personalised medicine. We can expect to see improved disease screening and treatment methods through the use of quantum computers as a diagnostic tool to estimate disease patterns and the spread of diseases.

Longer term, quantum cryptography could also lead to the protection of patient data in the most secure computers that exist, which no ordinary computer would be able to decrypt.

In conclusion, quantum computers are still in the development stage. By some estimates, a useful quantum computer could be up to 10 years away. Even the technology to create a quantum computer effectively is a subject of debate. Among the contenders are superconductors, atoms, and trapped ions. Furthermore, because quantum computers work in a fundamentally different manner, the method of programming is very different from a classical computer, hence a new era of programming and programmers needs to evolve.

The main companies to watch in the development of quantum computers are currently IBM, Google, Honeywell, Alibaba, Microsoft, Intel, D-Wave, CQC, 1Qbit, and IonQ.

Digital Twins

The Birth of the Twin

Like artificial intelligence and quantum computing, the "digital twin" idea was born earlier than might be expected. In 1991, the term was coined by computer scientist David Gelernter, an associate professor at Yale, in his book *Mirror Worlds: or the Day Software Puts the Universe in a Shoebox—How It Will Happen and What It Will Mean*,[10] where in a not-so-distant future he predicted that, "You will look into a computer screen and see reality." He called this a "mirror world", which "is fed by a steady rush of new data pouring in through cables". More importantly, he described how it could be achieved through technology, both computer hardware and software. In this new world, digital twins are mirror images of physical objects constructed by data.

Similar to the "AI winters", the digital twin simply remained an idea until late in 2010, when John Vickers brought the concept to NASA's roadmap—the first real-world application.[11] NASA's application did not come out of thin air or scientific imagination. As early as 2003, Michael Grieves introduced the concept of "a virtual, digital equivalent to a physical product" in an executive course on Product Life

---

[10] Gelernter DH. Mirror worlds: or the day software puts the universe in a shoebox—how it will happen and what it will mean. Oxford; New York: Oxford University Press. 1991. ISBN 978–0195079067. OCLC 23868481.

[11] Piascik R. et al. Technology Area 12: materials, structures, mechanical systems, and manufacturing road map. NASA Office of Chief Technologist. 2010.

Cycle Management at the University of Michigan.[12] At the time, the technology was immature and the data "was limited, manually collected, and mostly paper-based", but, he argued, with the development of new technologies, digital twins could become "virtually indistinguishable from their physical counterparts".

What technological advancements in the last decade have pushed the digital twins into adolescence? Let's take a look at the enabling conditions.

Nurturing Growth: The Enabling Conditions

Many technology advances were made between 1991, the birth of digital twin idea, and 2010, when it was featured in NASA's roadmap. Among the most memorable are the World Wide Web, e-commerce (e.g. Amazon and eBay), DVD and DVR, the Personal Digital Assistant (e.g. Apple Newton, Palm Pilot), the iPhone, 2G connectivity, and many more. Development in specialised fields such as bioscience and medicine include the complete sequencing of human genome, the synthesis of the first artificial chromosome, the development of GeneChip, approval of the first monoclonal antibody for cancer therapy, and the list goes on.

How can we understand which technologies contributed to the materialisation of the digital twin?

One way is to look at the technological requirements for a digital twin. As mentioned previously, the *Mirror World* that hosts the digital twins, according to Professor Gelernter, relies on "a steady rush of new data pouring in through cables" to construct a realistic world behind the computer screen. Taking the key words from that depiction and mapping them to the related technology development, we can start to understand the enabling conditions for the digital twin's adolescence.

- *New data*: Sensor and imaging technologies, among others, allow the collection of new and interesting data. For example, ultra-red sensors can accurately detect body surface temperature without physical contact. When we watch a still or video advertisement, high-resolution cameras can accurately track movements of the iris that help us understand where and how we focus our attention.
- *A steady rush*: The accurate and dynamic reconstruction of physical objects in the digital world requires the accurate collection of data in real time. The development and commoditization of Internet of Things (IOT) make it possible to collect steady streams of real-world data through connected sensors. For example, connected sensors could be installed on various parts of a deep-ocean oil

---

[12] Grieves M. Digital twin: manufacturing excellence through virtual factory replication. 2015. https://www.researchgate.net/publication/275211047_Digital_Twin_Manufacturing_Excellence_through_Virtual_Factory_Replication

Grieves M. Virtually intelligent product systems: digital and physical twins, in complex systems engineering: theory and practice, Flumerfelt S. et al., Editor. American Institute of Aeronautics and Astronautics; 2019. p. 175–200. https://www.researchgate.net/publication/334599683_Virtually_Intelligent_Product_Systems_Digital_and_Physical_Twins

platform. The collection and monitoring of real-time data can reduce the need for human presence in extreme conditions.

- *Pouring through cables*: Funnily enough, although David Gelerntner's predictions were accurate, he missed a minor detail: that less than two decades later, wireless combined with Cloud technologies could stream and store data through wavelengths rather than cables. Beyond freedom from cables, these technologies allow highly centralised data hosting, which means we can access a huge variety of data without the need to lay cables into all the data centres.
- *Behind the computer screen*: Continuous advances in hardware such as microchip technologies have enables the improvement and commoditization of processing power. The increase in computing power, according to Moore's Law,[13] opens the possibility of analysing the large volume of data needed to construct the digital twin. For example, IBM Deep Blue, the first supercomputer that beat the world chess champion Garry Kasparov in 1997, performed at 11.38 billion floating-point operations per second (FLOPS), or 11.38 gigaflops (GFLOPS). Samsung Galaxy S5, released in 2014, can output 142 GFLOPS at your fingertip.
- *Construct*: Advances in machine learning and AI technology (see Chap. 2) have enabled the efficient processing of data. More important than processing, these algorithms help humans gain insights from large volumes of data ('big data'). For example, computer vision can analyse infrastructure, traffic and pedestrians in real-time, which enables autonomous cars to drive themselves (e.g. Google, Uber and Tesla).
- *Realistic world*: The integration of these technologies completes the data cycle from collection, transmission and storage to processing, analysing and recommending. The volume, variety, velocity, and veracity of data, known as the IBM 4Vs, made it possible to represent the real world through digital and in the form of data.

The young and energetic digital twin quickly entered many fields of business and society. Here are just a few examples.

Digital Twins in Maritime

The Damen Group is a family-owned shipyard that build large marine vessels including patrol tankers, logistic supporting vessels, fishing boats, ferries and many more.[14] To meet the demand for on-vessel management, the company collaborated with Tata Consultancy Services to build connected vessels and digital twins. The construction of digital twins has changed many aspects of Damen's business. For example, the rich data presented by the digital twins can help Damen understand how their vessels perform under different conditions, such as extreme weather, crew

---

[13] https://www.intel.com/content/www/us/en/silicon-innovations/moores-law-technology.html
   https://en.wikipedia.org/wiki/Moore's_law
[14] https://www.damen.com/

operations, and maintenance quality and frequency. These insights help them improve product design and manufacture. The real-time data collected by the digital twins helps Damen monitor their vessels in real-time. Should the algorithm detect any abnormality, Damen and the ship operator can inform the crew and provide maintenance instructions. When necessary, they can even send maintenance crew or spare parts to reduce the risks of costly accidents. The historical data hosted across the digital twins became even more meaningful for Damen. Insights from these data could inform the ship maker how frequent their vessels went to maintenance and what type of maintenance was performed over time. These were the foundation for Damen to transform the business from ship manufacturer to vessel management provider.

Digital Twins in Manufacturing

Now consider a leading chemical manufacturing company which operates multiple chemical processing plants that produce one of their proprietary products. The founder invented the production process a few decades ago and this unique product has always been in high demand in the market. However, the production process is highly dangerous. The plant operators need to keep the large chemical reactors at a specific temperature: too high and the reactor will produce a chemical mixture that can take days to clean up, which will shut down the entire production line. Worse, the chemical reactor could explode if the temperature is kept high for too long. Therefore, the plant operators and managers work around the clock, monitoring their reactors to maintain this narrow temperature range for production. Despite the digital control systems, this monitoring and responding process remains largely manual and relies heavily on the managers' experiences, which adds workload and safety risks to the plant workers.

To improve this process, the company upgraded one of their production lines. They installed IoT technologies to the entire line and built a digital twin. The plant manager was impressed by the results in just a few weeks. The digital twin incorporates all their historical data and provides a model to predict temperature movements. The model can alert plant managers and operators before the temperature reaches a critical level. Moreover, the digital twin can also make recommendations on how to maintain the reactor temperature within the narrow window to avoid reaching a critical level. The plant is working on building digital twins for all their production lines in this factory and extended functions for the algorithm to recommend the optimal production line to increase productivity.

Digital Twins in Hybrid Healthcare

For a variety of reasons, digital twin applications in healthcare are still in their infancy. Although we have not seen the full application, many meaningful experimentations have been on their way. Here we provide a few examples that try to build digital twins from different angles. First, Microsoft HoloLens 2, among other augmented reality tools, experimented to build 3D visualisations of real-life objects. For healthcare, it can provide a 3D reconstruction of a patient's organs based on imaging technologies such as ultrasound. The digital reconstruction could help surgeons to design and simulate different surgery plans for complicated procedures ahead of the actual operations, which may help reduce risks. Second, the UK BioBank by the National Health Services (NHS) has already started to track genetic and health information from 500,000 participants.[15] These longitudinal studies in various disciplines will not only help advance our understanding of genetic and epigenetic influences on health. The variety of data can help us ultimately construct the "digital health twins" to better understand our bodies and behaviours. Third, national electronic health record (EHR) systems were implemented by many countries including Australia and China. These EHR systems, for the first time, integrated distributed individual healthcare records at the central location. Everyone who opts into the programme will be able to "carry" their complete medical history with them.

It is expected that in a hybrid healthcare system, treatments (both preventative and reactionary) can be first tried on a digital health twin prior to being administered in the physical world. Moreover, our health data can be further enriched by combining with our behaviour data, such as e-commerce purchasing data. E-commerce giants, including Alibaba and JD.com in China and Amazon in the US, are working on building databases for both through their e-commerce and digital health platforms. The collection of such data can be very powerful in constructing the "digital twins" that can help us better understand our health and form the cornerstone of a future hybrid healthcare system.

A Perfect Marriage: Physical and Digital

Far beyond the glow as a digital wonder, the construction of digital twins represents a perfect integration of the physical and digital worlds. Not just a mirror image of the physical world on the other side of the computer screen, the digital twin is a translation of the physical properties to the information and insights that govern them. The wonder of the digital twin signifies the advancement of human knowledge and our understanding of the physical world that we live in. More importantly, the digital twins open new doors for us to deepen those knowledge and our understanding even further.

"Dry" experiments, or computer simulated experiments, have helped us advance our knowledge in physics, chemistry, biology, and medicine. For example, pharmaceutical research and development uses computer models to design or modify molecules to fit in certain target configurations. The process significantly reduced

---

[15] https://www.ukbiobank.ac.uk/

various search costs, such as material costs and labour for laboratory "wet" experiments, time, and safety risks. Bioinformatics has also been instrumental in advancing our understanding of the molecular mechanisms at the system level, such as genomics, proteomics, and more. By reconstructing our physical bodies into digital twins and tracking the data over time, we may be able to connect more dots between currently independent research areas. We may establish more causal relationships between our behaviours and health. We may uncover new mechanisms to manage our health.

If we apply the lessons from the digital twins in manufacturing, maritime and energy sectors to healthcare, we can start to appreciate the power of the digital twins in health. Let us use e-commerce giants as examples to examine the potential benefits from their digital data.

First, Amazon and AliHealth both have e-pharmacy services. These data can help them build more complete consumer profiles from various aspects of life, including entertainment (e.g. Blu-Ray, Prime Video, and Prime Music), book (e.g. books and Kindle Store), toys and games (including video games), fashion, cosmetics, electronics, home and household, and many more. "The Everything Store" correctly identified Amazon's vision and ambition. Adding pharmacy business to their portfolio, Amazon can start to identify correlations across categories and try to answer the question how lifestyle choices relate to health outcomes. For example, the data may be able to test the correlation between "couch potato" or heavy streaming behaviours and obesity.

Second, AliHealth and JD Health have additional services in addition to pharmacy. For example, both sites provide telemedicine and teleconsultation. During COVID pandemics, both sites also offer early triage services through chatbot, machine learning algorithm, and teleconsultation. These additional services, plus the additional categories in groceries, provide the possibility for these Chinese e-commerce giants to build an even more complete picture of their customers. These data may provide additional insights on how consumers interact with the healthcare system, for example what triggers visits to physicians, whether and how soon patients fill prescriptions, whether patients follow up with physicians after treatments, and much more. Such additional insights can help the healthcare system interpret and improve the current patient outcomes. These insights can also help underwriting health insurance plans. For example, for diabetic patients, the app may help analyse whether the frequency of physician visits, compliance to the treatment, and adjustment to daily behaviours such as diet and exercise have impact on their treatment or health outcomes.

Third, Alibaba Group does not only own e-commerce (e.g. Taobao.com, T-Mall, etc.) and AliHealth. Their supper APP connects to many other services including mobile payment (AliPay), finance (Ant Finance programmes), entertainment and content (e.g. Youku.com, Tudou.com, etc.), and food delivery services (e.g. ele.me). As you could see, the integration of all these consumer data across categories, combined with Alibaba's dominant market position, will enable Alibaba to build digital twins that are close to the complete picture of the consumers' behaviours. These data may further advance medical research and finally link our behaviours to our health conditions. For example, mental health may be caused by multiple factors including physical (e.g. hormone), behavioural, and social. Digital twins may host data in all these areas. AliHealth may host medical data from physician visits and laboratory tests for physical conditions; AliPay and e-commerce may host purchase histories for purchasing behaviours; entertainment and gaming apps may have data on content consumption behaviours; ele.me may have data on dietary behaviours; and chat and payment apps will have information on social interactions. Thus, studies of the digital twins of mental health patients may help us identify patterns of abnormality and even early signs. We can apply these insights to generate predictions in the undiagnosed population and test the effectiveness of the predictions. Based on this new knowledge from digital twins, we may even develop new treatment regimens for early stages or even methods of prevention.

The development of digital twins makes it possible for hybrid models to advance. The combination of digital and physical in the hybrid model can be pushed beyond simple complementarity. A naïve version of the hybrid model has already been put into practice in the automotive industry by Tesla, the hybrid of the digital and physical twin means both are in dynamic synchronisation. This integration allows the real-time monitoring, predictive maintenance, and periodic upgrade on both sides. When applied to health, the digital twins can become a cornerstone of the hybrid healthcare model.

Progenies: Future of Twins?

Like the adolescent stage, the diffusion of digital twins technology will rely one multiple factors, including but not limited to:

- *The continuous development of enabling technologies.* The further advancement and commoditization of sensor technologies, IoT, machine learning algorithm, computing power (including quantum computing), wireless technologies, cloud technologies, consumer electronics, and more.
- *The articulation of value through healthcare use cases.* From inside or outside of the healthcare system, experimentation with digital twins can help discover new use cases and evolve the current business models.
- *The consumer and societal demands.* Consumers' fundamental demand for high-quality, personalised, and preventative care, combined with the need to reduce healthcare cost at the societal level will continue to push for new ways of organising the health system and delivering care.
- *The shared mission of healthcare players.* Despite the competitive dynamics in healthcare, players in the ecosystem share a strong mission to deliver the best patient outcomes. This shared vision may help to overcome the challenging process of developing and adopting digital twins.
- *The readiness of adoption.* The road to adoption will be face with economical, practical, social, and geopolitical challenges. Beyond the maturity of digital twin

technologies and the articulation of their values, healthcare needs to be open-minded to the next evolution.

- *The sensitivities of data.* The core of a digital twin is data. As we explore and experiment to adopt digital twins, the healthcare system and all the players need to pay close attention to challenges around data and data processes, and more importantly, around data rights, privacy, and security.

In conclusion, digital twins are digital reconstructions of physical objects from dynamic and comprehensive data sets. From concept to realisation, the application of digital twins relied on the advancement in many enabling technologies, including IoT, Cloud, computing power, machine learning algorithm, and more. Many industries, including manufacturing, transportation, energy, among others, have recognised the potential of digital twin technology and started to experiment with its real-world applications. The pilots in manufacturing plants, maritime, and offshore drilling start to uncover the new value created in improving both efficiency and effectiveness. Although the digital twin applications can be equally powerful in health, current development remains fragmented and slow due to concerns on technology maturity, costs, and risks in data privacy and security. At the same time, disruptive forces may come from outside of the healthcare system. Technology and e-commerce giants have invested in building comprehensive consumer profiles, or digital twins, that integrate consumer data from multiple sectors. These novel experiments may push our hybrid healthcare system to accelerate the speed and scale of exploration. We are encouraged to see multiple projects by different players in the healthcare system such as digital start-ups, medical research institutions, and health authorities. The future of digital twins in health depends on collaborative efforts and these efforts can significantly improve the patient outcomes.

Chapter 15
Strategic Implications of Hybrid Healthcare on Patient, Medicine, Services, and Society

Chengyi Lin

Abstract A hybrid health model that integrates digital and physical care has a broad impact on our healthcare system and beyond. In this chapter, we will use the Apple Heart Study as an anchor example to analyse the various strategic implications of the hybrid health model. Based on the foundational knowledge and analysis of various technologies from previous chapters, we aimed at expanding our understanding of the potential impact on various participants in healthcare and society at large. With the continuous development of technologies and the application in health, we will see a range of new combinations of hybrid delivery models. We will focus on four areas that these innovations could change how we design and deliver care, namely the evolutions in human-machine, human-human, life-heath, and individual-public interfaces. We will also present an integrative framework to help our readers navigate these evolving interfaces of the health system.

The unleash of data can be powerful in changing our healthcare landscape and its integration with society. It may present new opportunities to improve health outcomes and reduce costs. At the same time, it may also present threats to our existing system and even introduce new risks, such as privacy and security. Importantly for all players in the health system, from patient to practitioners and from private to public sectors, we need to continuously reflect on our actions and determine our strategic actions on this transformational journey.

Keywords Hybrid health · Strategic impacts · Strategic implications · Societal impacts · Digital twin(s) · Apple heart study · Digital wearables · Human-machine Interface · Human-human Interface · Life-health Interface · Individual-public Interface

C. Lin (✉)
INSEAD, Fontainebleau, France
e-mail: chengyi.lin@insead.edu

© The Author(s), under exclusive license to Springer Nature Switzerland AG 2022
M. Al-Razouki, S. Smith (eds.), *Hybrid Healthcare*, Health Informatics, https://doi.org/10.1007/978-3-031-04836-4_15

Let us start this Chapter by rolling back in time to the year 2017. The year endured the Trump inauguration, North Korea missile launch, Las Vegas shooting, wildfires across the globe, and a total solar eclipse. The same 2017 also saw many social and cultural movements including Me-too and NFL kneeling protest against racism. And adding to the list, the US declared opioid pandemic a public health emergency and Artificial Intelligence came into spotlight due to its potential dangers to society.[1] Quietly hidden under these tidal waves was the launch of a study by Apple, commonly known as the Apple Heart Study with Stanford Medicine, that attracted great attention in the medical world. Tech giants are coming to healthcare.

Previous chapters explored various digital technologies and their use cases in medicine and healthcare. In this chapter, we will venture beyond the practice of medicine itself and try to explore the many implications of digital transformation of our health system and society in general. We will follow the Apple heart study to illustrate its ripple effects, which can help us systematically understand the strategic impacts of a hybrid healthcare model.

First, let us take a brief look at the Apple Heart Study itself. On November 29, 2017, Stanford Medicine joined started a clinical study using the Apple Watch data to "identify irregular heart rhythms, including those from potentially serious heart conditions such as atrial fibrillation".[2] This collaboration aimed at improving the digital technologies embedded in the Apple Watch that can detect and analyse potential heart conditions.

The study concluded on February 21, 2019 and generated a series of publications including an article in the *New England Journal of Medicine.*[3] Here we will not discuss and debate the results and interpretation of the data from these clinical studies. Instead, we will focus on the implications of this study outside of clinical research and analyse its potential future impact together.

First and foremost, the Apple Heart Study could be viewed as an important initial step towards a hybrid healthcare model. There are potentially three ways to look at this study at a strategic level. First, the Apple Watch could be a "new device" that replaces the EKG machine. This view can lead to a simple conclusion that at the current stage, the sensitivity and reliability would not position Apple Watch as a meaningful "replacement". Second, Apple Watch is just another consumer wearable that can provide additional healthcare benefits. Applying this view, one would put Apple Watch back into the consumer product category based on the results, granting it some premium functionality after this public relationship flair. Third and maybe the most important view is that the Apple Watch can become the bridge, or a hybrid healthcare model, that connects physical devices and digital data. Moreover, it also connects the episodic occurrence of illness with the continuity of healthy living.

Although the clinical trial data showed that the technology still needs time to mature, the promise of the new hybrid healthcare model should not go unnoticed even at its infancy. To fully appreciate the impact of such a new model on the

---

[1] https://www.history.com/topics/21st-century/2017-events

[2] http://med.stanford.edu/appleheartstudy.html

[3] https://www.nejm.org/doi/full/10.1056/NEJMoa1901183

healthcare industry and beyond, we need to analyse how it can potentially affect the various elements both inside and outside the healthcare system. To do so, we will focus our analysis on a few critical interfaces.

- The human-machine interface

  The hybrid healthcare model created two important human-machine interfaces, one between the patient and the front end of the digital app, and the other between the healthcare practitioners and the data back end. The second interface can also extend to other stakeholders in the healthcare ecosystem, such as insurance and government.
- The human-human interface

  The data generated from the hybrid healthcare model does not only benefit the patients and the healthcare practitioners, but also changes the dynamics within the healthcare ecosystem. These data could improve many critical steps in the healthcare delivery process, from drug discovery to supply chain optimisation to personalised medicine. As a result of these improvements, the dynamics within the ecosystem may shift as the technology advances.
- The life-health interface

  Tech giants, including Apple, Amazon, and Google, entering healthcare have more profound strategic impacts beyond digital products, revenues, and supply chain. The data at the backend of these digital solutions starts to connect our life—how we live, what we eat, and how much we work—with our interactions with the healthcare system. These data can enrich our understanding of the correlations and causations between our behaviours and our health outcomes.
- The individual-public interface

  As our world becomes more connected, we are also exposed to increasing public health challenges. Recent pandemics, caused by infectious diseases such as Ebola and COVID-19 or behaviours such as obesity and opioid, have demonstrated the speed and scale they could affect us. Digital technologies have shown promises in helping us anticipate and manage these challenges. Hybrid healthcare can take its part to reimagine the individual-public health interface.

The Human-Machine Interface

Anthropologists, historians, and evolutionary biologists would point to the ability to make tools as a key characteristic of human intelligence. The relationships between humans and the tools we made, or technologies we invented, have defined and redefined human society throughout the course of human evolution. From the early agricultural evolution, to scientific evolution, from the first to now the fourth industrial revolution, each time the development of new technology generated a new interface between humans and the machines humans created.

In the current digital era, the new interface is between human and the electronic devices that hosts our individual and collective information. In medicine, these electronic devices are not limited to the medical devices in the physicians' offices, the medical laboratories, or the hospitals. New generations of such devices could very well be in our pockets, handbags, on our desks and in our living rooms. Smart phones, tablets, desk-top and laptop computers, connected gym equipment, smart household appliances and many more. Many of these connected consumer devices have sensors that can collect and keep records of various information, from our chats to images, and from our physical movements to our choices (e.g. food, music, movies, and written media). After we can read our emails from anywhere on our mobile phone and tablets, the human-machine interface for "work" has moved from office to everywhere with a wireless or mobile data connection. Similarly, the human-machine interface for medicine starts to move out of physicians' offices, laboratories, and hospitals.

What could the movement of the human-machine interface mean?

Before we discuss the implications from Apple Watch and Apple Heart Study, let us go back a couple of decades in time. For diabetic diagnoses, the first blood glucose home test device, Dextrometer, was launched in 1980. Combined with Dextrostrix, it allowed continuous monitoring of glucose level by diabetic patients at home.[4] Around the same time, pharmaceutical companies also competed to develop the first commercial insulin pumps. Autosyringe, also known as "Big Blue Brick" was among the pioneer devices to be launched in 1978.[5] The devices to monitor glucose level and regulate insulin kept evolving over the years. After the launch of the iPhone and its App Store, many companion apps also sprouted to help diabetic patients manage their devices.

Beyond the physical movement out of the medical facilities, the human-machine interface evolution changed how diabetes was treated. Both patient outcome and quality of life have improved as they could live a normal life with the help of the device. These improvements also mean less physician and hospital visits, which can reduce costs to the healthcare system and release some healthcare capacities.

The evolution did not stop at adding companion apps to the pumps. In 2020, University of Cambridge and Cambridge University Hospitals NHS Foundation trust announce the first artificial pancreas app.[6] The app integrates glucose monitoring and insulin delivery systems. Moreover, it uses an algorithm to analyse data from a glucose monitor and automatically deliver insulin through a pump.

A true hybrid healthcare model is brought to life—digital enabled data analytics plus digital control of the physical devices. Without eliminating human intervention completely, the app-device hybridisation maximised the utilisation of digital technologies. What are the benefits?

---

[4] Clarke SF, Foster JR. A history of blood glucose meters and their role in self-monitoring of diabetes mellitus. Br J Biomed Sci 2012;69:83–93.

[5] Alsaleh FM, Smith FJ, et al. Insulin pumps: from inception to the present and toward the future, Journey of Pharmacy and Therapeutics, 2010. https://doi.org/10.1111/j.1365-2710.2009.01048.x

[6] https://www.cambridgeindependent.co.uk/news/artificial-pancreas-app-for-type-1-diabetes-patients-launched-after-university-of-cambridge-research-9102950/

First, potential increase of patient outcomes through increased accuracy. The real-time data entry combined with algorithms generated from clinical data sets may increase the accuracy of insulin delivery, therefore increasing the safety and efficacy. It could reduce risks for both the patients and the healthcare practitioners.

Second, improvement of quality of life. According to Cambridge Independent among other sources, patients have reported to "feel free." The device may further reduce the burden on patients for continuous treatment and restore normalcy of life and enjoyment.

Third, reduce costs. Accurate delivery of insulin may reduce the consumption or waste of the pharmaceutical, and improved management of the disease may reduce potential complications and visits to emergency rooms.

Fourth, enriching clinical data sets. These hybrid healthcare models can enable continuous collection of data, anonymous or in aggregation, to deepen our understanding of the diseases and the effectiveness of the treatments.

Examples of hybrid healthcare go beyond devices moving out of the hospitals. Many mobile apps start to complement physical therapeutics with digital elements. Apps often use machine learning algorithms to analyse multiple data sets beyond medical data.

We can find an abundance of examples in the field of allergy management as well. WebMD Allergy[7] and Allergy Alert[8] are just two examples of the many allergy management apps that patients can find in the App Store or Android App market. These apps often offer multiple functions from symptom tracking to predictions and from alerts to recommendations. The way these apps generate predictions and recommendations can be through analysing multiple data sets using machine learning algorithms.

The analysis across multiple data sets are beneficial, because allergy symptoms often develop based on the environment patients are in contact with. Beyond medical data, some allergy algorithms employ data sets such as weather patterns, forestry and botany, and air pollution, to name a few. We will discuss additional examples of the industry convergence between health and retail in the "life-health interface" segment. These allergy apps provided additional human-machine interfaces beyond the allergy tests in the laboratories. In addition, the app can handle many allergy-related "dialogs" 'outside of the physician's office. Moreover, this new interface could support patients 24/7 and make recommendations based on both individual and population data.

Of course, none of these are perfect and many, including the first artificial pancreas app, are still at their experimental stage. Nonetheless, the promise of these evolved human-machine interfaces is worth noticing.

Now let us bring back the Apple Heart Study. The pioneer nature of the study is demonstrated in its attempt to combine the benefits of both examples we mentioned above. First, similar to the Cambridge artificial pancreas, AHS tried to take a device,

[7] https://apps.apple.com/us/app/webmd-allergy/id588509171
[8] https://www.pollen.com/tools/iphone

an EKG machine, out of the physicians' office or hospital. Using the sensors, a consumer electronic device and start to collect pulse signals and track them over time. Moreover, the computational power of the Apple Watch can enhance the signal to noise ratio and derive a baseline for each individual. All these digital technologies present the possibility to detect and predict small abnormalities. Second, similar to the allergy management apps, AHS aggregates data over the cloud. Using machine learning algorithms, the app can improve the detection sensitivity and predictive accuracy over time. Combined with other data stored in the Apple Watch, such as sleep time and quality, exercise habits, among others, the algorithm may also develop the ability to predict health risks in the future.

In summary, hybrid healthcare models may not only move the human-machine interface physically out of medical facilities, but also change the interface temporarily from episodic monitoring after the diagnostics to real-time tracking to reduce certain health risks.

How could the movements of the human-machine interface impact the health systems?

While the full implications remain to be seen, we can already expect some benefits and downsides for the various stakeholders. For patients, especially patients with chronic conditions, the hybrid healthcare model could help them better manage their condition, gain more autonomy and reduce risks and costs. For healthcare practitioners, the hybrid healthcare model could provide a window into the longitudinal data they have been missing and gain additional insights into the effectiveness of the therapeutic regimens. For payers, both insurers and public sectors, the hybrid healthcare model may help improve cost management as well as patient outcomes. And for regulators, the hybrid healthcare model may encourage a new way to construct the standard of care beyond pharmaceuticals.

Since the 2010's, FDA and EMA have constantly increased the approval of *in vitro* companion diagnostics.[9] These diagnostic tools became increasingly critical, many as prerequisite, for the appropriate treatments. In the same period, studies and papers on the relevance and effectiveness of the medical use of AI/ML algorithms also started to rise.[10] We can expect the continued increase of importance to these algorithms in processing and analysing medical data, both structured and unstructured, in order to generate the best recommendations for treatments. As hybrid healthcare models, for example combinations of pharmaceuticals and devices or pharmaceuticals and algorithms, continue to improve their effectiveness, regulators also need to update the methods of evaluations on their cost-benefit trade-offs and potential risks.

---

[9] https://www.fda.gov/medical-devices/vitro-diagnostics/list-cleared-or-approved-companion-diagnostic-devices-vitro-and-imaging-tools

[10] https://www.nature.com/articles/s41746-020-00324-0

The Human-Human interface

When digital technologies helped medical devices move out of medical facilities and found new homes in patients' daily lives, they did not but shift the machine-human interface. Subtly and gradually, they also impact the human-human interfaces in different ways.

WebMD[11] gained its popularity in the early 2000's after its founding in 1998 and later merged with Sapient Health Network, Direct Medical Knowledge and Healtheon. Rising with Google the search engine, Facebook the social media, and iTune the music store, WebMD joined an era of information democratisation and digital consumption. Public became increasingly excited about obtaining and consuming all kinds of information online, from product information to scientific knowledge, from theoretical works to practical know-hows. There is no exception for health. Patients can find additional information about their diagnostic results, search diseases by symptoms, and get answers to medical questions they may have.

When patients started to obtain medical information on WebMD, this new practice had non-trivial implications to the healthcare system. For example, patients may start to self-diagnose and request more visits to the doctors. Patients may want to spend more time with their doctors and ask questions. Patients may even challenge their doctors' diagnostics and ask for additional tests. All these could add additional burden to the healthcare system.

Around 2000, many physician practices, clinics and hospitals were under huge financial pressure. Patient throughputs were of great importance to their financial solvency. Physicians found themselves spending more time with each patient and laboratories found themselves doing more tests. The change in human-human interface as a result of the shifts in machine-human ones had real impacts on the financial performances of the system.

These impacts were before the acceleration of wearable data and the development of machine learning algorithms. To date, WebMD remains an information database, *fortunately*. What if WebMD can "recommend" diagnoses based on your symptoms or your personal data?

To help us imagine this unlikely scenario, we can examine a distant yet close example—the Amazon recommendation system, aka "The Amazon Recommender". It has been a critical turning point in Amazon's early development. Dreaming to revolutionise retail through e-commerce, Jeff Bezos has launched many innovations to improve online shopping experience in order to change consumer habits. The Amazon recommender is one of the crown jewels because it reduced search costs, improved product visibilities, facilitated trust building, and increased "basket size" or the amount of purchase per transaction.

What is behind the Amazon Recommender? For computer scientists, it was equally exciting. A machine learning algorithm can keep integrating the real-world data collected from Amazon's transaction histories, connecting them to the

---

[11] https://www.webmd.com/

consumer profiles, generating product associations, and predicting consumer preferences. The ever-growing data will not only continuously fuel the algorithm but also make it more and more accurate in its predictions.

The Amazon Recommender, through its novelty and effectiveness, has helped Amazon attract and retain more e-commerce shoppers, which eventually lead to its dominant position in the US e-commerce market.

Could a similar phenomenon happen in healthcare? If we introduce a similar machine learning algorithm to process the ever-growing medical data and link them to patient profiles, what could happen? Would we have a "pocket doctor" who can recommend personalised medicine for you? Many digital health start-ups have started working on this problem. We may not see a "digital GP" before 2025, but the various developments of machine learning algorithms for specific disease areas are promising. For example, Nabta Health started to work on a machine learning algorithm that can suggest a treatment path based on diagnostic results. These could be useful for both the patients and physicians. Once a patient consents to share her diagnostic and treatment history data with the physician, the physician can leverage the suggestion from the machine learning algorithm. Similarly, the patient-app could track patient behaviours, such as whether the patient follows up with the physician after diagnostics and whether she takes her prescribed medicine. Based on these behaviour data, the algorithm can send notifications to increase patient compliance during the treatment process.

The important question is what would become the role of the physicians if these "recommender apps" 'were introduced? Would they enhance or diminish your role as medical experts? How would you redesign your interface with the patients?

One potential implication of this human-human interface change could be the redesign of the patient journey. If we take the view that machine learning algorithms combined with patient data could enhance both the efficiency and effectiveness of the healthcare practitioners, then we could design a different personalised treatment journey. One additional benefit is that the machine learning algorithm can analyse medical research and clinical study data in greater details than the current analysis. Many startups have started using detailed patient data, including genetic sequence, metabolic analysis, blood analysis, urine analysis, and other information to analyse clinical trial data of certain disease areas such as oncology. Such new development could help us better understand drug efficacy and pharma kinetics in order to recommend more personalised treatment regimen.

Now, if we take a step further, the human-human interface can become even more complicated. Let us explore an additional dimension: peer-to-peer interactions, or P2P. In recent years, the rise of peer-to-peer sharing platforms has made it possible for individuals to directly share with each other their photos and videos through Instagram, youtube.com, and TikTok, crafts and products through Etsy.com and Kickstarter, as well as ideas and thoughts through LinkedIn and Facebook. These peer-to-peer interactions give voices to many new "influencers" or "web celebrities", who created communities of followers from thousands to millions around certain subjects. An interesting example comes from the Facebook P2P community. The famous "Ice Bucket Challenge (IBC)" drew attention from many celebrities, business tycoons, and politicians to bring awareness to amyotrophic lateral sclerosis, or Lou Gehrig's disease, and donate to ALS Association in 2014. Bill Gates, LeBron James, Taylor Swift, former US President George W. Bush, and many more have all participated in the IBC challenge.[12] According to the New York Times, ALS collected $41.8 million in less than 1 month from July 29, more than doubling the total donations in 2012-13. With the increased donations, ALS Association supported nearly 120 global research projects, 21 of which were newly financed in 2014.[13] More importantly, the campaign increased ALS awareness among the general public. People have shared more than 1.2 million videos on Facebook in less than 6 months, and IBC has received more than 2.2 million Twitter mentions in less than 2 weeks.

Similarly, P2P communities are also rising in more professional contexts. For example, in computer programming communities, Github and Stack Overflow are two of the many digital platforms on which individual programmes can collaborate on projects and answer each other's programming questions. These P2P communities go beyond simply sharing insights, they can serve an important function of improving the knowledge of the field. An important example for the medical field can be found in COVID long haulers. During the 2019 global pandemic, many COVID patients displayed lasting symptoms even without detectable COVID virus by PCT tests. They were turned away by medical professionals as the mechanism was not understood. The patients self-organised stand-alone online communities, such as Survivor Corps[14] and Facebook Groups, including COVID-19 Long-Haulers Discussion Group,[15] Long COVID-19 Support Group,[16] to name a few. They shared experiences and home-developed remedies with each other to provide medical and psychological support. As the number of long haulers grew, medical field started to pay closer attentions and research these long-term effects.[17]

Many functions of the P2P platforms and the traditional patient communities are alike. Consumers or patients can directly share their needs—medical conditions, products—medical treatments, experiences—effects, product knowledge—insights from medical research and development, and product "hacks"—patient-driven innovations. For example, we have seen the many patients hack their glucose monitor or develop DIY algorithm to determine their insulin intake (see an example article[18]). These patient communities are not only powerful but can also be very helpful to medical research and development. Digital and digital platforms can provide additional tools to enrich these P2P interactions by increasing information

---

[12] https://www.nytimes.com/2014/08/18/business/ice-bucket-challenge-has-raised-millions-for-als-association.html?_r=1

[13] https://www.nytimes.com/2014/08/22/business/media/ice-bucket-challenge-donations-for-als-top-41-million.html?partner=rss&emc=rss&smid=tw-nytimes&_r=0

[14] https://www.survivorcorps.com/

[15] https://www.facebook.com/groups/COVIDLongHaulers/

[16] https://www.facebook.com/groups/longcovid/

[17] https://www.nature.com/articles/d41586-020-02598-6

[18] https://globalnews.ca/news/6517053/diabetes-hack-insulin-pumps-health-tech/

transparency and timely flow, providing multiple perspectives and fact-checking, and gathering large amounts of patient information. Of course, these interactions have their inherent weaknesses, such as inaccurate information, confirmation bias, and group think. Nonetheless, when used appropriately, these P2P interactions can provide increasing values to the medical community.

Now we can bring back AHS. How can AHS help us imagine the human-human interface evolution?

Without conducting a comprehensive analysis, we can highlight a few potential effects on the patient-physician and patient-patient interfaces.

- Patient-physician interface

    Scenario 1: Apple watch data can provide longitudinal data for physicians. Combined with machine learning algorithms, Apple watch data can provide insights on patient baseline information, behaviour patterns, and outlier episodes. The algorithm can also compare across patients and make recommendations to both patients and physicians. These additional information could: (a) reduce unnecessary physician visits, (b) make direct appointment when emergencies rise, (c) ensure both patient and physician are informed about the data and the situation, (d) improve the quality of the patient-physician conversation, (e) make it salient that the responsibility of treatment is shared by patient and physician.

    The historical data on Apple watch or Apple cloud can also be provided to ER physicians. This critical information can reduce the time for gathering EMR data and present the most relevant data for the episode.

    Scenario 2: Apple watch can facilitate a community for the patients' emergency contacts and caregivers. This community can also be supervised by physicians to provide medical advice. The emergency contacts and caregivers can share their experience and insights on how to handle urgent situations. With the help from medical professionals, they could also develop new or enhance existing protocols.

- Patient-patient interface

    The Apple Watch users can also form a community digitally or physically. They can choose to discuss their experience of using the product (Apple watch) and the service (algorithm) with their peers. Such discussions may also lead to recommendations on potential hardware improvements and further development of software. These support communities can also engage with medical professionals and collaborate on medical research. They may also play an important role in advocating for patient data rights and appropriate usage.

The Life-Health Interface

The evolution in human-machine and human-human interfaces mostly modifies the current medical practices through enhancement and replacement. A potential larger transformation may come from the third dimension: blurring the life and health interface. For over a decade, our healthcare industry has been continuously trying to transition from a "sick care" model to a "health management" model. The benefits are clear: increase patient outcomes and reduce costs to the system. This transition is especially important for many chronic conditions, such as diabetes. Effectively managing patients' habits including diet, exercise, and stress may help reduce the potential risks of life-threatening conditions that also require expensive ambulant services and ER visits.

The journey to managing health from treating illness has not been easy. The difficulties partly come from patient behaviours, physician mandates and lack of data. For patient behaviour, we have been heavily relying on patients to detect their own conditions and be the first line triage to decide whether to visit a medical professional. These actions require disease awareness, awareness of body, decision-making, foundational level of knowledge, and resources to seek medical attention, among others. For physician mandates, the healthcare system has been set up to educate, require, measure, and incentivise physicians to "treat diseases". Physicians are evaluated based on patient outcomes, throughputs, and cost management. For data, the healthcare system has accumulated high quality and volume of clinical data on "diseases". These data are detailed and comprehensive, and yet are mostly collected around certain episodes. In addition, within the health system, some of the existing data were scattered across different entities and some are difficult to match to the same patient over time. Beyond the health system, there exists a strong divide between the medical world and the everyday life we live in.

Now, digital health may start to bring changes to all three aspects and hopefully accelerate the transition from treating illness to managing health.

First, consumers start to pay more attention to their overall health, including diets, exercises, and daily routines. For example, with increasing awareness of type II diabetes, obesity, and heart attacks, many consumers changed to high fibre, low carbon, and low cholesterol diets from organic sources. With increasing education on brain health and mental health, many consumers started to pay attention to their daily rhythm, such as time to bed, and their quality of sleep. Consumer electronics, especially digital wearables including Apple watch and Fitbit, started to provide data to help consumers monitor these activities and routines.

Digital health start-ups were fast to jump on these trends. Many digital apps were developed to help consumers monitor and manage these data, such as diet, exercises, and sleep. Many health insurance players also jumped into "digital play". For example, VitalityHealth[19] is one of the early movers to track exercise data through digital wearables. They have developed a unique healthcare plan to incentivise exercise and reward consumer behaviours through tracking wearable data.

However, the most important disruption may have just started. AHS is one of these attempts, in which the continuous monitoring of all daily activities may lead to early and potentially preventative care before critical episodes rise. In addition to Apple, other tech giants, including Microsoft, Huawei, and Google, and e-commerce

---

[19] https://www.vitality.co.uk/

giants, including Alibaba, JD.com, and Amazon, are all coming into healthcare through their own experimentations (see below).

Second, digitalisation calls for changes in the roles and requirements of physicians and other medical professionals. With the potential evolutions we have explained in this chapter, our hybrid healthcare system needs to reflect on some new questions, including but not limited to the following.

- Should physicians and other medical professionals continue to be measured on patient throughputs?

    - If not, how can we meaningfully measure patient outcomes? How can digital help?
    - In addition, how can we set up the incentive system to reward patient outcomes instead of throughputs (e.g. in forms of revenue)?

- If the hybrid healthcare system shifts to a "health management" model, how can the system handle the inherent dilemma that increased health means reduced illness?

    - If the answer is around increasing quality of life and life span, how does that challenge the current business model of the healthcare system?
    - Is it the responsibility of the healthcare system to monitor and measure quality of life? How can we enable such monitoring and measurements? How can digital help?
    - How can we set up the appropriate incentive system to reward the effective management of health?

Third, consumer electronics and E-commerce started to blur the boundary between healthcare and healthy living. These new movements provide additional data, in both high quality and quantity, to finally help us understand our living habits. The combination of both health and illness data could finally help us make direct connections, both correlational and causal, between behaviours and medical conditions. For example, NHS started UK BioBank initiative[20] from 2006, which creates medical databases to track up to 500,000 patients over a decade. AHS and other initiatives started to connect consumer data with medical data.

Since their inceptions, Amazon and Alibaba have been tracking consumer purchasing behaviours. Now, Amazon Health and AliHealth started to add consumer health data to their record, which can further complete their profiling of individual consumers or segments (see Chap. 14).

What are the broader implications as we transition in all three areas, patient behaviours, physician mandates and data?

We may find our answers when we take a deeper look at the business model of the healthcare system. Currently, the healthcare system is organised around therapeutic areas. Pharmaceutical companies develop drugs for various medical conditions and engage with physicians, including Key Opinion Leaders or KOLs, in those

---

[20] https://www.ukbiobank.ac.uk/

areas for clinical trials and product distribution. Hospitals arrange their facilities and services according to those therapeutic areas with medical devices and services companies supporting those activities. Health authorities and insurance companies approve and reimburse the costs based on the standard of care in each therapeutic area as well. The organisation based on therapeutic areas put physicians at the centre of the system. When one follows the money, the incentives are usually set up to pay for "activities" conducted—patient throughput, number of tests, volume of prescription, etc. Although patient outcomes are a shared mission for all players and therefore the system, the tracking mechanism within the system remains focused on activities.

When the system evolves from treating illness to managing health, the centre of focus may shift from physicians to patients. Although the organisation based on therapeutic areas remains relevant, the practice may need to shift the thinking towards "individual health experience". What does this look like? First, with consent, individual consumers may obtain analysis of their entire genome. Algorithms may use the information to identify disease vulnerabilities and make dietary, exercise, daily routine, among other behaviour recommendations. Second, consumer wearables may monitor various individual health parameters through sensors and digital apps may analyse those data to build health models for individual consumers. Moreover, these apps may draw data from other data platforms such as e-commerce to analyse other behaviour data, such as food consumption and exercises. Third, some consumer apps may start to serve some basic triage functions for medical interventions. For example, if any irregularity or abnormality was detected by the wearables, the algorithm may make recommendations to seek medical attention or even trigger direct alert to medical facilities. In such a way, the apps may start to serve an important function of suggesting, recommending or even selecting physicians or medical facilities based on a combination of criteria, such as expertise, distance, availability, and insurance coverage, among others. This new organisation will put consumer plus technology at the centre, while medical professionals and services remain important to serve designated functions.

This change may seem drastic and scary to some yet subtle and non-controversial to others. What may come with the reorganisation is the change in measuring and rewarding based on patient outcomes. For example, for insurers such as Vitality. The new model could mean better ability to price health risks, less medical procedures thus less costs, reduced premium and less or even automated claim processing. At the first glance, this may reduce the total revenue and growth of the business. At the same time, counter arguments could be made that the revenues will simply be shifted to a later stage in life. With the aging population, total revenue will continue to grow.

This analysis leads us to an important point, how likely and when will this new hybrid model be put in place? Like other disruptive forces, business model shifts in the healthcare system are difficult to predict. Efforts on accurately predicting the time, scale, and speed of transformation will more likely lead to wrong results. Instead, it is more important to consider the following question: What impact could the business model shift have on my part of the healthcare system? How can I prepare my part for evolution? Do I want to be a leader or a follower in the process? What are the signals I need to pay attention to in order to "see" evolution?

Healthcare system is not alone in the journey from health to life. Many other industries are observing similar transformations. For example, the automobile industry is struggling to transition from manufacturing and selling cars to re-organising around total mobility experiences. The transition may involve a fundamental business model shift from car ownership to "mobility as a service". It will shift the current focus on automobile manufacturers to the new centre around consumer experience—curating and creating the multi-modality of mobility. Along with the business model shift, the industry is likely undergoing a re-organisation to redefine each player's role and power within the system.

The Individual-Public Interface

Last but certainly not the least, is the potential evolution of the individual-public interface. In this segment, let us analyse this evolution from two perspectives: health benefits and data.

- *The Health Benefit Dilemma*

We have analysed the potential evolutions in the three interfaces, human-machine, human-human and health-life. The combined effects can lead to personalised and preventative medicine with great experience that significantly benefit individual consumer-patient. In addition, the cost efficiency gained from digital transformation can expand healthcare access to a broader population in our society.

What About Public Health?

In most cases, individual and public interests were aligned on critical issues such as patient outcome, quality of life, cost, and access. However, under certain circumstances, individual and public interest on population health may not be perfectly in sync. For example, many such misalignments were on display in 2020. The first example can be found in "the US opioid crisis" or the global opioid epidemic. The crisis illustrated the danger of a maleficent incentive system and weak morality combined with behaviour challenges, among other factors. Pharmaceutical companies, including Purdue Pharma, aggressively and deceptively marketed and pushed the sales of opioid drugs.[21] Physicians were misguided and incentivised to prescribe the drugs to satisfy patient needs. And patients were ill-informed and overly rely on pharmaceuticals. The combinatorial effects of individual cases were more than significant at the populational level. WHO reported that opioid overdose caused an estimated 115,000 death in 2017.[22]

---

[21] https://www.newyorker.com/magazine/2017/10/30/the-family-that-built-an-empire-of-pain; https://www.npr.org/sections/health-shots/2019/03/26/706848006/purdue-pharma-agrees-to-270-million-opioid-settlement-with-oklahoma

[22] https://www.who.int/news-room/fact-sheets/detail/opioid-overdose

Another example can be found in the 2020 COVID19 global pandemic. Although the health risks for the 30–40 age group is lower than those for age over 60, the potential asymptomatic spread between the populations could increase COVID exposure to the latter group can cause significant challenges to the healthcare system, including lack of ICU, hospital bed, and medical staff capacities.

Hybrid health could potentially help with these situations in multiple ways. First, tracking, analysing, and monitoring aggregated data to understand and anticipate such events. For the opioid crisis, improved tracking of prescriptions, patient compliance, and dosage effects combined with longitudinal studies could inform us the possibilities of misuse and overdose, and may even suggest ways to change behaviours. Second, tracking, informing, and nudging individual behaviours could help manage some public health crises. For COVID, the effective contact tracing through mobile app and digital wearables has enabled many countries including Singapore, South Korea, and China to control the spread of COVID. Low adoption of such digital technology in countries including France, 2% coverage of the StopCOVID app by June 2020, has impacted their ability to reduce the spread.[23] Third, collecting and analysing the effectiveness of healthcare policies, including how individuals comply with the policies, can inform future healthcare guideline-setting and policy making. During the COVID pandemic, the availability of data, especially real-time data through digital means, has enabled analysis on different effects of healthcare policies.[24]

Health is a human right that everyone should be entitled to. Healthcare data, an artifact of this important right, has always been viewed as part of our individual right. As digital transformation brings additional challenges around privacy and security to many other industries, the digital healthcare data also becomes more pronounced. As a result, the digitization process in healthcare was accompanied by scepticism, resistance, and even fear.

Digital, and even more so, hybrid health can be beneficial for all players in the healthcare system; patients, pharmaceutical companies, device manufacturers, physicians and other medical professionals, hospitals and clinics, service providers, insurers, public health authorities, and others. Stopping or slowing down the progress also means denying the benefits. A more meaningful question is how can we govern and use data more responsively as a system?Hybrid health models heavily rely on the consumer-patient data, which means we need to approach it with caution and care. Although the actual answers can only be developed through the transformation process, I propose a more comprehensive way to consider the various data challenges. By clearly dividing the entire data challenge into distinct and manageable areas, we can develop concrete, practical, and innovative solutions for each area.[25] Here is one way to think about the data challenge based on the various stages of usage.

---

[23] https://www.lemonde.fr/pixels/article/2020/06/10/l-application-stopcovid-connait-des-debuts-decevants_6042404_4408996.html

[24] https://www.sciencedirect.com/science/article/pii/S2211883720300940#bib0048; https://www.sciencedirect.com/science/article/pii/S2211883720300812

[25] https://hbr.org/2020/10/building-health-care-ai-in-europes-strict-regulatory-environment

Conclusion

We began this chapter by introducing the Apple Hearth Study, a collaboration between Apple watch and Stanford Medicine. Through this experimental study, we expanded our scope and explored how digital health, more specifically our hybrid health model, can impact the healthcare system beyond the advancement of medicine. We walked through four critical areas of impacts: the evolutions of human-machine, human-human, health-life, and individual-public interfaces. These four areas of impact are enabled by the applications of digital technology, but the ultimate evolutions come from the changes to medical practices and the overall healthcare system. Furthermore, these new practices can shift the strategic focus of the healthcare system and change the business models for both the individual players and the entire system. For example, from treatment focused to prevention focused or from physician centred to patient centred. Some of these evolutions may also invite new players into the healthcare system and may even merge multiple industries. For example, e-commerce provides healthcare products and services, including telemedicine consultation and pharmacy services.

The evolutions of human-machine, human-human, health-life, and individual-public interfaces are also inter-related. Some may provide pre-requisite for others, while some are interdependent. For example, the improved experience from the human-machine interface may push how we re-imagine the human-human interface. Between 2018 and 2020, online scheduling and telemedicine became more widely adopted by many partly thanks to the improvement of digital experiences. For another example, the human-machine and health-life interfaces may be interdependent. Whether data and algorithms can be effective in helping individual consumers manage their health, or at least part of their health, may depend on the quality and quantity of data gathered from increasing consumer adoptions. At the same time, consumers are waiting for the demonstrated effectiveness of the digital products, for example apps that have unique algorithms to process data, before adopting them. The good news is many companies large or small, including Microsoft, Google, Alibaba, and start-ups such as Babylon Health and Nabta Health, have been experimenting with new approaches to develop digital and hybrid approaches to health.

Finally, the objectives of this chapter are not to provide answers or projections. Far from them, and more importantly, we want to raise awareness to these important topics and explore together what are the potential opportunities and challenges the health system may face during our transition. We are at an exploration stage to define the collective future for health, and the hybrid healthcare model. How to do it? AHS has shown us, only through bold yet rigorous experimentations, we can continue to push the frontier. As a continuation of AHS, Johnson & Johnson has launched a new Heartline™ study to explore the effectiveness of Apple Watch and an iphone app.[26]

We encourage you, and your colleagues, to develop your strategic thinking abilities. These ways of considering, analysing, and anticipating the potential impacts on the health system will help us effectively manage this important healthcare evolution. Turn threats into new opportunities.

---

[26] https://www.jnj.com/johnson-johnson-launches-heartline-the-first-of-its-kind-virtual-study.-designed-to-explore-if-a-new-iphone-app-and-apple-watch-can-help-reduce-the-risk-of-stroke

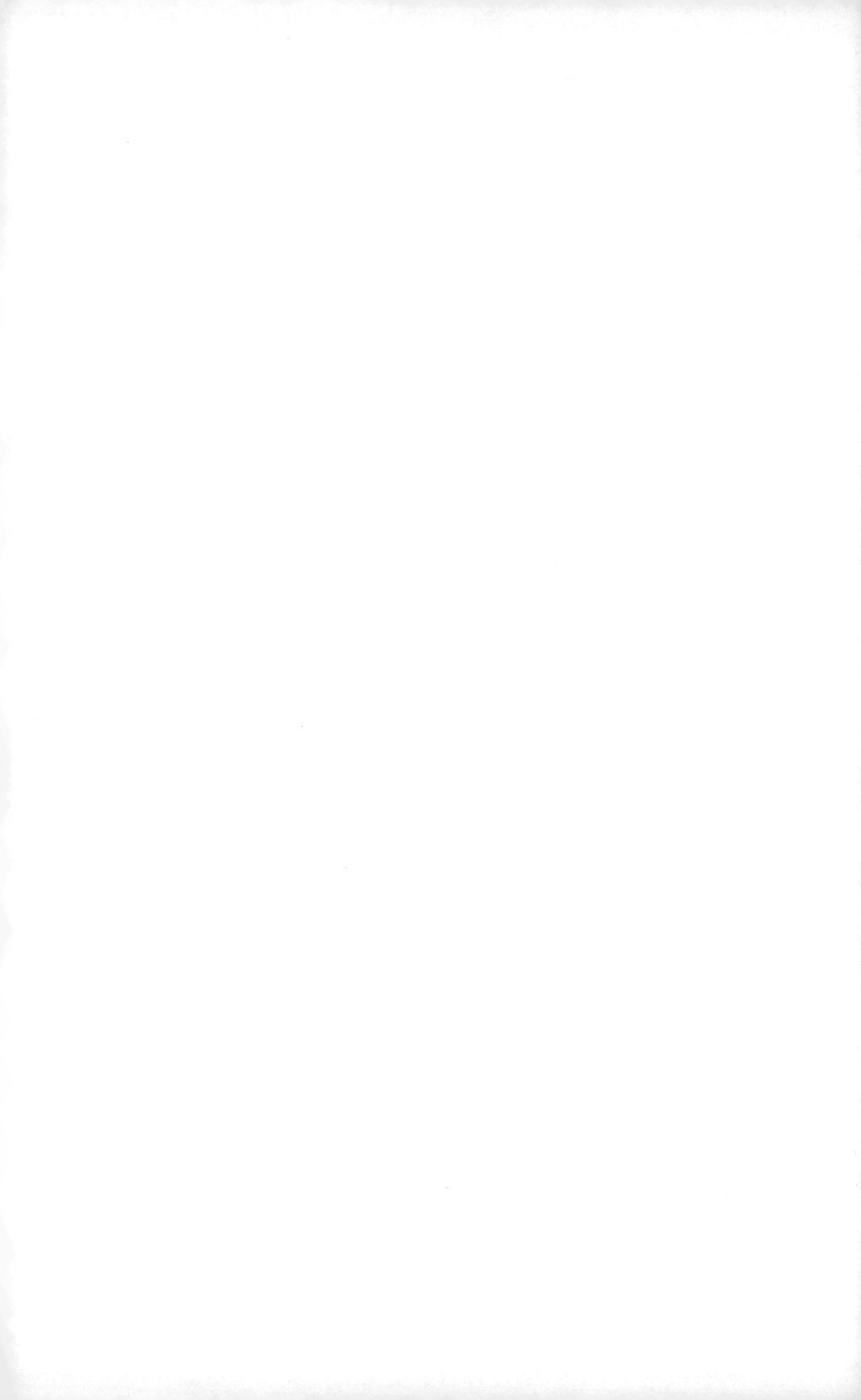

Chapter 16
Future Directions and Funding of Hybrid Healthcare

Mussaad Al-Razouki

Congratulations! You are now a burgeoning expert in Hybrid Healthcare. You have covered a wide variety of health and technology concepts that aim to intertwine the psychosocial, physical, and digital into an accountable, high quality and sustainable service.

In Chaps. 2, 3 and 4 we covered the ABC's of hybrid healthcare where we learned how breakdawn technologies such as Artificial Intelligence, Blockchain, and the Cloud will enable hybrid healthcare platforms to scale rapidly in the most cost efficient manner while also providing added prescriptive (and predictive) powers to clinicians via big data analysis.

In Chap. 5 we covered the hardware enabled Remote Patient Monitoring technologies (via both wearables and implantables) that will provide hybrid healthcare platforms with never-before-seen insight into patient performance, both in terms of prevention as well as ongoing post procedure/treatment (or chronic disease) monitoring.

In the next section, we covered the hybridization of traditional healthcare starting with the disruption of existing delivery mechanisms of provider health services (Chap. 6) followed by more specialized niche (yet fast growing) healthcare services such as home care (Chap. 7), maternal care (Chap. 8), mental health (Chap. 9) and chronic disease management (Chap. 10).

Chapter 11 then covered the different regulatory hurdles that exist and must be upgraded to enable these hybrid healthcare platforms to thrive.

The final section covered various future applications of hybrid healthcare technologies in novel specialties such as genomics (Chap. 12), consumerization (Chap. 13), and quantum computing (Chap. 14). We then covered the strategic implications

M. Al-Razouki (✉)
Business Development, Kuwait Life Sciences Company, Kuwait City, Kuwait
e-mail: mussaad@klsc.com.kw

© The Author(s), under exclusive license to Springer Nature Switzerland AG 2022
M. Al-Razouki, S. Smith (eds.), *Hybrid Healthcare*, Health Informatics, https://doi.org/10.1007/978-3-031-04836-4_16

of hybrid healthcare on its different stakeholders (Chap. 15); namely the patient, the medical establishment, the healthcare industry and the society overall, as well as a final look at the implications of data security of the increasing amount of patient data and digital access as well the impact on that important bond of trust between a patient and the clinical establishment.

Funding the Future of Hybrid Healthcare

The path to disrupting the healthcare industry starts with an idea; an idea to solve a particular problem or pain point that usually tackles either improving access, improving quality or decreasing costs. The founder must usually then invest in imprinting the idea on his or her initial team of co-founders as well as most likely a group of early financial partners known as angel investors. Together, this group of risk-seeking individuals expand on the idea into a practical application that would ideally involve both a humanistic and digitally enabled approach. Founders may also choose to seek grant funding as well through various government agencies or private non-for profit foundations. It is very rare these days for a startup to scale rapidly by depending on its initial revenues. This is especially true in healthcare where the capital expenditure (CAPEX) is high and regulatory timelines are long.

Nevertheless, it is important for founders not to raise further capital until they have proven their revenue model. In a hybrid healthcare world this means initially deciding on a B2B or B2C or B2G or sometimes B2B2C marketplace. In case you are unfamiliar, B = business, C = consumers or patients and G = government, usually the dominant financier of healthcare in most countries around the world. Hybrid health entrepreneurs most also typically navigate a few other business model acronyms such as SaaS, PMPM and P4P. SaaS or software as a service, might be interpreted differently depending on your region or school of thought, but for the purposes of this book on hybrid healthcare, we look to SaaS models as a way for entrepreneurs to spread out their revenue stream across future timelines without creating a cumbersome startup cost or fee (although many companies still charge those) thereby allowing their clients to better appreciate the value add of their service. PMPM stands for Per Member Per Month and is similar to the SaaS model and is perhaps more applicable to hybrid healthcare as we are not just focusing on digital software tools. A great example of this is concierge or retail medicine clinics such as One Medical (more on this company later) where members pay a monthly fee to access both in clinic and digital healthcare services. Finally P4P or Pay For Performance is quite unique to the healthcare industry and perhaps the most important component of any business model since quality in healthcare is a must and not a purchasing choice. Many third party payors or insurance companies are incorporating P4P models and so are some drug companies. A great example of the latter is the world's most expensive drug Kymriah (tisagenlecleucel) produced by Novartis. Kymriah is also the world's first "living drug" since the treatment (also known as CAR-T cell therapy) involves removing T cells from the patient's immune system and then genetically modifying the cells in the laboratory to attack and kill leukemia cells. It is a 22-day process that is customized for each patient. With innovation in therapeutics, so too comes innovation in pricing as Novartis has priced the one-time treatment at $475,000 per positive response. This means that patients who do not respond to Kymriah within a month would not be charged, meaning that their T cell's do not express a chimeric T cell receptor ("CAR-T") that is able to target a protein called CD19 that is common on the B cells of acute lymphoblastic leukemia (ALL). To its credit, Novartis has taken additional steps to make sure everyone who needs the drug can afford it.

As unit economics are tested and revenue models become real, a commercially active startup would typically seek further private rounds of funding from either individuals or institutions (known as venture capital) in the common alphabet rounds known as Series A, B, C, etc. until the company is ready to go public via three different routes we will cover later. It is essentially in this private funding era for entrepreneurs and investors to build the internal processes and frameworks needed to ensure the long term sustainability i.e. they must operate with the mentality of a public company beholden to society's trust. As of the publication of this book, there are just over 800 unicorns or private companies worth over $1 billion. Around 10% of these companies are working on healthcare, the majority of which are employing hybrid healthcare models. The bubble of this blessing of unicorns signifies the preference of founders to stay private longer due to the willingness of large pools of institutional finance to fund innovation and disruption, a great sign for any burgeoning hybrid healthcare entrepreneurs.

The 2020s have also seen the rise of a formerly obscured method of public market finance known as the Special Purpose Acquisition Company or simply SPAC. The other two main routes to the capital markets are the traditional IPO or Initial Public Offering as well as the Direct Listing. The major difference between an IPO and a Direct Listing is that an IPO involves selling additional shares that are usually marketed by third parties to the public which involves higher fees to underwriters and investment banks as well as the exchanges themselves. In a direct listing the company is selling only existing shares which also usually means there is no 6 month lock up period preventing the original private investors (and founders/employees) from selling their shares immediately.

The year of COVID-19 (2020) saw 227 SPACs top traditional IPOs for the first time in history, raising $76 billion compared to $67 billion raised from traditional IPOs. After the first quarter of 2021 generated a record 144 SPACs raising $44 billion, the SPAC market slowed down as regulatory pressure increased with the supply of SPACs reaching unsustainable levels. SPAC issuance fell 87% in the second quarter of 2021 to a relatively low total of $13 billion. Nevertheless, the current pipeline of pending SPAC IPOs remains high at over $70 billion. Digital and hybrid health platforms have certainly ridden the SPAC wave of 2020, with yet a few more splashes yet to come, but most of the 2021 SPAC class has failed to maintain last year's momentum.

As of the writing of this book, there are just over 620 SPACs at various levels of development chasing a blessing of 800+ unicorns. Note that since a SPAC has

2 years to find an acquisition target, many of the earlier SPACs were listed as far back as 2019. The typical process after a listing is for the SPACs management team to announce a potential acquisition target. Usually, the announcement must be unanimously approved by both management teams and boards of the SPAC and the private target company. The stockholders of the SPAC must then vote on the acquisition, which is usually unanimous and done quite quickly. The final step involves the close of the combination and completion of the merger resulting in a ticker change; symbolizing the start of the once private company officially becoming public. The following is an analysis of twelve of 2020 and 2021s most sought after hybrid health SPACs:

As seen in Fig. 16.1, the SPACs took, on average, 168 days or (5 months, 2 weeks and 4 days) for the merger to be announced, the longest timeline belonging to Oaktree Acquisition Corp (OAC) merging with Him & Hers (HIMS) in 384 days and the shortest belonging to Virgin Group Acquisition Corp (VGAC) merging with 23andMe (ME) in 74 days (2 months and 4 days). On average, it took 2 days for the merger to be approved by the SPAC shareholders, with the longest approval taking 5 days for D8 Holdings (DEH) merging with Vicarious Surgical (RBOT). Furthermore, it is important to note that despite it taking an average of 168 days and 126 days respectively from listing to merger and merger to approval, the process of approval to completion took a lot less time, averaging only 2 days.

As seen in Fig. 16.2, the SPACs popped, on average, around 1.70% when the merger was announced and actually dipped −3.01% when the merger was approved. The date of the ticker changing resulted in a significant 5.38% average increase. The largest positive move on the day the merger was announced belongs to Longview

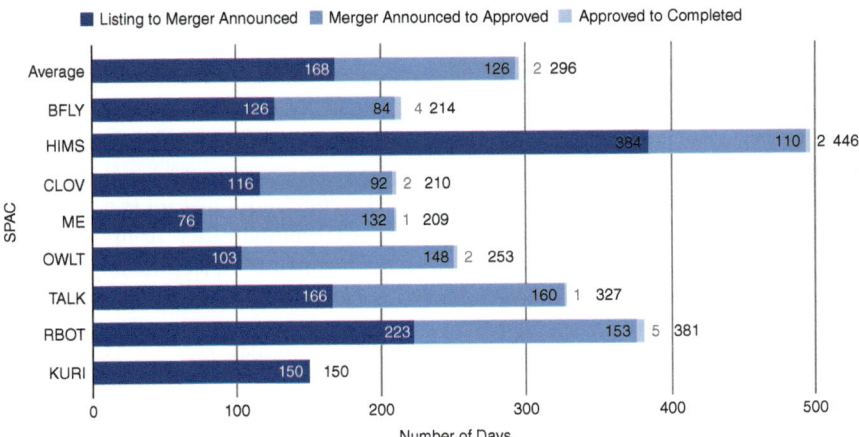

Timeline Chart of Days to Achieve Milestones

Fig. 16.1 Timelines of SPAC mergers—from announcement to approval to completion

Timeline Chart of Stock Bounce at Milesones

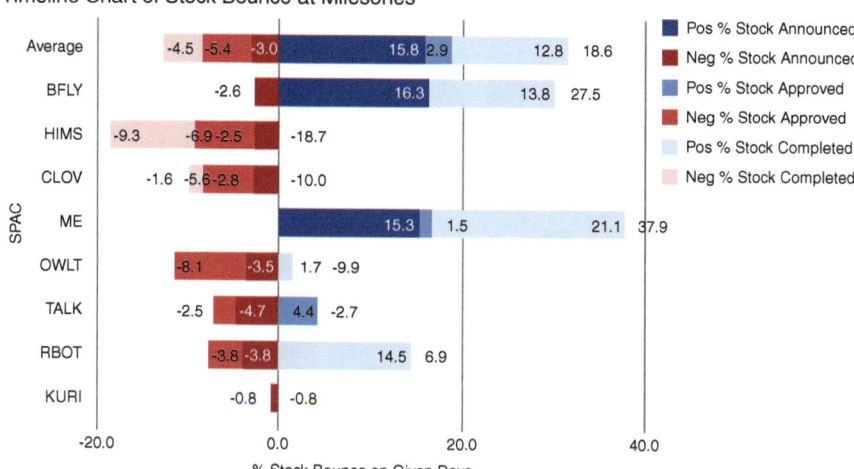

Fig. 16.2 Timeline chart depicting the highest movement in stock price during key SPAC milestones

Acquisition Corp (LGVW) which popped 16.30% on 11/20/2020 when the announcement was made for it to merge with Butterfly Network Inc. (BFLY). The largest positive move on the day the merger was approved belongs to Hudson Executive Capital LP (HEC) when it was approved to merge with Talkspace (TALK) on 06/22/2021, rising 4.41%. The largest positive move on the day the ticker changed belonged to Virgin Group Acquisition Corp (VGAC) when its ticker was changed to 23andMe (ME) on 06/17/2021 rising an astonishing 21.1%.

The largest negative move on the day the merger was announced belongs to Hudson Executive Capital LP (HEC) merging with Talkspace (TALK) on 01/13/2021, which dropped −4.66%. The largest negative move on the day the merger approval belongs to Sandbridge Acquisition Corp (SBG) merging with Owlet Health (OWLT) on 07/14/2021 and dropping −8.07%. The largest negative move on the day the ticker changed belongs to Oaktree Acquisition Corp (OAC) when its ticker was changed to Him & Hers (HIMS) on 01/21/2021, dropping −9.29%.

Furthermore, an interesting analysis that stands out is that initial market reaction to the announcing of the merger, be it positive or negative, correlated, to a strong decree, to future market reaction to both the approval and the completion of the merger. As a matter of fact, when SPACs experienced strong positive reactions to the announcing of the merger, they also generally grew strongly during the following announcements whereas every single negative initial reaction to the announcing of the merger led to an overall negative market reaction for the two subsequent milestone announcements. In other words, strength begets strength and weakness leads to weakness. Furthermore, with SPACs that experience overall positive stock

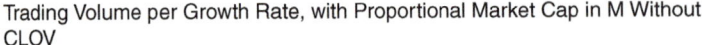

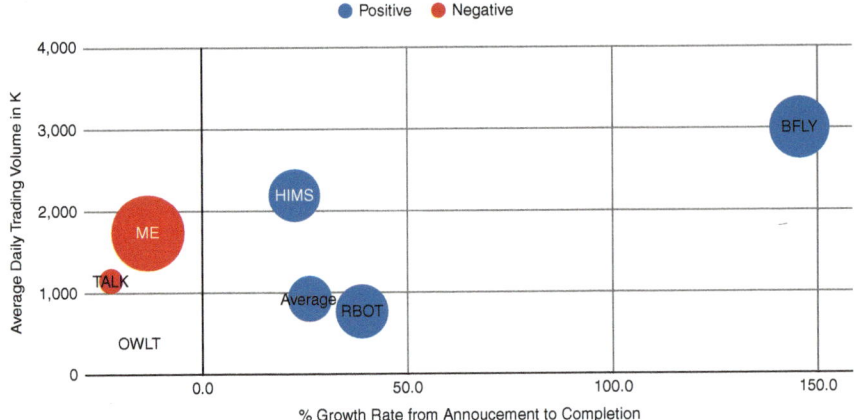

Fig. 16.3 Chart comparing average daily trading volume to the growth rate and market capitalization of the SPAC

bounces during key milestones, the biggest changes occurred when the merger was announced and completed, as opposed to the seemingly more important milestone of shareholder approval.

As seen in Fig. 16.3 and when it comes to mapping the overall growth rate to the average trading volume, we notice that, barring CLOV from the analysis due to its distorting effect, there is a positive correlation between averaging trading volume and growth rate even though the causal direction of such correlation, assuming it exists, cannot be determined. Furthermore, Butterfly Network Inc. (BFLY) stands out at experiencing the biggest growth rate of 146.0% with Talkspace (TALK) experiencing the biggest negative change rate of −22.4% from the time of their listing until the end of Q2 2021. Furthermore, and as referenced above, Clover Health Investments, Corp. (CLOV) saw by far the biggest average trading volume of 34,656 thousand with Owlet Health (OWLT) seeing the smallest average trading volume of 380 thousand. Lastly, it is interesting to note that of the seven selected SPACs, four of them grew whereas three have so far recapitulated in terms of stock price, with the average nonetheless standing at a positive 26.6%.

As seen in Fig. 16.4, when analyzing the market cap (as of the end of Q3 2021) of the selected digital health SPACs, the average stands at $1.28 billion. Along those lines, Clover Health Investments, Corp. (CLOV) stands as the company with the highest market cap of $3.36 billion whereas MedTech Acquisition Corporation (MTAC) has the lowest market cap of 309 million dollars.

The following is a list of select shell companies that have either merged with or are planning to merge with a hybrid health company as well as their relative performance:

Market Cap

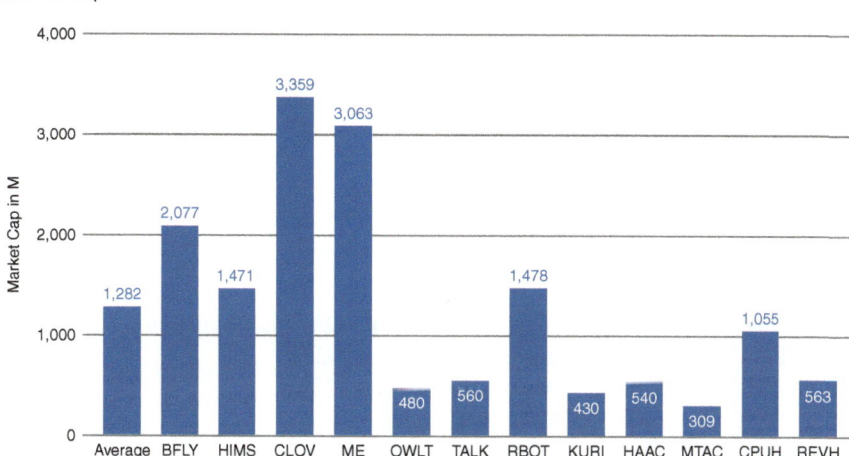

Fig. 16.4 Chart comparing market capitalization of the SPAC at the end of Q3, 2021

Merged

1. Longview Acquisition Corp. (LGVW)
   Date of Listing: 7/17/2020.
   Merged With: Butterfly Network Inc.
   Date Merger Announced: 11/20/2020.
   Date Merger Approved: 2/12/2021.
   Date Merger Completed: 2/16/2021 with LGVW ticker changing into BFLY.
   Performance of SPAC (as of Q1, 2021): +67.7%.
   Performance of SPAC (as of Q3, 2021): +2.0%.
   Performance of SPAC (as of Q1, 2022): −52.4%.

Longview started as an affiliate of leading healthcare investment firm Glenview Capital Management, which owned, along with its affiliates, 7.6% of the combined SPACs outstanding shares. Longview is Chaired by Glenview CEO, Larry Robbins. Leading institutional investors including Eldridge, Fidelity Management & Research Company LLC, Glenview, Ridgeback, Tenet Healthcare Corporation, UPMC Enterprises and Wellington Management had anchored a $175 million private investment in public equities (PIPE) at $10 per share, which is the usual floor price of a SPAC.

Butterfly Network is a medtech company that manufactures the Butterfly iQ, an ultrasound transducer that can perform "whole-body imaging" with a single hand-held probe using semiconductor technology. Connected to a mobile phone or tablet, it is powered by Butterfly's proprietary Ultrasound-on-Chip™ technology and harnesses the advantages of artificial intelligence (AI) to deliver advanced imaging that aims to improve patient outcomes and lower the cost of care.

All of Butterfly Network's existing investors, including Baillie Gifford, The Bill and Melinda Gates Foundation and Fosun Industrial Co., Limited, converted their equity into shares of the combined company.

2. Oaktree Acquisition Corp. (OAC)
   Merged With: Hims & Hers.
   Date of Listing: 9/13/2019.
   Date Merger Announced: 10/1/2020.
   Date Merger Approved: 01/19/2021.
   Date Merger Completed: 01/21/2021 with OAC ticker changing into HIMS.
   Performance of SPAC (as of Q1, 2021): +50.2%.
   Performance of SPAC (as of Q3, 2021): −24.7%.
   Performance of SPAC (as of Q1, 2022): −46.7%.

Oaktree Acquisition Corporation (OAC) is the first SPAC launched by Oaktree Capital Management, a global investment manager specializing in alternative investments, with ~$150 billion in assets under management. Oaktree Capital launched its second SPAC, Oaktree Acquisition II (OACB) in September of 2020, raising $225 mn in the process.

Originally focused on men's health, Hims & Hers prefers to now label itself as a telehealth company modernizing the delivery and accessibility of digital, consumer-focused healthcare services. The transaction will enable further investment in growth and new product categories that will accelerate Hims & Hers' plan to become the digital front door to the healthcare system.

The combined company to have an implied initial enterprise value of approximately $1.6 billion, with the company expected to have an estimated $330 million in cash after closing. Top-tier investors, including Franklin Templeton and clients of Oaktree, anchored a $75 million PIPE, again at a $10 floor price.

As with Butterfly, existing institutional backers of Hims & Hers, including Founders Fund, Forerunner Ventures, IVP, Redpoint Ventures, Thrive Capital, McKesson Ventures, and the Canadian Pension Plan Investment Board rolled 100% of their equity into the SPAC.

3. Social Capital Hedosophia Holdings Corp. III (IPOC)
   Date of Listing: 06/12/2020.
   Merged With: Clover Health Investments, Corp.
   Date Merger Announced: 10/6/2020.
   Date Merger Approved: 01/06/2021.
   Date Merger Completed: 01/08/2021 with IPOC ticker changing into CLOV.
   Performance of SPAC (as of Q1, 2021): −17.1%.
   Performance of SPAC (as of Q3, 2021): −26.0%.
   Performance of SPAC (as of Q1, 2022): −64.5%.

Social Capital Hedosophia Holdings Corp. III (IPOC) is one of several SPACs launched by Silicon Valley scion and erstwhile enfant-terrible Chamath Palihapitiya. The transaction valued Clover at an enterprise value of $3.7 billion and provided up to $1.2 billion in cash proceeds, including a fully committed PIPE of $400 million and up to $828 million of cash held in the trust account of Social Capital Hedosophia Holdings Corp. III. The PIPE was led by a $100 million investment from Chamath Palihapitiya and $50 million from Hedosophia, as well as commitments from Fidelity Management & Research Company and funds affiliated with Jennison, Senator Investment Group LP, Casdin Capital and Perceptive Advisors.

Clover is a next-generation Medicare Advantage insurance company offering best-in-class plans that combine wide access to healthcare and rich supplemental benefits with low out-of-pocket expenses. A unique model in health insurance, Clover partners with primary care physicians using its software platform, the Clover Assistant, to deliver data-driven, personalized insights at the point of care.

In Q1 of 2021, Clover Health revealed that it received a letter from the SEC "following the publication of an article by renowned short seller Hindenburg Research. Allegations included claims that Clover Health had not properly disclosed that its business model and its software offering, Clover Assistant, were under active investigation by the Department of Justice (DOJ). The DOJ is still currently investigating at least 12 issues ranging from kickbacks to marketing practices to undisclosed third-party deals.

4. Virgin Group Acquisition Corp (VGAC)
    Date of Listing: 11/20/2020.
    Merging With: 23andMe.
    Date Merger Announced: 02/04/2021.
    Date Merger Completed: 17/07/2021 with VGAC ticker changing into ME.
    Performance of SPAC (as of Q1, 2021): +9.2%.
    Performance of SPAC (as of Q3, 2021): −14.7%.
    Performance of SPAC (as of Q1, 2022): −61.7%.

Virgin Group Acquisition Corp (VGAC) is the first SPAC backed by ever-green entrepreneur Sir Richard's Branon's eponymous Virgin Group. No stranger to SPACs, Sir Richard's space startup, Virgin Galactic merged with Chamath Palihapitiya first SPAC back in the early days of April of 2020, somewhat sparking the current skyrocketing SPAC-mania.

23andMe is a leading consumer genetics and research company that offers a personalized health and wellness experience that has built a genetic database to unlock insights leading to the rapid discovery of promising new targets for drug development. The transaction will provide the capital to fund additional investment in key growth initiatives across 23andMe's consumer health and therapeutics businesses.

The transaction will value the outstanding shares of capital stock of 23andMe at an aggregate enterprise value of approximately $3.5 billion. It is important to note that the announcement was made a mere 2 months after 23andMe disclosed closing a $80 million venture financing round led by Sequoia Capital and NewView Capital.

Both 23andMe CEO and Co-Founder Anne Wojcicki and Virgin Group's Sir Richard Branson are each investing $25 million into a $250 million PIPE and are joined by leading institutional investors including Fidelity Management & Research

Company LLC, Altimeter Capital, Casdin Capital, and Foresite Capital. The pro forma cash balance of the combined company will exceed $900 million at closing and the current shareholders of 23andMe will own 81% of the combined company.

5. Sandbridge Acquisition Corp (SBG)
    Date of Listing: 11/5/2020.
    Merging With Owlet Baby Care.
    Date Merger Completed: 16/07/2021 with SBG ticker changing into OWLT.
    Performance of SPAC (as of Q1, 2021): −1.1%.
    Performance of SPAC (as of Q3, 2021): −44.1%.
    Performance of SPAC (as of Q1, 2022): −55.5%.

Launched in 2012 by a committed team of parents, Owlet has built a connected and accessible nursery ecosystem that brings technology and vital data to modern parenting. Owlet's flagship product, the Owlet Smart Sock baby monitor, uses proprietary and innovative pulse-oximetry technology to track a baby's real time heart rate, oxygen levels and sleep patterns to provide parents with invaluable peace of mind. The Owlet Smart Sock integrates seamlessly with Owlet's camera product, the Owlet Cam, enabling parents to see and hear their babies via Owlet's natively developed smartphone app.

The reverse merger with SBC values Owlet on a pre-transaction basis of $1 bn in equity value and values the post-transaction combined company at an enterprise value of approximately $1.074 bn. The SPAC is expected to deliver up to $325 million of cash to the combined company, after payment of estimated transaction expenses, through the contribution of up to $230 million of cash held in Sandbridge's trust account and a $130 million concurrent PIPE of common stock. PIPE participants include leading institutional investors such as funds managed by Fidelity Management & Research, Janus Henderson Investors, Neuberger Berman Funds, OrbiMed, private funds affiliated with PIMCO, and Wasatch Global Investors.

As part of the transaction, Owlet's current management and existing equity holders, including Eclipse Ventures and Trilogy Equity Partners, intend to roll nearly 100% of their equity into the combined company.

6. Hudson Executive Capital LP (HEC)
    Date of Listing: 7/31/2020.
    Merging with Talkspace.
    Date Merger Announced: 1/13/2021.
    Date Merger Completed: 16/07/2021 with HEC ticker changing into TALK.
    Performance of SPAC (as of Q1, 2021): 1.3%.
    Performance of SPAC (as of Q3, 2021): −62.5%.
    Performance of SPAC (as of Q1, 2022): −82.6%.

Hudson Executive Investment Corp. is a SPAC led by Doug Braunstein and Doug Bergeron of Hudson Executive Capital, which has an outstanding track record in healthcare and technology as both an investor and a strategic partner to public companies.

Talkspace targets a vast unmet need in behavioral health, improving access and outcomes while reducing costs via a telemedicine platform focused on mental health services. The transaction and partnership with Hudson Executive Investment Corp. is expected to help Talkspace grow its user base, add partnerships, and expand internationally. The pro-forma enterprise value of the transaction is approximately $1.4 billion including a 300MM fully committed PIPE anchored by leading investors including the Federated Hermes Kaufmann Funds, Jennison Associates, Woodline Partners, and renowned healthcare alternatives investor Deerfield.

7. D8 Holdings' acquisition (DEH)
   Date of Listing: 04/09/2020.
   Merged With: Vicarious Surgical.
   Date Merger Announced: 15/04/2021.
   Date Merger Approved: 15/09/2021.
   Date Merger Completed: 20/09/2021 with DEH ticker changing into RBOT.
   Performance of SPAC (as of Q1, 2021): −0.9%.
   Performance of SPAC (as of Q3, 2021): +38.4%.
   Performance of SPAC (as of Q1, 2022): −49.4%.

Hong Kong based D8 Holdings Corporation announced its merger with Vicarious Surgical Inc., a Waltham Massachusetts based next-generation hybrid healthcare technology company seeking to improve both cost and efficiency of surgical procedures as well as patient outcomes with a focus on virtual reality enabled robotics.

The business combination will provide approximately $220 million in gross proceeds to fund the further development and planned commercialization of the Vicarious' intelligent and affordable, single-incision surgical robot (the "Vicarious System") that virtually transports surgeons inside the patient to perform minimally invasive surgery. The Vicarious System is the first surgical robotic system to receive Breakthrough Device Designation from the U.S. Food and Drug Administration (the "FDA").

A total $142 million PIPE supporting the transaction is funded by multiple strategic investors including global medical technology company BD (Becton, Dickinson and Company) major hospital groups in the U.S. and Asia, and surgical robotics pioneer Roberta Lipson, founder of United Family Healthcare and its predecessor Chindex International Inc. and CEO of New Frontier Health Corporation Technology luminaries Bill Gates, Vinod Khosla's Khosla Ventures, Innovation Endeavors, Sun Hung Kai & Co. and Philip Liang's E15 VC have also invested.

Merger Announced

1. Alkuri Global Acquisition Corp (KURI.O)
   Date of Listing: 01/04/2021.
   Merging with Babylon Health.
   Date Merger Announced: 03/06/2021.
   Suggester ticker: BBLN.
   Potential Merger Date: Q4, 2021.
   Performance of SPAC (as of Q3, 2021): −0.2%.
   Performance of SPAC (as of Q1, 2022): −61.1%.

British online health startup Babylon Health has agreed to go public in the United States through a merger with a blank-check firm Alkuri Global Acquisition Corp (KURI.O) led by former Groupon chief Rich Williams and chaired by former Qatar Investment Authority (QIA) executive Sultan Almaadeed, at a pro-forma equity valuation of $4.2 billion. The deal will provide up to $575 million in gross proceeds to Babylon, including $230 million private placement from investors such as AMF Pensionsförsäkring and cyber security pioneer Palantir Technologies.

Founded in 2013, Babylon provides video medical appointments and AI-powered diagnoses. It has partnered with the UK's National Health Service and U.S. hospitals such as Mount Sinai Health Partners as it pushes for global expansion.

Babylon said it now covers 24 million patients around the world. It reported $79 million in revenue in 2020, a 394% year-over-year increase, and it expects that to swell to $321 million this year.

The company was last valued at $2 billion during a fundraising round in 2019, counting investors including Munich Re Ventures and Saudi Arabia's Public Investment Fund as backers.

Despite announcing financial results for the first half of 2021 via a press release, the movement in the stock price of Alkuri Global Acquisition Corp remained mostly unchanged, perhaps due to revenue not aligning with the previous guidance of $321 million for 2021 having only achieved 40% of the target in the first 6 months despite the H1 revenues of $128.8 increasing some 464% from the $22.5 million achieved during H1 2020 and despite Net loss improvement to $75.7 million in H1 2021 compared to a net loss of $90.8 million during H1 2020. In August 2021, Babylon completed a debt offering of $50 million which is due to be repaid at the completion of the transaction with Alkuri Global Acquisition Corp.

Still Searching

1. Health Assurance Acquisition Company (HAAC)
   Date of Listing: 11/13/2020.
   Performance of SPAC (as of Q1, 2021): +10.2%.
   Performance of SPAC (as of Q3, 2021): −2.2%.
   Performance of SPAC (as of Q1, 2022): −1.5%.

Founded by a triptych of venture capitalist from General Catalyst; Hemant Taneja, Evan Sotiriou, and Quentin Clark, HAAC aims to partner with leading healthcare businesses leveraging technology to create consumer-centric, data-driven, cloud-based solutions that can both bend the cost of care and improve wellness. The aim is to support the target company's efforts to become an iconic category winner that accelerates the digital transformation of existing healthcare into a new system of health assurance.

HAACU is supported by an independent board of directors that include digital health demigod.

Glenn Tullman who was the former CEO of Livongo and Allscripts as well as with Dr. Stephen Klasko, Dr. Jennifer Schneider, and Anita V. Pramoda.

2. MedTech Acquisition Corporation (MTAC)
   Date of Listing: 12/18/2020.
   Performance of SPAC (as of Q1, 2021): −0.3%.
   Performance of SPAC (as of Q3, 2021): −1.3%.
   Performance of SPAC (as of Q1, 2022): −2%.

MTAC was formed for the purpose of effecting a merger, capital stock exchange, asset acquisition, stock purchase, reorganization or similar business combination with a company primarily operating in the medical technology sector in the United States. The company is led by Medtech maverick and Chairman Karim Karti, who is the current COO of iRhythm Technologies and the former President and CEO of GE Healthcare's Imaging Business. MTAC's day to day management is led by Chief Executive Officer Christopher Dewey, Chief Financial Officer David Matlin, and Chief Administrative Officer Robert Weiss. In addition to Messrs. Karti, Dewey, and Matlin, the Company's Board of Directors includes Maurice Ferré, Martin Roche, and Ivan Delevic. with Michael Stansky as a special advisor.

3. Compute Health Acquisition Corp (CPUH.UN)
   Date of Listing: 2/5/2021.
   Performance of SPAC (as of Q1, 2021): −0.3%.
   Performance of SPAC (as of Q3, 2021): +0.1%.
   Performance of SPAC (as of Q1, 2022): −1%.

Compute Health Acquisition Corp. is a SPAC that raised just over $862 mn, making it the richest SPAC so far on our list. Before deducting. The units began trading on the New York Stock Exchange ("NYSE") under the ticker symbol "CPUH.U" on February 5, 2021. For a while, Compute Health Acquisition Corp was briefly known by the ticker CAHC. In a unique structure compared to the SPACs we have so far covered, each unit of CPUH.U consists of one share of Class A common stock and one-quarter of one redeemable warrant. Think of warrants simply as long term options to buy more stock. Each whole warrant may be exercised for one share of Class A common stock at a price of $11.50 per share following the later of 30 days after the completion of the Company's initial business combination and 12 months from the closing of the Company's initial public offering. Once the securities comprising the units begin separate trading, the shares of Class A common stock and warrants are expected to be listed on the NYSE under the symbols "CPUH" and "CPUH WS," respectively.

Like other blank check companies covered, CPUH is formed for the purpose of effecting a merger, capital stock exchange, asset acquisition, stock purchase, reorganization or similar business combination with one or more healthcare businesses that are already leveraging, or have the potential to leverage, computational power, with an emphasis on companies in the medical device space, including imaging and robotics, and companies operating in the virtual care space, including telehealth, care delivery and next-generation payor and provider models. The Company's management team is led by the former Medtronic Chairman and CEO and current Intel Chairman Omar Ishrak, Jean Nehmé and Joshua Fink.

In mid-February, it was disclosed that the Public Investment Fund (PIF), the $400bn sovereign wealth fund of the Kingdom of Saudi Arabia, had purchased a 8.7% stake in CPUH.U, while Medtronic PLC, a medical device giant with a current market value of about USD 155bn, had expressed interest in purchasing 1.5mn shares of CPUH in the offering, according to prospectus.

4. Revolution Healthcare Acquisition (REVH).
    Date Filed: 3/1/2021.
    Date of Listing: 14/05/2021.
    Performance of SPAC (as of Q3, 2021): −2.4%.
    Performance of SPAC (as of Q1, 2022): −1.9%.

Revolution Healthcare Acquisition is a blank check company to join the digital health SPAC race on Monday the first of March. It is formed by both General Catalyst (who are still actively searching for a target for their HAAC SPAC) and ARCH Venture Partners.

The Cambridge, MA-based company plans to raise $500 million by offering 50 million SAIL (Stakeholder Aligned Initial Listing) securities at $10. Similar to CPUH, each SAIL security consists of one share of common stock and one-fifth of a warrant, exercisable at $11.50. At the proposed deal size, Revolution Healthcare Acquisition would command a market value of $525 million, making it the second largest health SPAC after CPUH. The sponsors promote is only 5% due to the SAIL construct, which uses a performance-based incentive structure to create alignment.

The company is led by CEO Jay Markowitz, who is a Senior Partner at ARCH Venture Partners, and Chairman Jeff Leiden, the Executive Chairman of Vertex Pharmaceuticals. The company plans to target businesses at the intersection of health care, life sciences, and technology and plans to list on the Nasdaq under the symbol REVHU.

5. Blueprint Health Merger
    Date Filed: 2/26/2021.

Blueprint Health Merger is a blank check company that joined the SPAC race in February 2021. Formed by Blueprint Health, who has not selected a symbol yet, Blueprint Health Merger will be targeting digital healthcare businesses, plans to raise up to $200 million in the public offering.

The company is Providence, RI-based and led by CEO and Director Dr. Rajiv Kumar, the former President and Chief Medical Officer of Virgin Pulse who was also the co-founder and former CEO of ShapeUp, and Chairman Richard Harrington, the former CEO of The Thomson Reuters Corporation.

A Brown University and Brown Medical School Alumnus, Dr. Kumar is also the Co-Founder of Brown Angel Group; a global network of 700+ angel investors who leverage capital, connections, and community to support early stage startups founded by Brown University alumni. Their investments to date have been in wide-ranging industries including computer vision, robotics, consumer packaged goods, health & wellness, digital health, and talent recruitment. Brown Angel Group port-folio companies include RootAI, KineticEye, Jiant Kombucha, Pangea, CandooTech, Minded, Premama, and Siren Snacks.

Potential Hybrid Health IPO Candidates and SPAC Targets

Cera Care (see Chap. 7)

Cera Care is a London-based technology-enabled home-care company established to allow families to arrange, schedule and manage home care for elderly relatives. It uses an on-demand digital platform to match people seeking in-home assistance with professional caregivers, thus allowing them to stay updated on a patient's prog-ress. It also uses AI to predict potential health deteriorations.

Cera Care was formally launched in early 2016 by Dr. Mahiben Maruthappu, and since then has developed a £100 million M&A pipeline, including a robust diligence process for selecting acquisitions of traditional home care service providers.

Cera Care introduced a chatbot, Martha, created in partnership with Bloomsbury AI, as a virtual assistant able to review patients' digital records and answer ques-tions for both patients and caregivers, basing the answers on data points gathered by care workers and digitized care records.

Cera Care later developed a patient-care dashboard to provide patients with on-demand access to care, medications, transportation, food and doctors' services via tablet computer. It also claims to have developed a platform that predicts patient deteriorations by computing the risk of events such as hospitalizations based on caregiver input.

During the COVID-19 pandemic, Cera filled 10,000 jobs (from April 2020 to September 2021), supporting those who have lost roles due to the crisis. This mile-stone coincided with Cera's growing 100X-fold from 2019 to 2021 achieving ~$300 million revenues, and delivering over 40,000 healthcare visits every day to older and vulnerable people across the UK. Looking forward, Cera plans to create a further 5000 hybrid healthcare jobs throughout the UK, spanning frontline healthcare services and operational team members to technologists and data scientists.

CMR Surgical

CMR Surgical (formerly known as Cambridge Medical Robotics) is a British medical technology company based in Impington. It produces a robotic surgery system called Versius and could be a match-made-in-heaven target for medtech focused SPAC MTAC. It was incorporated in 2014 and in 2018 employs over 400 people.

Founded in 2014, CMR Surgical raised $100 million in the summer of 2018, in Europe's largest ever deal for a medical devices company, including investments by Cambridge Innovation Capital, the Zhejiang Silk Road Fund, Escala Capital Investments, LGT Group, and Watrium. The current valuation is considered to be around $1bn.

Biomimicking the human arm, the Versius gives surgeons the choice of optimized port placement alongside the dexterity and accuracy of small fully-wristed instruments. With 3DHD vision, easy-to-adopt instrument control and a choice of ergonomic working positions, the open surgeon console has the potential to reduce stress and fatigue and allows for clear communication with the surgical team. By thinking laparoscopically and operating robotically with Versius, CMR plans to help both patients and surgeons benefit from the value of robotic minimal access surgery (MAS).

Devoted Health

Devoted Health is a health care company serving seniors in the US aiming to launch Medicare Advantage plans. The firm's mission is to help its silver tsunami users navigate the healthcare system with personal guides. It can be considered a competitor to Clover Health.

Devoted Health's current valuation is $4.99 bn having raised $369 million from Andreessen Horowitz, F-Prime Capital, Oak HC/FT Partners, and Premji Invest amongst others.

Heart Flow

HeartFlow is a digital health company aiming to transform how heart disease is diagnosed and treated. HeartFlow provides a new approach to non-invasive diagnosis of coronary artery disease (CAD), which is considered one of the leading causes of death in the US. Leveraging deep learning and trained analysts, HeartFlow creates a personalized, digital 3D model of patients' coronary arteries based on data from CT scans.

Heart Flows current valuation is $1.77 bn and has raised funds from BlueCross BlueShield Venture Partners, US Venture Partners, Baillie Gifford & Co, Capricorn Investment Group, GE Ventures, HealthCor Management and Martis Capital amongst others.

Hinge Health

Hinge Health developed a digital care program to manage chronic back and joint pain. The company's software application combines sensor-guided exercise therapy with health coaching and education and collects real-time insight into clinically valid outcomes such as pain, stiffness, and functional ability.

Hinge Health's current valuation is $1.77 bn and has raised $453.9 mn from 11.2 Capital, Atomico, Bessemer Venture Partners, Coatue Management, and Heuristic Capital Partners amongst others.

Lyra Health

Lyra Health provides mental health benefits for employees and dependents. Lyra Health uses a proprietary matching technology and digital platform to connect companies and their employees-plus spouses and children-to therapists, mental health coaches, and personalized medication prescribing. Lyra can be considered as a direct competitor to Talkspace.

Lyra Health's current valuation is $2.3 bn having raised $284.1mn from Adams Street Partners Addition Breyer Capital Castlight Health and Casdin Capital amongst others, the latter of which are invested in both IPOC/CLOV and VGAC.

Modern Health

Modern Health is yet another technology play on mental health, but this time as a benefits platform for employers. The company covers the full spectrum of mental well-being needs through both evidence-based technology and professional support from either a coach or therapist.

Modern Health's current valuation is $1.17 bn raising $94.1 mn from 01 Advisors, Afore Capital, Battery Ventures, Felicis Ventures, and Founders Fund amongst others, the latter of which are invested in HIMS.

Ro

Formerly known as Roman, Ro is a patient-driven telehealth company that aims to put patients in control of their health. The company builds technology to make healthcare accessible, affordable and enjoyable. Ro powers three digital health clinics—Roman for men's health (its original focus that was similar to HIMS), Rory for women's health, and Zero for fighting smoking cessation—and Ro Pharmacy, a simple and affordable online pharmacy where every generic medication is priced at the attractive rate of $5 per month.

Ro's current valuation is $1.5 bn and has raised $476.5mn from 3 L, Aaron Harris, BoxGroup, FirstMark Capital, and Forbes Media amongst others.

ZocDoc

Although patient booking pioneer ZocDoc recently raised $150 million earlier this month in a round led by Francisco Partners, the New York based firm has been rumored to be a strong target of multiple technology focused SPACs. Expanding beyond its core patient booking service, ZocDoc added a vaccine finder feature and a telehealth scheduler in 2020 as a response to the COVID19 pandemic. In December of last year, a lawsuit by former co-founder and CEO, Cyrus Massoumi was dismissed by the New York State Supreme court allowing current CEO and cofounder Dr. Oliver Kharraz to completely focus on continuing the company's rapid expansion into telehealth.

ZocDoc's current valuation is $1.77 bn having raised a total of $383mn from Atomico, Baillie Gifford & Co. Bezos Expeditions, DST Global, Founders Fund, Khosla Ventures, Goldman Sachs amongst others.

Mergers and Acquisitions

Once companies are public (or sometimes even as private companies) they usually fund innovation and growth by either developing intellectual property and new business models in house (organically) or merging with / acquiring other businesses (inorganic). A great example of this is hybrid primary care pioneer One Medical's acquisition of Medicare-focused provider Iora Health in June of 2021.

Both One Medical and Iora Health offer brick-and-mortar provider clinics as well as digital tools, with Iora more focused on the 65-and-older population. Iora's business model involves assigning each of its members either a doctor, nurse/caregiver and health coach, all connected to through the company's platform.

Unlike publicly listed One Medical, Iora was a private company that had closed several rounds of funding totalling $350 million, the latest of which occurred in February 2020, when Iora raised $126 million to build a new Medicare Certified EHR system.

One Medical plans the acquisition to help expand its full-risk models, as well as expand into new patient populations both in terms of geography and demographics and leveraging its existing digital platform to drive profitable membership growth, engagement with members, improve health outcomes and lower costs.

One Medical and Iora Health aren't the only unicorn companies with hybrid healthcare models. Emilio Health, which focuses on pediatric behavioral health, offers in-person and digital tools and both Carbon Health and Kindbody also use a similar hybrid approach.

A Final Word from the Editors

It is important to understand that the fundamental difference between building a hybrid healthcare company and a traditional or digital only healthcare company is the realization that efficiencies exist in leveraging both the real touch dynamic of the physical world with the scalability and logarithmic automation of digital tools. Moreover, we must take the socioethical dimension of the patient as the primary architect of their own healthcare within the confines and as part of a broader community into consideration.

While healthcare's past has been prone to human error, healthcare's present provides us with the hope of digital solutions and evidence-based medicine. Healthcare's future must certainly be hybrid.

Index

© The Editor(s) (if applicable) and The Author(s), under exclusive license to
Springer Nature Switzerland AG 2022
M. Al-Razouki, S. Smith (eds.), *Hybrid Healthcare*, Health Informatics,
https://doi.org/10.1007/978-3-031-04836-4